Kazuyoshi Endo • Toshihiro Kogure
Hiromichi Nagasawa
Editors

Biomineralization

From Molecular and Nano-structural Analyses to Environmental Science

Editors
Kazuyoshi Endo
Department of Earth and Planetary Science
The University of Tokyo Graduate School
of Science
Tokyo, Japan

Toshihiro Kogure
Department of Earth and Planetary Science
The University of Tokyo Graduate School
of Science
Tokyo, Japan

Hiromichi Nagasawa
Department of Applied Biological Chemistry
Graduate School of Agricultural and Life
Sciences
The University of Tokyo
Tokyo, Japan

https://doi.org/10.1007/978-981-13-1002-7

Preface

Biomineralization is a process by which organisms form mineral-like inorganic substances inside or outside their bodies. Biominerals are diverse in terms of structure, composition, morphology and role, depending on organisms. The research area of biomineralization is really interdisciplinary in methodology, ranging from microscopic observation to molecular biology. It includes not only basic researches mainly focusing on the mechanisms and evolutionary processes of biomineral formation but also applied researches including medical, dental, agricultural, environmental and materials sciences. Therefore, the society of biomineralization research constitutes a group of researchers with a variety of background. It is a good stimulation for us to get together and exchange ideas for new developments.

The International Symposium on Biomineralization began in 1970 and was held irregularly up to the 10th symposium but thereafter regularly every 2 years. This volume was planned as a record for the proceedings of the 14th International Symposium on Biomineralization (BIOMIN XIV): From Molecular and Nanostructural Analyses to Environmental Science. The symposium was held during October 9–13, 2017, at Tsukuba International Congress Center in Tsukuba, Japan. A total of 210 participants, including four accompanying persons, from 18 countries and areas attended this symposium. The participants included 157 regular researchers and 49 students, who contributed to the 106 oral presentations, including 10 keynote lectures, and 84 poster presentations. The presentations were classified into the following 8 topics:

1. Structure and analysis of biominerals
2. Molecular and cellular regulation of biomineralization
3. Genome-based analysis of biomineralization
4. Evolution in biomineralization
5. Biomineralization in medical and dental sciences
6. Bio-inspired materials science and engineering
7. Biominerals for environmental and paleoenvironmental sciences
8. Mollusk shell formation

This volume consists of 42 articles which are arranged in the order of the above topics. Most of them are original articles, and a few are reviews. The contributors were those who chose to submit their manuscript. All articles were peer-reviewed. Although the volume does not necessarily represent the whole contents of the symposium, it contains articles from all 8 topics. Thus, we are able to understand the present status of the cutting-edge of various aspects in biomineralization research from this volume. The volume has an appendix, which comprises valuable SEM and TEM images taken and left unpublished by late Dr. Hiroshi Nakahara, a distinguished researcher majoring in electron microscopy of biominerals. This appendix was arranged by Dr. Mitsuo Kakei, who selected the photographs from about 160 slides, which were shown on the screen during the lunch times in the symposium.

The symposium and the publication of this volume were supported by a number of Japanese scientific societies, to which we extend our gratitude. We express our sincere thanks to the Naito Foundation, Tokyo Ouka Foundation for the Promotion of Science and Technology, Kato Memorial Bioscience Foundation, Inoue Foundation for Science, Suntory Foundation for Life Sciences, Life Science Foundation of Japan, Tsukuba Tourism and Convention Association, and Tsukuba City for their financial support. Thanks are also due to Japanese Fossil Museum, Kouchiken Nihonkei Hozonkai, K. MIKIMOTO & Co. Ltd., Mikimoto Pharmaceutical Co., Ltd., Kao Corporation, LOTTE Co., Ltd., and Kotegawa Sangyo Co., Ltd., for their kind donations.

Tokyo Japan
April, 2018

Kazuyoshi Endo
Toshihiro Kogure
Hiromichi Nagasawa

Contents

Part I
Structure and Analysis of Biominerals

Chapter 1
On the Transition Temperature to Calcite and Cell Lengths for Various Biogenic Aragonites

Taiga Okumura, Masahiro Yoshimura, and Toshihiro Kogure

Abstract In order to understand the mineralogical difference between biogenic aragonites and their geological or synthetic ones, the transition temperature from aragonite to calcite by heating and the cell lengths of a number of biogenic aragonites have been measured using conventional and high-temperature XRD, as well as those of abiotic ones. Among 21 specimens, most biogenic aragonites showed a transition temperature 60–100 °C lower than that for abiotic ones. However, the shells of land snails showed almost similar transition temperatures. The temperature range from the beginning to the completion of the transition was also varied among the biogenic aragonites. On the other hand, the axial ratios (*a/b* and *c/b*) of aragonites in marine molluscan species were considerably larger than those of abiotic ones. However, aragonites in freshwater molluscan species and land snails showed axial ratios similar to abiotic ones. X-ray microanalysis suggested that the origin of such abnormal cell lengths was sodium incorporated in the aragonite crystals, not due to lattice distortion induced by the intracrystalline organic molecules proposed in previous researches.

Keywords Aragonite · Calcite · Transition temperature · Cell lengths · Axial ratio · Sodium

1.1 Introduction

Aragonite is one of the polymorphs of anhydrous calcium carbonate ($CaCO_3$) and thermodynamically slightly less stable than calcite at the ambient temperature and pressure in which organisms are alive. However, aragonite commonly occurs by biomineralization processes. It has been often reported that biominerals possess distinct characteristics and properties which are not observed in their geological or

T. Okumura · M. Yoshimura · T. Kogure (✉)
Department of Earth and Planetary Science, The University of Tokyo, Tokyo, Japan
e-mail: okumura@eps.s.u-tokyo.ac.jp; Masahiro.Y@eps.s.u-tokyo.ac.jp; kogure@eps.s.u-tokyo.ac.jp

K. Endo et al. (eds.), *Biomineralization*,
https://doi.org/10.1007/978-981-13-1002-7_1

synthetic counterparts. Biogenic aragonite is not the exception. For instance, Koga and Nishikawa (2014) investigated the transition from coral aragonite to calcite by heating in a thermogravimetric (TG)-differential thermal analysis (DTA) apparatus. They found that when the temperature was increased at a certain rate, the temperature at which the aragonite-calcite phase transition occurred was around 100 °C lower for the coral aragonite than the geological ones. Please note that this temperature is not corresponding to that at which the thermodynamic stability between aragonite and calcite is reversed. They ascribed such a low temperature for the transition to the existence of interstitial water between aragonite crystals, which was released during the transition.

On the other hand, the crystallographic parameters of biominerals have been also reported to be specific, compared to abiotic minerals. Pokroy et al. (2004, 2007) found that the cell lengths of aragonite in the shells of three molluscan species were slightly different from those of abiotic minerals; the *a*- and *c*-lengths are longer, and the *b*-length is shorter. They suggested that this "distortion" was induced by intracrystalline organic molecules, namely, a biological effect.

These two examples as the specific characters of biogenic aragonite are interesting to consider, for instance, the diagenetic effect on biominerals to form fossils. However, it is not certain whether such characters can be observed ubiquitously in biogenic aragonite formed by other species, families, etc. The present study investigated more than 15 specimens for biogenic aragonite as well as geological and synthetic ones, with respect to their temperatures for aragonite-calcite transition by heating and cell lengths.

1.2 Materials and Methods

The aragonite specimens investigated are listed in Table 1.1. In general, all specimens except the synthetic ones were powdered using an agate mortar and pestle for X-ray diffraction (XRD). The two synthetic aragonite specimens (Syn-PVA and Syn-Mg) were prepared according to Kim et al. (2005) and Kitano (1962) using polyvinyl alcohol (PVA) and $MgCl_2$, respectively. In case of multilayered shells with a calcite layer, the calcite layer was removed by grinding with a micro drill, and then the remaining aragonite layer(s) was crushed into powder using an agate mortar and pestle. They were washed with distilled water and ethanol and then dried in an oven.

In the present study, we used an X-ray diffractometer (Rigaku SmartLab) with a high-temperature specimen holder (Rigaku DHS 900), to measure the temperature for the transition from aragonite to calcite. A copper X-ray tube was used and CuKα was selected by Ni filter. X-ray was detected using a silicon strip detector (Rigaku D/teX Ultra 2). The powdered specimens were processed into a disk of 3 mm in diameter and 0.5 mm thick by a press and placed on the high-temperature specimen holder. The temperature was raised at a rate of 5 °C, and 2θ was scanned repeatedly

Table 1.1 Aragonite specimens investigated in this study

Geological aragonite		
Specimen name	**Morphology**	**Occurrence**
Sefrou, Morocco	Hexagonal prism	Unknown
70087[a]	Lath	Veins in serpentinite rock
70096[a]	Aciculum	Deposit from hot spring
Synthetic aragonite		
Syn-PVA		Precipitated with PVA
Syn-Mg		Precipitated with Mg
Molluscan shells (freshwater)		
Microstructure	**Class**	**Species**
Nacre	Bivalvia	*Anodonta cygnea*
		Hyriopsis schlegelii
		Unio douglasiae
Prism	Bivalvia	*Anodonta cygnea*
Otolith		
		Oncorhynchus mykiss
Molluscan shells (terrestrial)		
Microstructure	**Class**	**Species**
Cross-lamellar	Gastropoda	*Coniglobus mercatorius*
		Acusta despecta
		Zaptychopsis buschi
Molluscan shells (brackish water)		
Microstructure	**Class**	**Species**
Cross-lamellar	Gastropoda	*Pythia pantherina*
Molluscan shells (salt water)		
Microstructure	**Class**	**Species**
Cross-lamellar	Gastropoda	*Murex pecten*
		Acanthopleura japonica
		Lottia dorsuosa
Nacre	Cephalopoda	*Nautilus pompilius*
	Bivalvia	*Pinctada fucata*
	Gastropoda	*Haliotis discus*
Coral		
		Galaxea fascicularis

[a]Collection of The University Museum, The University of Tokyo

from 25.5° to 30.5° at a rate of 5°(2θ)/min. One hundred eleven reflection of aragonite and 104 reflection of calcite were recorded in the 2θ range.

The XRD measurement to refine the cell lengths of aragonite was conducted using a Rint-Ultima$^+$ diffractometer (Rigaku) with CuKα radiation monochromated with Ni filter and a silicon strip detector (Rigaku D/teX Ultra 2). The 2θ range was 10°–90° with continuous scan and a rate of 1° (2θ)/min. Data was collected at every 0.02° (2θ). The powder specimens were mounted in a shallow dimple on a nonreflective plate made of silicon. The cell lengths (*a*, *b*, and *c*) of aragonite were calculated from the 2θ values of around 48 reflections, using PDXL software (Rigaku).

Finally, the chemical composition, particularly the concentration of sodium and chlorine, in aragonite was analyzed using an electron-probe microanalyzer (EPMA, JEOL JXA-8530F). The specimens for EPMA were prepared by embedding fragments of the minerals or shells in epoxy resin, polishing with diamond paste and colloidal silica. Finally amorphous carbon was coated by vacuum deposition for electron conductivity.

1.3 Results and Discussion

Figure 1.1 represents an example of the high-temperature XRD measurement. The temperature at the right of each pattern indicates the temperature at the beginning of the scanning. Please note that it took only 1 min for the 2θ scan, and the rate to increase temperature was 5 °C/min. The peaks from aragonite were gradually decreased, and conversely 104 peak of calcite was increased, indicating the progress of the phase transition. We estimated by extrapolation the beginning temperature at which 104 peak of calcite had the integrated intensity and the ending temperature at

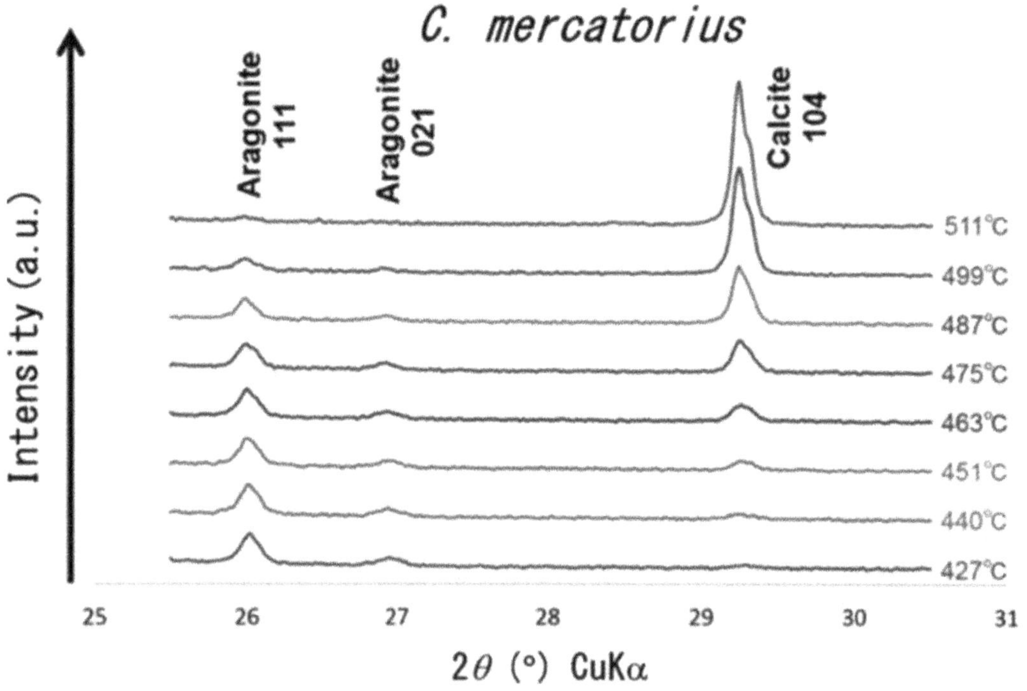

Fig. 1.1 An example of in situ high-temperature XRD pattern to determine the temperature for the aragonite-calcite transition

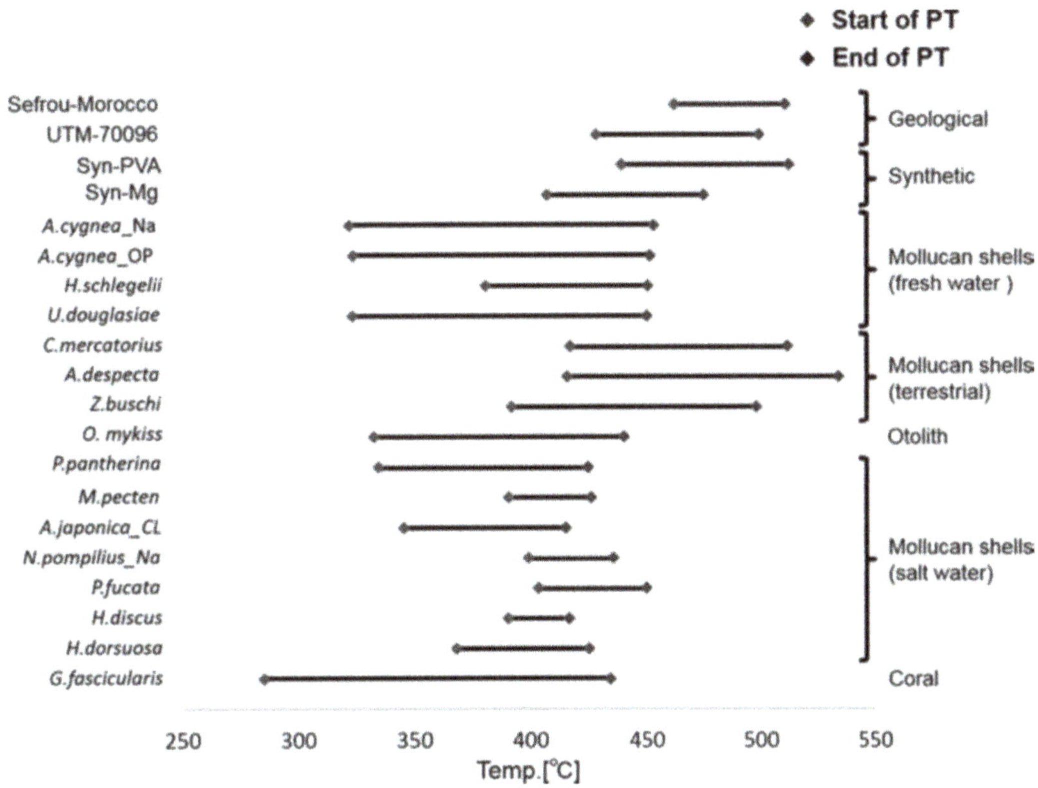

Fig. 1.2 The beginning and ending temperatures of the transition for aragonite specimens of various origins. PT indicates phase transition

which 111 peak of aragonite completely lost the intensity. The two temperatures for all biogenic aragonites of several geological and synthetic aragonites are shown in Fig. 1.2. As reported in the previous work (Koga and Nishikawa 2014), biogenic aragonite showed lower beginning and ending temperatures for the transition than geological and synthetic aragonites. Particularly, the beginning temperature for the coral was extremely low. However, the transition temperatures for terrestrial molluscan shells, or land snails, were similar to those for abiotic aragonite, suggesting that biogenic aragonites are not always less stable than abiogenic ones. The origin of the difference of the temperature for the transition is not clear at present. Koga and Nishikawa (2014) proposed that the origin is intercrystalline water in the coral aragonite because water molecules were detected by mass spectroscopy at the transition. However, this is not convincing because the release of water may not be the origin of the transition but the accompanied phenomenon of the transition. It should be revealed by further investigations in the future.

The cell lengths of most of the samples are shown in Fig. 1.3. In the figure, the cell lengths are expressed with the ratio to those of geological aragonite from Sefrou, Morocco ($a = 4.9629\ (10)$ Å, $b = 7.9690\ (15)$ Å, $c = 5.7430\ (11)$ Å), according to Pokroy et al. (2007). As Pokroy et al. (2007) reported, a- and c-lengths are considerably larger, and b-length is shorter for some aragonites in molluscan shells,

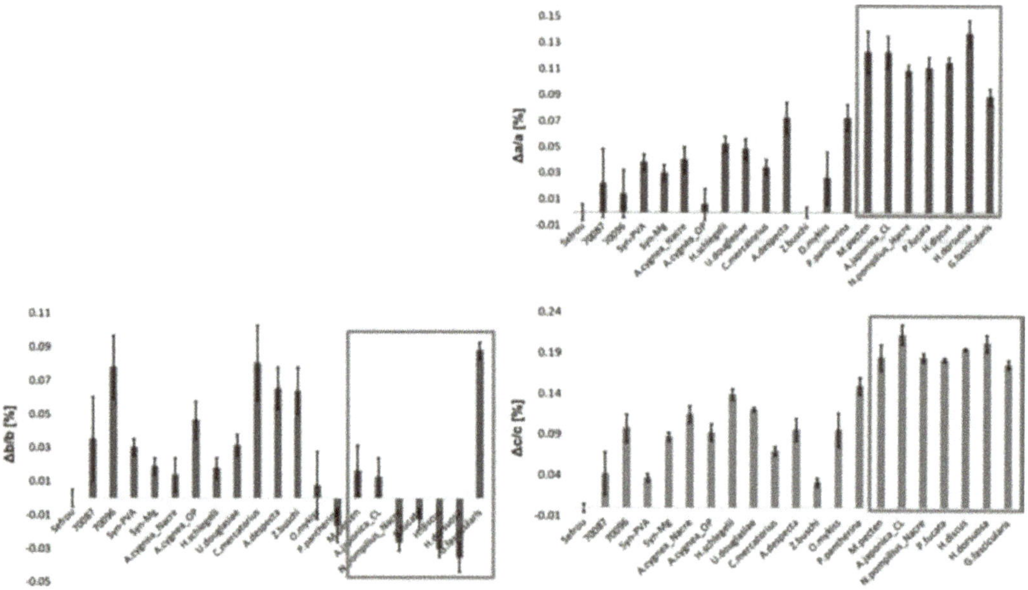

Fig. 1.3 The differences of the cell lengths of various aragonites from that of a geological sample (Sefrou, Morocco). The specimens surrounded with the rectangle are marine molluscan shells and coral

but this trend is not true for all biogenic aragonites. Among all samples investigated, the trend was distinctly observed only for marine molluscan shells. From this result, we supposed that salinity or incorporation of sodium and/or chlorine in the aragonite structure may have resulted in such a systematic change of the cell lengths. Hence, we conducted quantitative analysis of sodium/chlorine concentrations in the samples using EPMA. It was revealed that the content of chlorine was extremely low for all samples and not related to the cell lengths. On the other hand, the concentration of sodium was considerably varied, probably depending on the environments where the aragonites were formed. Considering the origin of the samples, the relationship between the axial ratio (*a*/*b* and *c*/*b*) and the sodium concentration was summarized as shown in Fig. 1.4. From the figure, it is apparent that distinct cell lengths or anisotropic *lattice distortions* observed in some biogenic aragonite compared to geological and synthetic ones are originated from the incorporation of sodium in the crystal structure of aragonite. We insist that the abnormality is not owing to intracrystalline organic molecules as proposed in the previous works (Pokroy et al. 2004, 2007).

Pokroy et al. (2004) considered Na-substitution in biogenic aragonite to change the cell lengths, but they denied its possibility because the ionic radii of Na^+ and Ca^{2+} are so close that a small substitution of Na^+ in aragonite cannot change its cell lengths significantly. It is probably true if we suspect only the isomorphic substitution, but the charges of the two cations are different, and some substitution for anions must be accompanied. As stated above, chlorine was not sufficiently detected

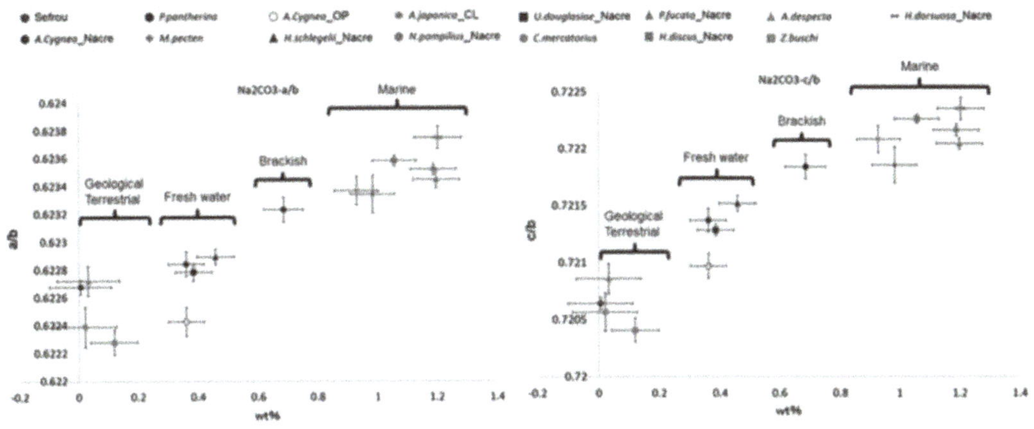

Fig. 1.4 The axial ratios (*a*/*b* in the upper and *c*/*b* in the lower figure) vs. concentration of Na in the aragonites of various origins. The concentration of Na is expressed as wt.% of Na_2CO_3

in the sodium-bearing aragonites. One possibility is the incorporation of proton or hydroxyl (OH^-) which substitutes O^{2-} or HCO_3^- instead of CO_3^{2-}. Probably Na^+ and OH^- reside closely in the aragonite structure, and they locally modify the atomic arrangement around the substitution, which may affect the cell lengths. Of course it is not clear why the *a*- and *c*-lengths were elongated and *b*-length was shrunk by such substitutions, but the idea of intracrystalline organic molecules also cannot explain the anisotropic change. Pokroy et al. (2007) reported that when the biogenic aragonites were heated to 350 °C in air, the cell lengths became identical to those of geological aragonite, which they proposed the evidence for organic molecules as the origin of the lattice distortion. However, our preliminary experiment revealed that when a marine molluscan shell (*N. pompilius*) was annealed at around 350 °C, the concentration of sodium was significantly decreased, probably by diffusing away from the aragonite structure. Accordingly, the Na-substitution can also explain the annihilation of abnormality of the cell lengths by heating.

Acknowledgments We are grateful to Prof. A. Checa (Univ. Granada) and Prof. T. Sasaki (Univ. Tokyo) for donating valuable shell samples, Prof. M. Suzuki (Univ. Tokyo) for instructing the preparation of the synthetic aragonite, Mr. K. Fukawa (Univ. Tokyo) for assisting XRD measurement, and Mr. K. Ichimura (Univ. Tokyo) for assisting EPMA analysis.

References

Kim W, Robertson RE, Zand R (2005) Effects of some nonionic polymeric additives on the crystallization of calcium carbonate. Cryst Growth Des 5:513–522

Kitano Y (1962) The behavior of various inorganic ions in the separation of calcium carbonate from a bicarbonate solution. Chem Soc Jpn 35:1973–1980

Koga N, Nishikawa K (2014) Mutual relationship between solid-state aragonite–calcite transformation and thermal dehydration of included water in coral aragonite. Cryst Growth Des 14:879–887

Pokroy B, Quintana JP, Caspi EN, Berner A, Zolotoyabko E (2004) Anisotropic lattice distortions in biogenic aragonite. Nat Mater 3:900–902

Pokroy B, Fieramosca JS, Von Dreele RB, Fitch AN, Caspi EN, Zolotoyabko E (2007) Atomic structure of biogenic aragonite. Chem Mater 19:3244–3251

Chapter 2
TEM Study of the Radular Teeth of the Chiton *Acanthopleura japonica*

Mitsuo Kakei, Masayoshi Yoshikawa, and Hiroyuki Mishima

Abstract The radula chiton teeth, *Acanthopleura japonica*, were examined using transmission electron microscopy (TEM). After cutting into segments corresponding roughly to three developmental stages from the onset of tooth development, the middle and the fully matured stages, toluidine blue staining has given the posterior side three different color patterns, colorless, reddish-brown, and black colors, respectively. At the colorless stage, the microvilli attached along the surface of the tooth cusp appeared to be dissembled and convert into the lamellar structure in the tooth interior. At the reddish-brown stage, the electron density between fibrous layers increased. A complex of tiny clusters of grains appeared along the fibrous layers. They seemed to aggregate each other to become larger. At the black stage, multiple layers consisting of irregular-shaped and various size of iron minerals were formed. After treating with an aqua regia solution, organic substances have remained between iron minerals, suggesting the abrasion-resistant role at the posterior side of chiton teeth during feeding. In addition, these minerals were randomly arranged. The lattice intervals of the ion minerals varied at an approximate range from 4.8 to 10.2 Å. Also, we have confirmed clearly the lattice fringe of apatite crystal in the core region.

Keywords Chiton · Transmission electron microscopy · Iron minerals · Apatite crystal

---

The original version of this chapter was revised. A correction to this chapter is available at https://doi.org/10.1007/978-981-13-1002-7_44

M. Kakei (✉)
Tokyo Nishinomori Dental Hygienist College, Tokyo, Japan
e-mail: mkakei@jcom.home.ne.jp

M. Yoshikawa
Division of Orthodontics, Meikai University School of Dentistry, Sakado, Japan
e-mail: ym-ortho@dent.meikai.ac.jp

H. Mishima
Department of Dental Engineering, Tsurumi University School of Dental Medicine, Yokohama, Japan
e-mail: mishima-h@tsurumi-u.ac.jp

K. Endo et al. (eds.), *Biomineralization*,
https://doi.org/10.1007/978-981-13-1002-7_2

2.1 Introduction

The lateral teeth of the radula exhibit a sequential series of tooth developments along with the production of iron biominerals from the organic stage to the fully mineralized stage. Regarding the iron biominerals in the radula teeth of the chiton, the teeth were composed of multilayers of iron oxide, predominately in the form of magnetite, but also in other forms of ferrihydrite and lepidocrocite (Lowenstam 1967). Therefore, many studies have focused mainly on these iron biominerals in the tooth cusp (Lowenstam 1967; Kim et al. 1986; Weaver et al. 2010; van der Wal 1989; Martin et al. 2009; Han et al. 2011). The tooth cusps of posterior side are mainly reinforced by the mineralization of magnetite at the matured stage. Due to its hardness, TEM study conducted by making thin sections has not been available in particular for the fully matured chiton teeth so far. On the other hand, the presence of a calcium phosphate mineral in the tooth core region has been examined using various techniques for a considerable time (Lowenstam and Weiner 1985; Kim et al. 1986; Evans et al. 1992; Evans and Alvarez 1999; Lee et al. 2000). Although a study using electron microscopy has been tried to demonstrate the presence of apatite crystal (Evans et al. 1992), the precise structure of apatite crystal has not yet fully elucidated. In this study, we have conducted the present study to demonstrate the unique iron mineral deposits and verify the detailed structure of apatite crystal mineral using an electron microscope.

2.2 Materials and Methods

Samples of the chiton *Acanthopleura japonica* were collected at Hachijojima's coastal area, Tokyo, Japan. Radulae were extracted from the chiton. After the removal of the soft tissue, radulae were cut into segments corresponding roughly to the three developmental stages of radula teeth from the onset of tooth development, the middle, and the fully matured stages, by using a razor blade. Then samples were subjected to examine using transmission electron microscope. They were fixed with 2% glutaraldehyde in 0.1 M cacodylate buffer at pH 7.4 for 1 h at 5 °C, post-fixed with 1% osmium tetroxide in the same buffer for 1 h at 5 °C, dehydrated by passage through a series of ascending ethanol concentrations, and then embedded in Araldite 502. Thick sections were stained with toluidine blue solution. Based on different color patterns at the posterior side of ralular teeth, these developmental stages tentatively called the initial stage with colorless, the middle stage with reddish-brown, and the fully matured stage with black color were examined. Thin sections were obtained with a Porter Blum MT2 ultra-microtome (SORVALL) equipped with a diamond knife. Sections were stained with saturated uranyl acetate and lead citrate, and some were left unstained. Also, some treated with an aqua regia solution were subjected to study. Then, they were examined under a JEM 100CX electron microscope (JEOL) at an accelerating voltage of 80 kV.

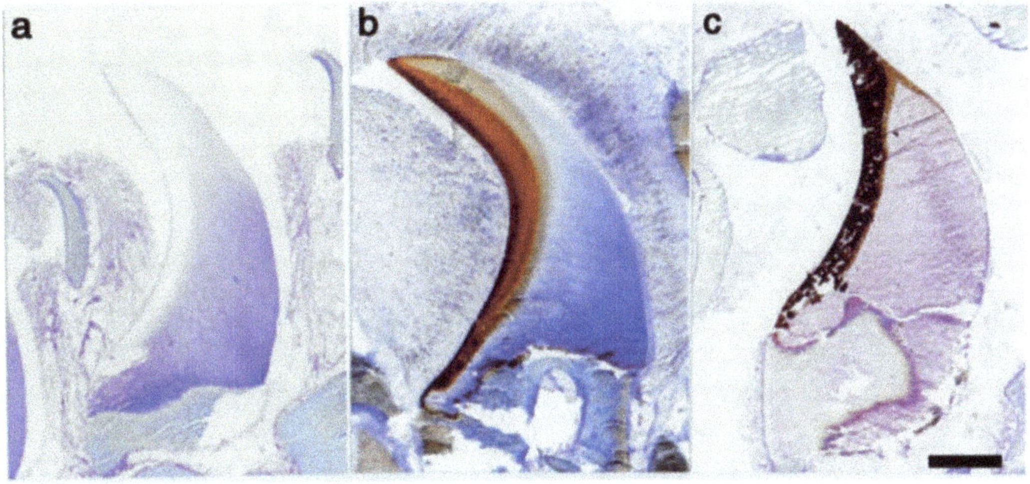

Fig. 2.1 Toluidine blue staining of the radula chiton teeth at three different stages. The change of color patterns at the posterior side reflects the degree of iron mineralization process. (**a**) The initial stage, (**b**) the middle stage, and (**c**) the fully matured stage. Toluidine blue-stained sections. Bar = 150 μm

2.3 Results and Discussion

Toluidine blue staining showed three different color patterns at the posterior side of three developmental stages from the initial stage with colorless, the middle stage with reddish-brown, and the fully matured stage with black color, respectively (Fig. 2.1).

At the colorless stage of the onset of tooth development, the internal structure of tooth cusps was filled with fibrous layers arranging in relatively parallel to the tooth surface at the anterior side (Fig. 2.2a). On the other hand, at the posterior side, fibrous layers bent upward adjacent to the inside of tooth cusp and run through toward the tooth tip (Fig. 2.2b).

At the reddish-brown stage of horizontal section, it was noted that higher magnifications of unstained sections have demonstrated that the deposits of ion mincrals appeared immediately and grew more quickly at the posterior side than at the anterior side. So, it is suitable to examine the mineral deposits at the anterior side of the tooth cusp. A comparison between stained and unstained sections showed that the electron-dense zones were sandwiched by electron-lucent fibrous layers (Fig. 2.3). This suggests that the electron-dense zones might store mineral ions. At this stage, fibrous layers were altered to be the plume structure (Fig. 2.4a). Double-stained section showed the small and discrete particles were developed along fibrous layers. Also, it have been observed that a complex of tiny clusters of fine grains showing different electron density, which looked like a bunch of grapes, developed associating with the plume structure (Fig. 2.4b). The developed fine grains showing different electron densities seemed to aggregate each other and increase its size to create larger nonuniform grains.

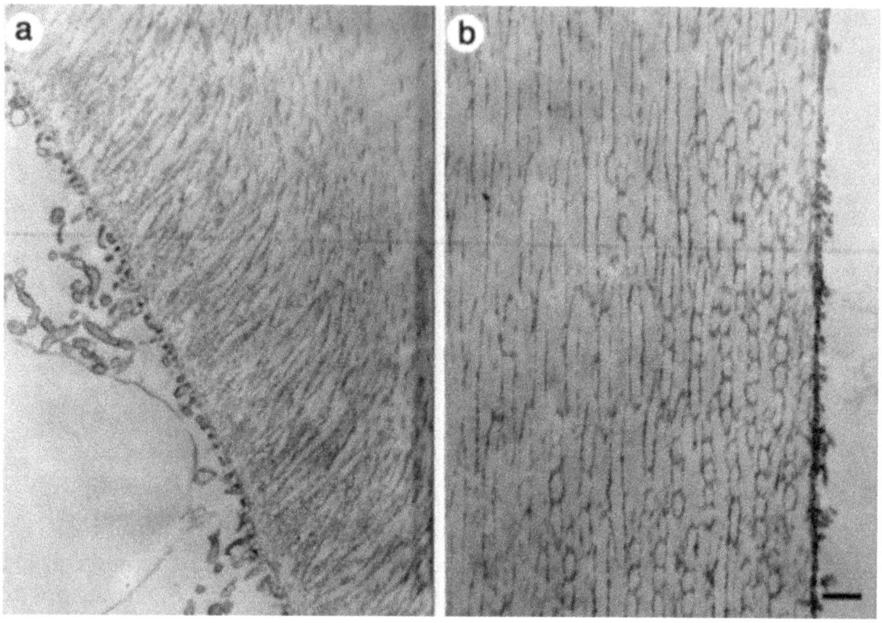

Fig. 2.2 TEM observations of the initial stage of chiton tooth. The arrangement of fibrous layer in the anterior side is different from posterior side of tooth cup. Double-stained sections. Bar = 0.5 μm

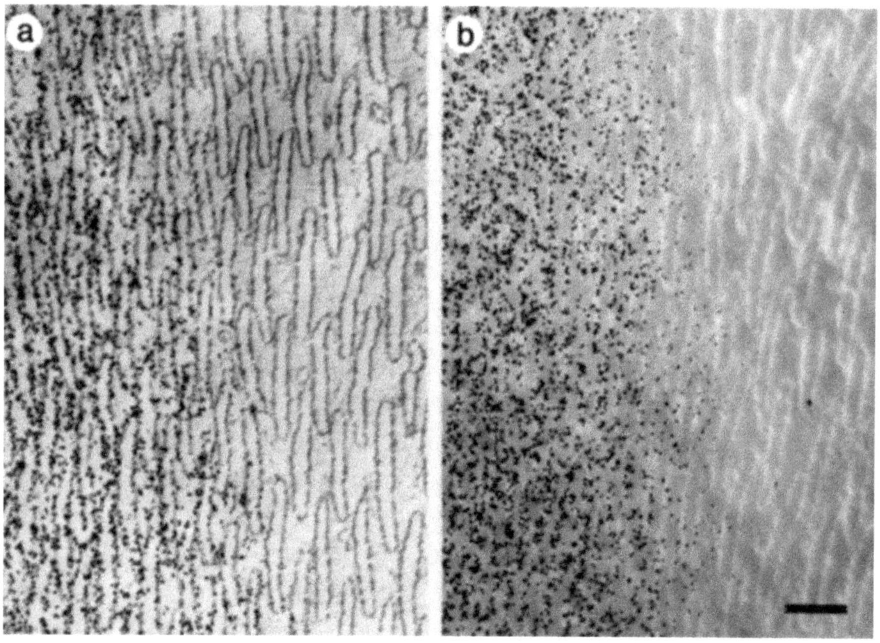

Fig. 2.3 TEM observations of the middle stage. By comparing stained with unstained sections, the space between organic layers shows a relatively high electron density. Double-stained (**a**) and unstained (**b**) sections. Bar = 1.0 μm

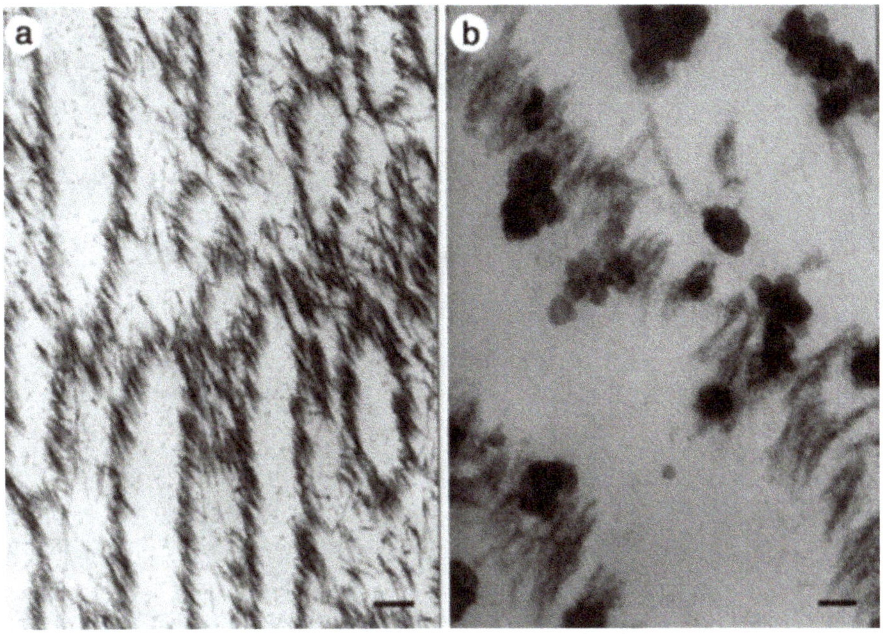

Fig. 2.4 High magnification of the plume structure (**a**) and the development of iron mineral grains (**b**) at the middle stage. The fine grains of iron minerals develop along the plume structure (**b**). Double stain. Bars = 100 nm (**a**), 2.0 μm (**b**)

At the black color stage of longitudinal sections, TEM study has demonstrated that the multilayers of iron minerals at the posterior side showed a brick-like or veneer-like wall structure (Weaver et al. 2010) (Fig. 2.5a). Each iron layer seemed to be comprised of relatively large minerals (Fig. 2.5b). Also, it was noted that small minerals were scattering in distribution. After treating with an aqua regia solution, organic substances remained between iron minerals (Fig. 2.6a, b). Although the role of organic matrix is not fully elucidated, it has been considered that the organic matrix may control the mineralization processes (van der Wal et al. 2000; Nemoto et al. 2012) and contribute to resist crack and increase the tensile strength and flexibility during the feeding by the teeth (Evans et al. 1990; van der Wal et al. 2000).

Iron minerals observed near the core (Fig. 2.7a, b) and in the magnetite (Fig. 2.7c, d) regions are shown in Fig. 2.7. Regarding the lattice fringes of iron minerals, the estimate of lattice intervals of these iron minerals was ranging from 4.8 to 10.2 Å, approximately. On the basis of the observation at a high magnification of Fig. 2.5b, it has been considered that small iron minerals might gather together to create a lump of iron minerals. It is also considered that random arrangement of iron minerals could prevent the radula teeth from becoming magnetic and attracting ion sand which comes from the sandy beach.

TEM observation has clearly demonstrated the crystal fringe of apatite crystal in the core region (Fig. 2.8). Whether the crystals are fluorapatite have been discussed previously (Lowenstam 1967; Kim et al. 1986; Evans et al. 1992; Evans and Alvarez 1999; Lee et al. 2000). To our knowledge, the biologically induced apatite crystals are divided into central dark line (CDL)-free and CDL-bearing types (Kakei et al. 2016). Viewing from the CDL-free type of crystal structure in the core region of the chiton teeth, we assumed that fluorapatite was formed.

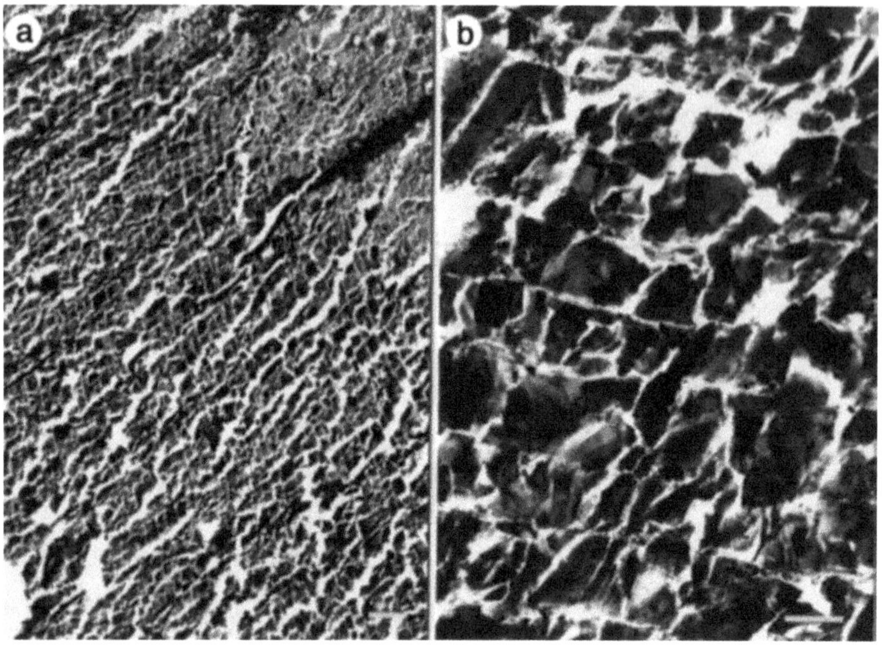

Fig. 2.5 TEM observations of the posterior region at the fully matured stage. The mineral layers consist of a brick-like wall or so-called veneer structure at the posterior side (**a**). Each mineral layer consists of both large angular and small minerals (**b**). No stain. Bars = 1.0 μm (**a**), 200 nm (**b**)

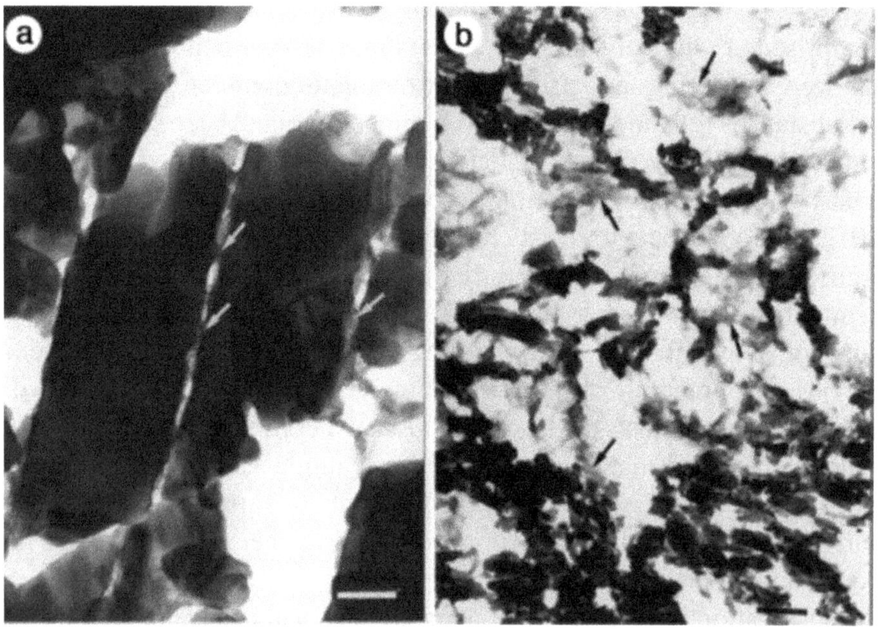

Fig. 2.6 TEM observations of aqua regia solution-treated sections. Treating with an aqua regia solution shows organic substances remained between iron minerals and suggesting a possible role of glue. (**a**) 5 min treatment, (**b**) 3 min treatment. Arrows indicate organic substances. Double-stained sections. Bar = 100 nm (**a**), 20 nm (**b**)

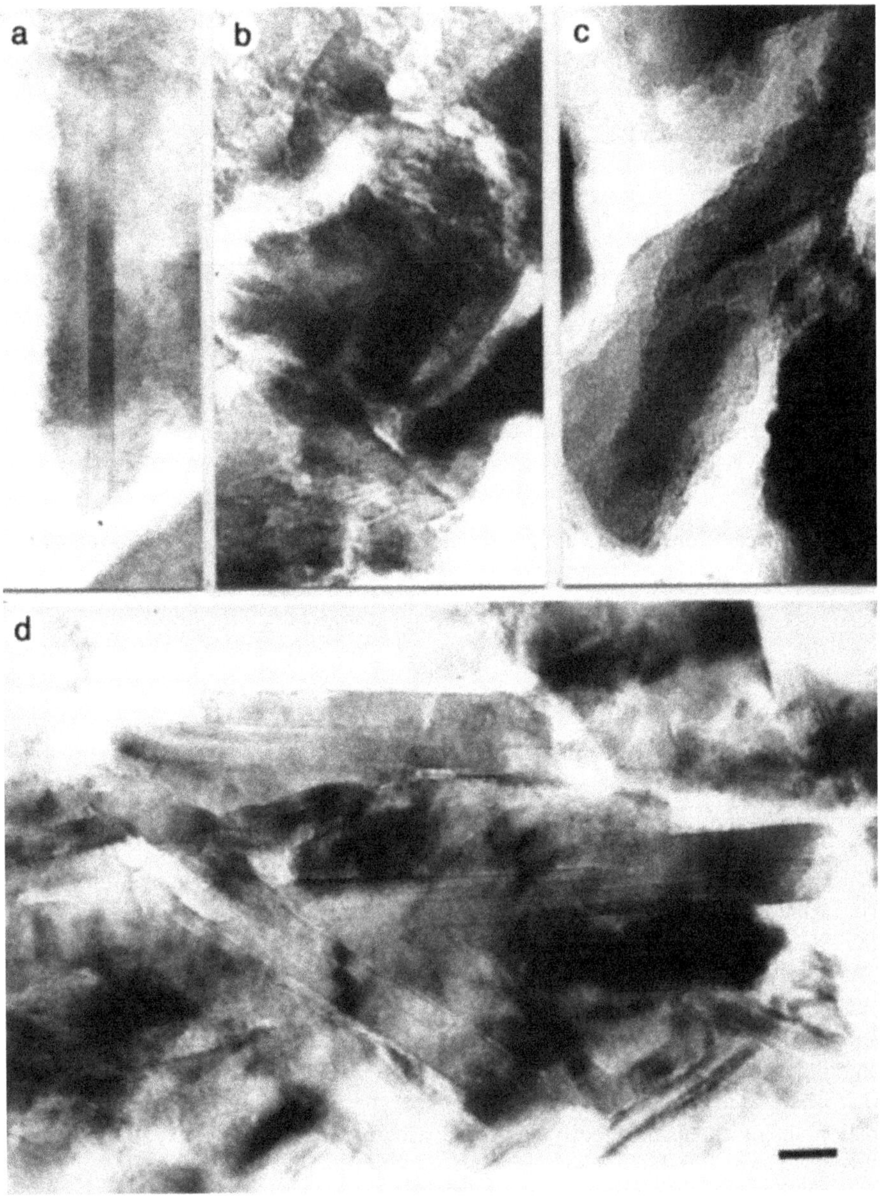

Fig. 2.7 TEM observations of iron minerals in the posterior region. Lattice fringes of iron minerals are recognized (**a–d**). Iron minerals are randomly arranged (**d**). No stain. Bar = 10 nm

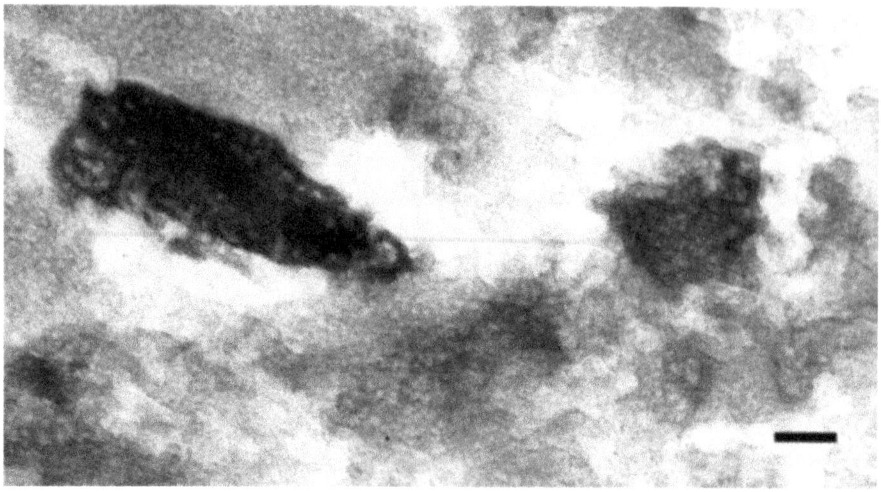

Fig. 2.8 TEM observations of calcium phosphate mineral in the core region. Two apatite crystals are confirmed. No stain. Bar = 10 nm

References

Evans LA, Alvarez R (1999) Characterization of the calcium biomineral in the teeth of chiton *Pellisepentis*. JBIC 4:166–170

Evans LA, Macey DJ, Webb J (1990) Characterization and structural organization of the organic matrix of the radular teeth of the chiton *Acanthopleura hirtosa*. Philos Trans R Soc Lond B 329:87–96

Evans LA, Macey DJ, Webb J (1992) Calcium biomineralization in the radula teeth of the chiton, *Acanthopleura hirtosa*. Calcif Tissue Int 51:78–82

Han Y, Liu C, Zhou D, Li F, Wang Y, Han X (2011) Magnetic and structural properties of magnetite in radular teeth of chiton. Bioelectromagnetics 32:226–233

Kakei M, Yoshikawa M, Mishima H (2016) Aspects of the apatite crystal: two pathways for apatite formation, the mechanisms underlying crystal structure defects, and the pathological calcification event. J Fossil Res 48(2):53–65

Kim K-S, Webb J, Macey DJ, Cohen DD (1986) Compositional changes during biomineralization of the radula of the chiton *Clavarizona hirtosa*. J Inorg Biochem 28:337–345

Lee AP, Brooker DJ, Macey DJ, van Bronswijk W, Webb J (2000) Apatite menralization in teeth of the chiton *Acanthopleura echinata*. Apatite mineralization in teeth of the chiton *Acanthopleura echinata*. Calcif Tissue Int 67:408–415

Lowenstam HA (1967) Lepidocrocite, an apatite mineral, and megnetite in teeth of chiton (Polyplacophora). Science 156:1373–1375

Lowenstam HA, Weiner S (1985) Transformation of amorphous calcium phosphate to crystalline dahllite in radular teeth of chitons. Science 227:51–53

Martin S, Kong C, Shaw JA, Macey DJ, Clode P (2009) Characterization of biominerals in the teeth of the chiton, *Acanthopleura hirtosa*. J Struct Biol 167:55–61

Nemoto M, Wang Q, Li D, Pan S, Matsunaga T, Kisailus D (2012) Proteomic analysis from the mineralized radular teeth of the giant Pacific chiton, *Cryptochiton stelleri* (Mollusca). Proteomics 12:2890–2894 van der Wal P (1989) Structural and material design of mature mineralized radula teeth of *Patella vulgata* (Gastropoda). J Ultrastruct Mol Struct Res 102:147–161

van der Wal P, Gleasen HJ, Videler JJ (2000) Radular teeth as models for the improvement of industrial cutting device. Mater Sci Eng C Biomim Supramol Syst 7:129–142

Weaver JC, Wang Q, Miserez A, Tantuccio A, Stromberg R, Bozhilov KN, Maxwell P, Nay R, Heier ST, DiMasi E, Kisailus D (2010) Analysis of an ultra hard magnetic biomineral in chiton radular teeth. Materialstoday 13 (1–2):42–52

Chapter 3
Experimental Cremation of Bone: Crystallite Size and Lattice Parameter Evolution

Martina Greiner, Balazs Kocsis, Mario F. Heinig, Katrin Mayer, Anita Toncala, Gisela Grupe, and Wolfgang W. Schmahl

Abstract In this study we investigate pristine and experimentally incinerated bovine bone material with differing annealing times and temperatures from 100 to 1000 °C to analyse the crystallographic change of natural bone mineral during cremation. We used X-ray powder diffraction (XRPD) and Fourier transform infrared (FTIR) spectroscopy as complementary methods. We observe a structural change of bone mineral during cremation. Our study highlights that there are only few or even no hydroxyl ions in pristine bone mineral (bioapatite), which is a carbonate-hydroapatite rather than a hydroxyapatite. A significant recrystallization reaction from bioapatite to hydroxyapatite takes place at elevated temperatures from 700 °C (after 30 min cremation time). This process is associated with a significant increase of crystallite size, and it involves an increase of hydroxyl in the apatite lattice that goes along with a depletion of water and carbonate contents during cremation. Our first results highlight the importance of both time and temperature on the recrystallization reaction during cremation.

Keywords Carbonated apatite · Calcium phosphate · Bioapatite · Bone · X-ray diffraction · FTIR · Rietveld refinement

---

M. Greiner (✉) · B. Kocsis · M. F. Heinig · W. W. Schmahl
Department für Geo- und Umweltwissenschaften, Ludwig-Maximilians-Universität, Munich, Germany
e-mail: martina.greiner@lrz.uni-muenchen.de; wolfgang.schmahl@lrz.uni-muenchen.de

K. Mayer · A. Toncala · G. Grupe
Fakultät für Biologie, Anthropologie und Humangenetik, Ludwig-Maximilians-Universität, Martinsried, Germany
e-mail: katrin.mayer@mnet-online.de; G.Grupe@lrz.uni-muenchen.de

K. Endo et al. (eds.), *Biomineralization*,
https://doi.org/10.1007/978-981-13-1002-7_3

3.1 Introduction

The Forschergruppe FOR 1670 project on human transalpine mobility in the Late Bronze Age to Early Roman times performs isotope studies on archaeological bone finds. During that age, cremating the deceased was the primary burial custom (Grupe et al. 2015). To understand bone alteration by cremation, we study the evolution of bone crystallography and crystallite size as a function of cremation temperature and annealing time for bovine bone by FTIR and X-ray diffraction. Mammal bone mineral is a nanocrystalline material consisting of an apatite mineral that is chemically far more complex than hydroxyapatite and can be approximated as $(Ca,Mg,Na)_{10-x}((PO_4)_{6-x}(CO_3)_x)(OH_{1-y-z}, (CO_3)_y, (H_2O)_z)_2$ (Elliott 2002; Rey et al. 2007). It comprises between 5 and 8 wt% carbonate, which substitutes in the $[OH]^-$ site (A-type substitution) as well as the $[PO]_4^{3-}$ site (B-type substitution) of the apatite structure (LeGeros et al. 1969; Wopenka and Pasteris 2005; Pasteris et al. 2012; Yi et al. 2013). Previous studies showed that recrystallization of the bioapatite and crystallite growth mainly sets in from about 600 °C (Piga et al. 2009; Schmahl et al. 2017), but small changes are already apparent at low temperatures of 100 °C (Harbeck et al. 2011). In this study, we want to define more precisely the cremation temperature and annealing time where hydroxyapatite crystallization sets in.

3.2 Materials and Methods

Pieces of compact bone were cut from the tubular part of bovine femur; the endosteal and periosteal surfaces were mechanically removed. Samples were ultrasonically washed in deionized H_2O. After air-drying, the bones were defatted for 5 days with diethyl ether in a Soxhlet and air-dried. Finally, the samples were homogenized to a fine powder and passed through a 100 μm sieve.

Cremation experiments were carried out between 100 and 1000 °C in air (oxidizing conditions) in steps of 100 °C with 150 min annealing time. After data analysis of the initial results, we focussed on the temperatures of 650 and 700 °C and used shorter exposure times between 10 and 60 min in intervals of 10 min.

X-ray diffractograms were collected on a General Electric 3003 powder diffractometer in Bragg-Brentano reflection geometry. Cu-$K_{\alpha 1}$ radiation was selected with an exposure time of 1000s.

All samples were mixed with NIST 660b LaB_6 as internal standard (2–5 wt%). The FULLPROF code (Rodríguez-Carvajal 1993; Rodríguez-Carvajal and Roisnel 2004) was applied for data evaluation and Rietveld refinement (Rietveld 1969). The Thompson-Cox-Hastings method for convolution of instrumental resolution with size and isotropic microstrain broadening (Thompson et al. 1987) was applied. For refinement, a hexagonal symmetry model for carbonated apatite was used (Wilson et al. 2004).

Infrared spectra were measured on a Bruker Equinox FTIR instrument with a resolution of 4 cm^{-1} with 128 scans.

3.3 Results

3.3.1 X-Ray Diffraction: 100 °C Intervals

Figure 3.1a shows X-ray powder diffraction patterns of untreated and cremated bones up to 1000 °C. The untreated bone mineral displays extremely broadened peaks. The broadening decreases only little with 150 min heat treatment up until 600 °C, whereas the diffraction pattern sharpens considerably from 700 °C upwards.

Exemplary Rietveld refinements of samples cremated at 600 °C and 700 °C for 150 min annealing time are shown in Fig. 3.1b, c. Enlarged images of the 31–35° 2θ section show overlapping apatite diffraction peaks in Fig. 3.1b, whereas peaks in Fig. 3.1c can clearly be distinguished from each other. The lattice parameters and crystallite sizes obtained by Rietveld refinement of diffractograms measured at room temperature for the 150 min heat-treated samples are shown in Fig. 3.1d, e. Note the sharp rise of the crystallite size setting in at 700 °C. The lattice parameters show an initial increase with annealing treatment and then sharply drop at temperatures where the grain size sharply increases.

3.3.2 X-Ray Diffraction: 10 Min Intervals

The X-ray diffractograms of the bovine bone cremated at 650 °C from 10 to 60 min depict a steady narrowing of the diffraction peaks with increasing annealing time. Nevertheless, a broad peak shape remains after 60 min annealing (Fig. 3.2a). The unit cell parameters shrink (Fig. 3.2b, c) already after 20 min cremation. The crystallite size increases more or less steadily with elapsed annealing time, whereas the biggest change is between 30 and 40 min with an increase of the crystallite size of 99.4(2) Å to 126.6(3) Å (Fig. 3.2c).

X-ray diffractograms of bovine bone cremated at 700 °C from 10 to 60 min show a broad diffraction peak shape from 10 to 30 min annealing time. Samples annealed for 40 min or longer depict sharper peaks. Bovine bone incinerated at 700 °C shows a steady increase of the crystallite size up to 30 min experimental cremation. From 30 to 40 min elapsing time, we observe a significant jump from 117.85(2) Å to 294.8(3) Å (2.5 times larger) (Fig. 3.2f). Moreover, we observe a decrease of lattice parameters a and c until 40 min annealing times. This trend is reversed after 50 min annealing (Fig. 3.2e, f).

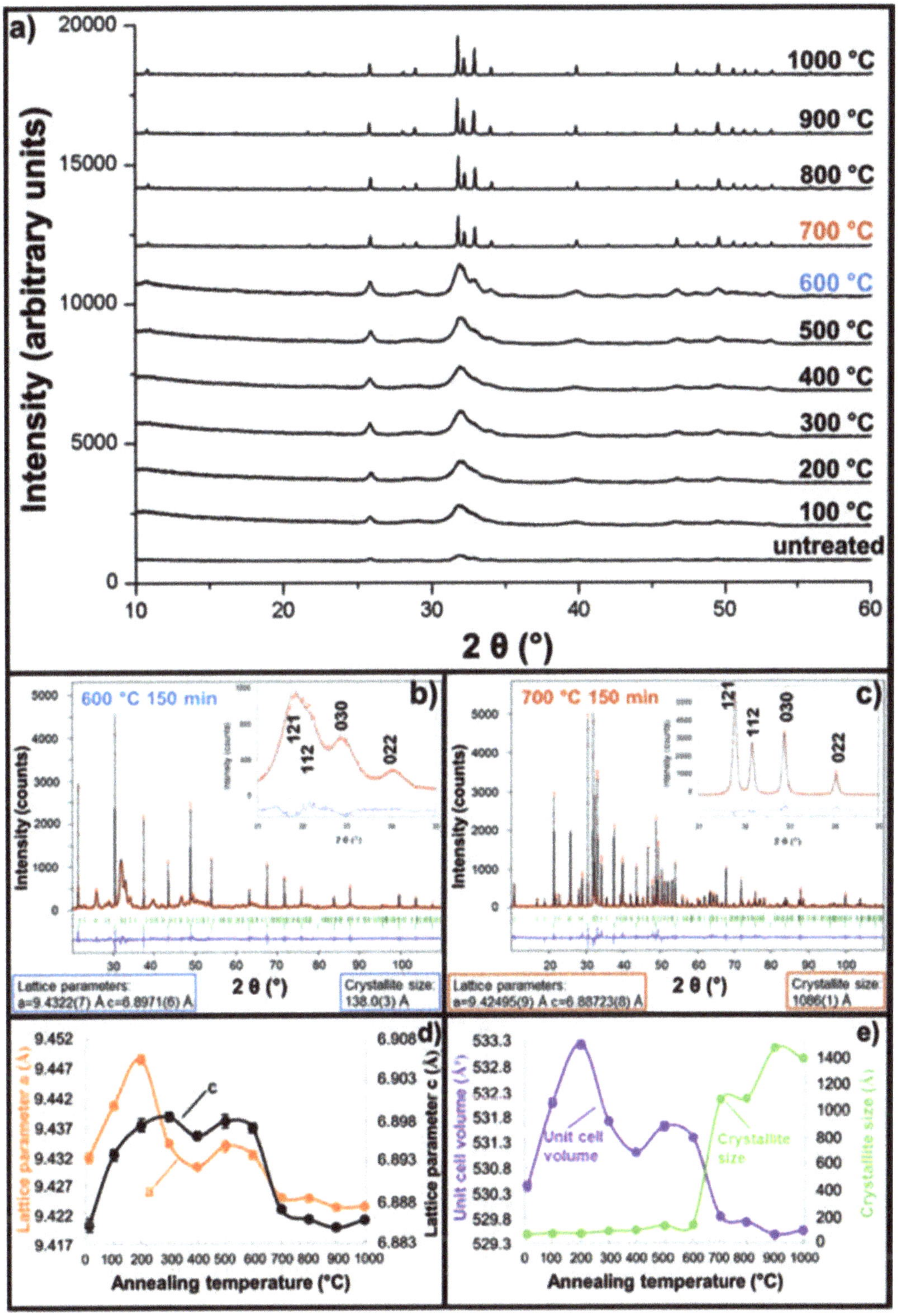

Fig. 3.1 (**a**) Comparison of the 10–60° 2θ range of X-ray diffractograms (Cu-$K_{\alpha1}$) of cremated bones from 100 to 1000 °C; (**b**) Rietveld refinement of bovine bone cremated at 600 °C, 150 min annealing. *Red dots*, observed data points; *black line*, calculated XRD profile; *bottom blue line*, difference of observed and calculated data; *green vertical bars*, positions of diffraction peaks; *top row*, bone apatite; *bottom row*, LaB_6 standard. Enlarged region shows 31–35° 2θ range with overlapping 121, 112, 030 and 022 peaks; (**c**) Rietveld refinement of bovine bone cremated at 700 °C after 150 min annealing. Enlarged region shows 30–35° 2θ range with clearly distinct 121, 112, 030 and 022 peaks; (**d**) Lattice parameters a (=b) and c of untreated and annealed bone material at temperatures from 100 to 1000 °C after 150 min annealing; (**e**) Unit cell volume and crystallite size of untreated and cremated bones from 100 to 1000 °C after 150 min annealing

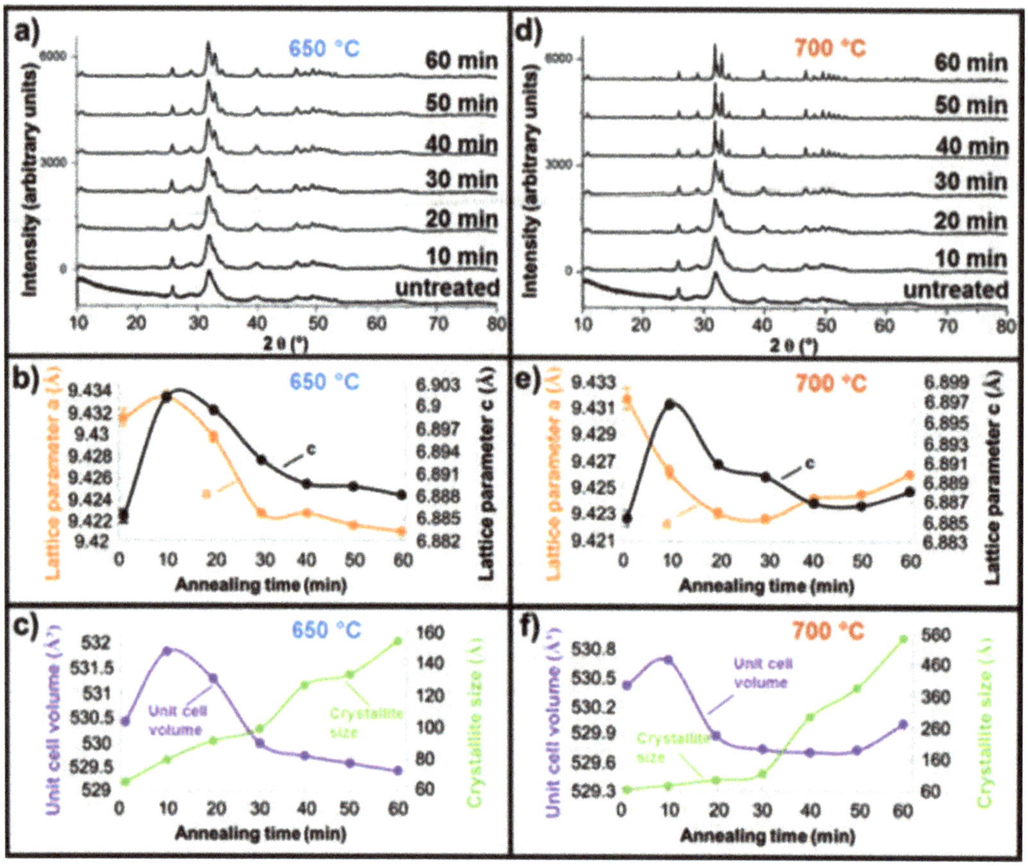

Fig. 3.2 (**a**) Comparison of the 10–80° 2θ range of X-ray diffractograms (Cu-$K_{\alpha 1}$) of untreated and cremated bones at 650 °C, 10–60 min annealing; (**b**) Lattice parameters a (=b) and c of untreated and cremated bones at 650 °C, 10–60 min annealing; (**c**) Unit cell volume and crystallite size of untreated and cremated bones at 650 °C, 10–60 min annealing; (**d**) 10–80° 2θ range of X-ray diffractograms of untreated and cremated bones at 700 °C, 10–60 min annealing; (**e**) Lattice parameters a(=b) and c of untreated and cremated bones at 700 °C, 10–60 min annealing; (**f**) Unit cell volume and crystallite size of untreated and cremated bones at 700 °C, 10–60 min annealing

3.3.3 FTIR

Figure 3.3a shows a comparison of IR spectra for different annealing temperatures. Characteristic phosphate group absorption bands at 470–480 cm^{-1} ($\nu_2 PO_4^{3-}$), 500–750 cm^{-1} ($\nu_4 PO_4^{3-}$), ~962 cm^{-1} ($\nu_1 PO_4^{3-}$) and 980–1120 cm^{-1} ($\nu_3 PO_4^{3-}$) were identified according to Destainville et al. (2003) and Raynaud et al. (2002). Annealed bone at 1000 °C shows a well-differentiated hydroxyl libration peak at ~632 cm^{-1} which is absent in the FTIR spectra of untreated bovine bone (Fig. 3.3b).

Absorption bands at 873–879 cm^{-1} and 1400–1458 cm^{-1} were attributed to $\nu_2 CO_3^{2-}$ and $\nu_3 CO_3^{2-}$ (Fleet 2009; Grunenwald et al. 2014; Rey et al. 1989). The intensity of carbonate bands begins to decrease from 400 °C with increasing annealing temperatures and can barely be observed for the sample cremated at 1000 °C (see Fig. 3.3a). For untreated bovine bone, we observe broad H_2O absorption bands from ~3000 to 3600 cm^{-1} (Brubach et al. 2005). These peaks lose intensity with heat treatment and disappear for the 700 °C and higher heat treatments (Fig. 3.3c).

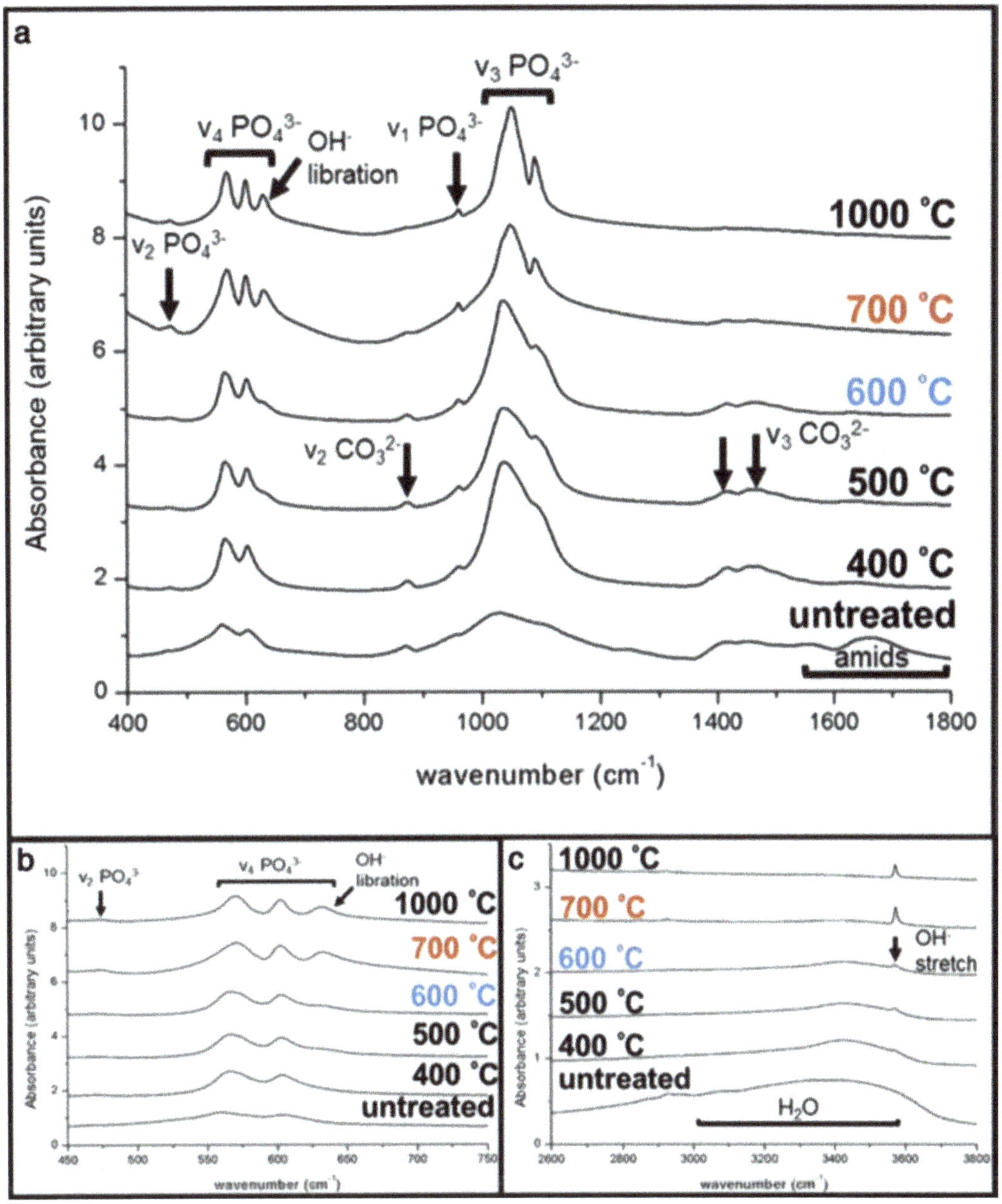

Fig. 3.3 (**a**) Comparison of the 400–1800 cm^{-1} FTIR spectra of untreated and cremated bovine bone at 400, 500, 600, 700 and 1000 °C (annealing time 150 min); (**b**) Enlargement of the 450–750 cm^{-1} region of Fig. 3.2a) with $\nu_2PO_4^{3-}$ and $\nu_4PO_4^{3-}$ vibration bands and emerging OH$^-$ libration band with increasing cremation temperature; (**c**) 2600–3800 cm^{-1} region of untreated and cremated bone (400, 500, 600, 700 and 1000 °C) indicating decreasing H_2O absorption bands and increasing OH$^-$ stretching mode with increasing cremation temperature

The OH$^-$ stretch vibration gives a sharp peak at 3570 cm^{-1} (González-Díaz and Hidalgo 1976; González-Díaz and Santos 1977; Vandecandelaere et al. 2012). The band at ~632 cm^{-1} was assigned to the OH$^-$ libration mode (Destainville et al. 2003). In the untreated bone spectra and for low annealing temperatures, neither the OH$^-$ libration peak near 630 cm^{-1} nor the sharp and distinct OH$^-$ stretching vibration peak at 3570 cm^{-1} is present. However, these OH^- signals emerge with annealing at 400 °C and significantly increase and become well-differentiated for samples annealed at temperatures of 700 °C or higher (see Fig. 3.3b, c).

3.4 Discussion

In the original bone, we observe broad diffraction peaks (Figs. 3.1a and 3.2a, b) due to the nanoscale dimension of the bone apatite crystallites. Further, the high intensity of the carbonate and H_2O vibration bands and absence of OH^- bands quite clearly indicate that bone apatite is a carbonate-hydro-apatite rather than a hydroxyapatite (Fig. 3.3a–c). Loong et al. (2000) using inelastic neutron scattering and Pasteris et al. (2004) using Raman spectroscopy came to similar conclusions.

With extended annealing treatment, the diffraction peaks of the bone mineral get sharper; the $(CO_3)^{2-}$ infrared signals decrease, while the OH^- infrared peaks increase. Within the broad water band, one can clearly see the rising of the OH^- stretching is a function of increasing annealing temperature (Fig. 3.3c). This indicates a reaction from bioapatite (carbonate-hydro-apatite) to hydroxyapatite with heat treatment, as the material approaches stoichiometric chemistry. This reaction is associated with growth of the crystallites; the growth becomes more rapid at temperatures from 700 °C and higher (Figs. 3.1a and 3.2d). At the same time, loss of carbonate and water and their replacement by OH^- in the structure lead to a decrease of unit cell parameters (Figs. 3.1d, e and 3.2b–f).

While observing these structural changes occurring, it cannot be simply concluded that the process occurs homogeneously within the apatite lattice. It is just as likely that the bioapatite decomposes and that hydroxyapatite is formed in a heterogeneous reaction at the expense of the decomposing bioapatite. It must be borne in mind that our techniques integrate over the whole volume of the sample, and the diffraction peak positions as well as IR frequencies of both mineral phases (bioapatite and hydroxyapatite) are very close and initially severely broadened. Thus our techniques might well record a superposition of the signals of both phases coexisting. Here it is important to note that the distinct increase of the crystallite size for temperatures of and above 700 °C sets in after 30 min of annealing time (Fig. 3.2e, f). This may be indicative of a heterogeneous rather than a homogeneous reaction from bioapatite to hydroxyapatite. For an increase of crystallite size of only one homogeneous apatite phase by Ostwald ripening, the evolution of crystallite size with time (Fig. 3.2f) should have the opposite curvature than observed.

The time dependence (Fig. 3.2) of the reaction process becomes important when concluding from bone crystallinity to cremation temperature. Up to 40 min cremation time, we see the same trend for lattice parameters when comparing 650 and 700 °C: a decrease of lattice parameters a and c and therefore a shrinkage of the unit cell coupled with an increase of the crystallite size (Fig. 3.2b–f). After more than 30 min annealing at 700 °C, we see more rapidly increasing lattice parameters, an effect which is not observable in the 650 °C temperature experiments. Moreover, at

700 °C after 30 min annealing, we observe also a significant change in crystallite size which we attribute to a progressive recrystallization reaction of bioapatite to hydroxyapatite. At that time, the decomposition products (essentially carbon) of organics such as collagen, which comprise about 35 wt% of the original bone material (Rogers and Zioupos 1999), are almost completely gone, and the hydroxyapatite crystallites can grow without being impeded by films of organics or their residues which separate the crystallites.

Note that bone annealed at 400 °C for 150 min displays essentially the same crystallite sizes as bone treated for 20 min at 700 °C (~97 Å), and bone annealed at 600 °C for 150 min displays similar crystallite sizes as bone treated at 650 °C for 50 min (~133 Å). Our experiments reveal that it is important to consider the influence of time when concluding from material state on cremation conditions.

Acknowledgement We thank the Deutsche Forschungsgemeinschaft (DFG) for funding the project in Forschergruppe FOR1670 under Schm930/12-1 and Gr 959/20-1,2.

References

Brubach JB et al (2005) Signatures of the hydrogen bonding in the infrared bands of water. J Chem Phys 122:184509

Destainville A et al (2003) Synthesis, characterization and thermal behavior of apatitic tricalcium phosphate. Mater Chem Phys 80:269–277

Elliott JC (2002) Calcium phosphate biominerals. Rev Mineral Geochem 48:427–453

Fleet ME (2009) Infrared spectra of carbonate apatites: v2-region bands. Biomaterials 30:1473–1481

González-Díaz PF, Hidalgo A (1976) Infrared spectra of calcium apatites. Spectrochim Acta A 32:631–635

González-Díaz PF, Santos M (1977) On the hydroxyl ions in apatites. J Solid State Chem 22:193–199

Grunenwald A et al (2014) Revisiting carbonate quantification in apatite (bio)minerals: a validated FTIR methodology. J Archaeol Sci 49:134–141

Grupe G et al (2015) Prähistorische Anthropologie. Springer, Berlin

Harbeck M et al (2011) Research potential and limitations of trace analyses of cremated remains. Forensic Sci Int 204:191–200

LeGeros RZ et al (1969) Two types of carbonate substitution in the apatite structure. Experientia 25:5–7

Loong CK et al (2000) Evidence of hydroxyl-ion deficiency in bone apatites: an inelastic neutron-scattering study. Bone 26:599–602

Pasteris JD et al (2004) Lack of OH in nanocrystalline apatite as a function of degree of atomic order: implications for bone and biomaterials. Biomaterials 25:229–238

Pasteris JD et al (2012) Effect of carbonate incorporation on the hydroxyl content of hydroxylapatite. Mineral Mag 76:2741–2759

Piga G et al (2009) The potential of X-ray diffraction in the analysis of burned remains from forensic contexts. J Forensic Sci 54:534–539

Raynaud S et al (2002) Calcium phosphate apatites with variable Ca/P atomic ratio I. Synthesis, characterisation and thermal stability of powders. Biomaterials 23:1065–1072

Rey C et al (1989) The carbonate environment in bone mineral: a resolution-enhanced Fourier Transform Infrared Spectroscopy study. Calcif Tissue Int 45:157–164

Rey C et al (2007) Physico-chemical properties of nanocrystalline apatites: implications for biominerals and biomaterials. Mater Sci Eng C 27:198–205
Rietveld HM (1969) A profile refinement method for nuclear and magnetic structures. J Appl Crystallogr 2:65–71
Rodríguez-Carvajal J (1993) Recent advances in magnetic structure determination by neutron powder diffraction. Physica B 192:55–69
Rodríguez-Carvajal J, Roisnel T (2004) Line broadening analysis using FullProf*: determination of microstructural properties. Mater Sci Forum 443–444:123–126
Rogers KD, Zioupos P (1999) The bone tissue of the rostrum of a *Mesoplodon densirostris* whale: a mammalian biomineral demonstrating extreme texture. J Mater Sci Lett 18:651–654
Schmahl WW et al (2017) The crystalline state of archaeological bone material. In: Across the Alps in prehistory. Springer International Publishing, Cham
Thompson P, Cox DE, Hastings JB (1987) Rietveld refinement of Debye–Scherrer synchrotron X-ray data from Al_2O_3. J Appl Crystallogr 20:79–83
Vandecandelaere N et al (2012) Biomimetic apatite-based biomaterials: on the critical impact of synthesis and post-synthesis parameters. J Mater Sci Mater Med 23:2593–2606
Wilson RM et al (2004) Rietveld structure refinement of precipitated carbonate apatite using neutron diffraction data. Biomaterials 25:2205–2213
Wopenka B, Pasteris JD (2005) A mineralogical perspective on the apatite in bone. Mater Sci Eng C 25:131–143
Yi H et al (2013) A carbonate-fluoride defect model for carbonate-rich fluorapatite. Am Mineral 98:1066–1069

Chapter 4
Effect of Carbonic Anhydrase Immobilized on Eggshell Membranes on Calcium Carbonate Crystallization In Vitro

M. Soledad Fernández, Betzabe Montt, Liliana Ortiz, Andrónico Neira-Carrillo, and José Luis Arias

Abstract The eggshell membranes (ESM) serve as the first interface with the inorganic phase during eggshell formation. During mineral growth, crystals nucleate on the outer side of the ESM at specialized sites called mammillae, mainly consisting of mammillan, a keratan sulfate proteoglycan together with the activity of carbonic anhydrase (CA).

In order to get insight into the mechanisms of chicken eggshell mineralization, ESM was used as a biotemplate for immobilizing carbonic anhydrase (CA) and study in vitro calcite crystallization. Here, we showed that when the eggshell membrane supplemented with immobilized or dissolved carbonic anhydrase is located at the gas-liquid interface, calcite nucleation and growth are sequestered by the ESM scaffold from solution, thus affecting the morphology and size of the crystals formed.

Keywords Eggshell membrane · Carbonic anhydrase · Biomineralization

4.1 Introduction

Biomineralization is a widespread phenomenon in nature leading to the formation of a variety of solid inorganic structures by living organisms, such as intracellular crystals in prokaryotes; exoskeletons in protozoa, algae, and invertebrates; spicules and lenses; bone, teeth, statoliths, and otoliths; eggshells; plant mineral structures; and also pathological biominerals such as gall stones, kidney stones, and oyster pearls (Lowenstam and Weiner 1989; Mann et al. 1989; Simkiss and Wilbur 1989; Heuer et al. 1992; Arias and Fernandez 2008). By this process living organisms precipitate inorganic minerals on organic matrices. The resulting biominerals are deposited in elaborated shapes and hierarchical structures by interaction at the organic-inorganic interface, where the rate of crystal formation is regulated by the

M. S. Fernández (✉) · B. Montt · L. Ortiz · A. Neira-Carrillo · J. L. Arias
Faculty of Veterinary Sciences, University of Chile, Santiago, Chile
e-mail: sofernan@uchile.cl; lbortizmendez@ug.uchile.cl; aneira@uchile.cl; jarias@uchile.cl

K. Endo et al. (eds.), *Biomineralization*,
https://doi.org/10.1007/978-981-13-1002-7_4

control of the microenvironment in which such mineralization events take place. One of the main biomineralization resulting mineral minerals is calcium carbonate ($CaCO_3$), especially the more stable form, calcite. The avian eggshell is a good example of multifunctional biomineral where an organic scaffold (or matrix), the eggshell membrane, plays a crucial role in regulating mineral nucleation and growth by incorporating inorganic precursors, such as ions, ion clusters, and amorphous phases (Rao et al. 2017); other organic matrices complete the formation of a calcified layer (i.e., palisade) composed of calcite columns (Panheleux et al. 1999). Structurally, the eggshell is a multilayered calcitic bioceramic. As the egg migrates through the oviduct, the biomineral matures under the influence of biomolecular additives and an extracellular matrix (Nys et al. 1999; Fernandez et al. 2001). The matrix, primarily composed of collagen fibers, constitutes the eggshell membranes (ESM) (Arias et al. 1991). Each fiber exhibits a core surrounded by a glycoproteinous material termed as the mantle. This serves as the first interface with the inorganic phase. During mineral growth, crystals nucleate on the outer side of the ESM at specialized sites called mammillae, mainly consisting of mammillan, a keratan sulfate proteoglycan together with the activity of carbonic anhydrase (CA). This metalloenzyme catalyzes the reversible hydration of carbonic dioxide to bicarbonate and a proton. In fact, it has been possible to mimic eggshell formation in vitro by adding the main organic components including CA, where an increase in calcium carbonate crystals growth and fusion was observed (Fernandez et al. 2004).

However, the use of enzymes in vitro is difficult, because of instability and the complexity for maintaining the catalytic function in chemical reactions (Lu et al. 2013). For that reason enzymatic immobilization on a solid substrate appears as a solution for this problem (Wanjari et al. 2013).

For in vitro biomineralization, a specific confined environment is needed, that means an inert scaffold which generates an almost two dimensional interface where the crystal nucleation takes place. Currently, many kinds of surfaces and/or supports are used for enzyme immobilization, and the ESM meets all the requirements to be used as a natural support for CA immobilization and in vitro biomineralization experiments.

In order to get insight into the mechanisms of chicken eggshell mineralization, ESM was used as a biotemplate for immobilizing carbonic anhydrase (CA).

4.2 Material and Methods

4.2.1 Carbonic Anhydrase (EC 4.2.1.1) Immobilization on ESM

ESM were obtained after 30 min incubation of an empty egg in 1% acetic acid to detach the membrane from de shell, and then ESM was incubated for another 48 h in 1% acetic acid to eliminate any remaining calcium carbonate crystals and then washed in deionized water three times (Arias et al. 2008).

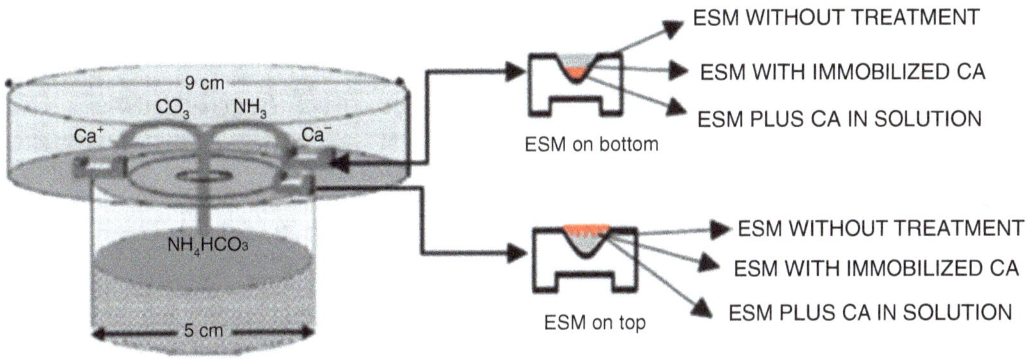

Fig. 4.1 Experimental setup used from growing in vitro $CaCO_3$ crystals showing the location of eggshell membrane strips either on the bottom or the top of the microbridges containers

For enzyme immobilization 1 mg of carbonic anhydrase (2500 units/mg, Sigma, St. Louis, MO, USA) in 1 mL deionized water was used; membranes were incubated for 1 h with 100 μL of this solution; then 20 μL of 2.5% glutaraldehyde for 30 min was used as cross-linking agent (Tembe et al. 2008). Then, membranes were washed with TRIS buffer solution pH 9 at 4 °C.

4.2.2 *Crystallization Experiments*

The crystallization assays were based on a variation of the sitting drop method developed elsewhere (Dominguez-Vera et al. 2000). Briefly, it consists of a chamber built with a 85 mm plastic petri dish having 18 mm in diameter central hole in its bottom, glued to a plastic cylindrical vessel (50 mm in diameter and 30 mm in height) (Fig. 4.1). The bottom of the petri dish was divided in 16 radii to assure an equidistant settling of odd number of polystyrene microbridges (Hampon Res., Laguna Niguel, CA). The microbridges were filled with 35 μL of 200 mM dihydrate calcium chloride solution in 200 mM Tris buffer, pH 9.0. The cylindrical vessel contained 3 ml of 25 mM ammonium carbonate. One strip of eggshell membrane with or without immobilized CA or with CA in solution was deposited on the bottom or on the top of each microbridge with the mammillary side facing up or upside down, respectively. Five replicates of each experiment were carried out inside the chamber at 20 °C for 24 h. After the experiments, eggshell strips were taken out of the microbridges, air-dried at room temperature, mounted on aluminum stubs with scotch double-sided tape, and coated with gold. Crystal morphology was observed and size estimated in an Hitachi TM 3000 scanning electron microscope.

4.3 Results

4.3.1 *ESM on Bottom of the Microbridge 24 H Incubation*

After 24 h incubation using ESM without treatment, rounded calcite crystals were observed deposited on the ESM (Fig. 4.2a), with an average size of 21.33 ± 1.97 μm (Table 4.1). By contrast, when ESM with immobilized CA was used, regular

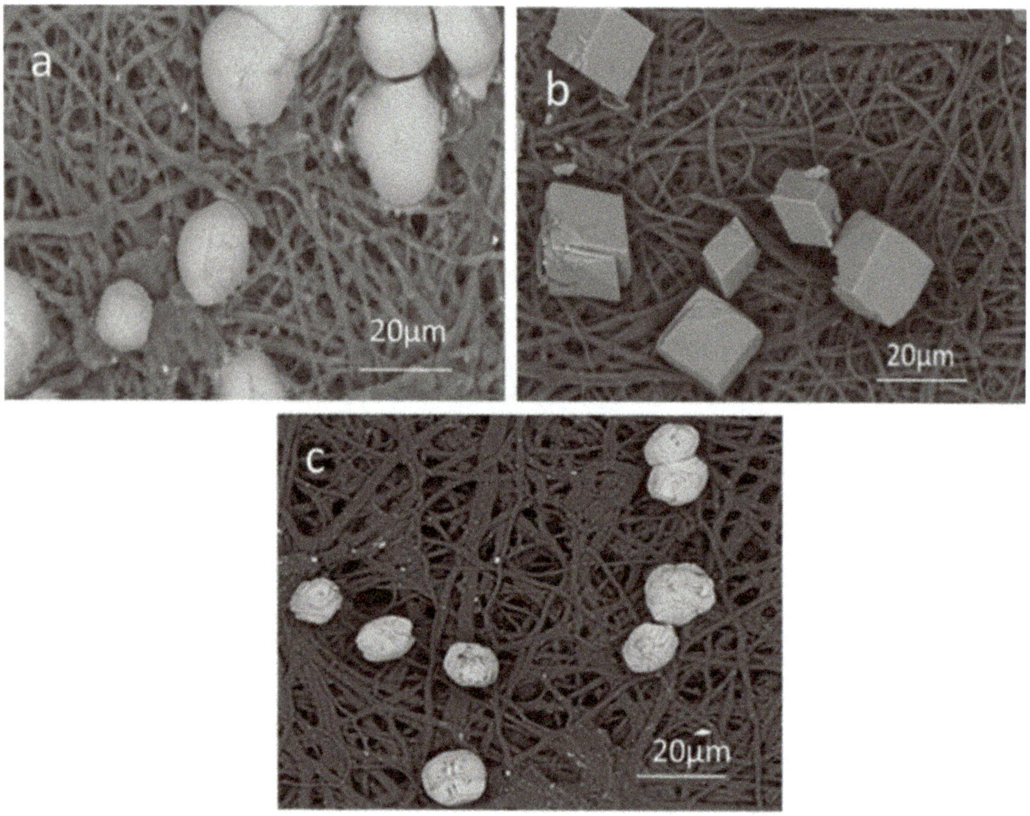

Fig. 4.2 Eggshell membrane (ESM) on bottom of the microbridge after 24 h incubation: (**a**) ESM without treatment, 1000X; (**b**) ESM with immobilized CA, 1000X; (**c**) ESM without treatment but with CA dissolved in the calcification medium 1000X

Table 4.1 Size of calcite crystals deposited on eggshell membrane (ESM) measured under different conditions

		Crystal size μm ± S.D
ESM at the bottom of the microbridge	Control	21.33 ± 1.97
	CA immobilized	31.0 ± 2.08
	CA in solution	20.0 ± 3.68
ESM at the top of the microbridge facing calcification solution	Control	22.1 ± 1.91
	CA immobilized	35.83 ± 3.53
	CA in solution	27.83 ± 2.47

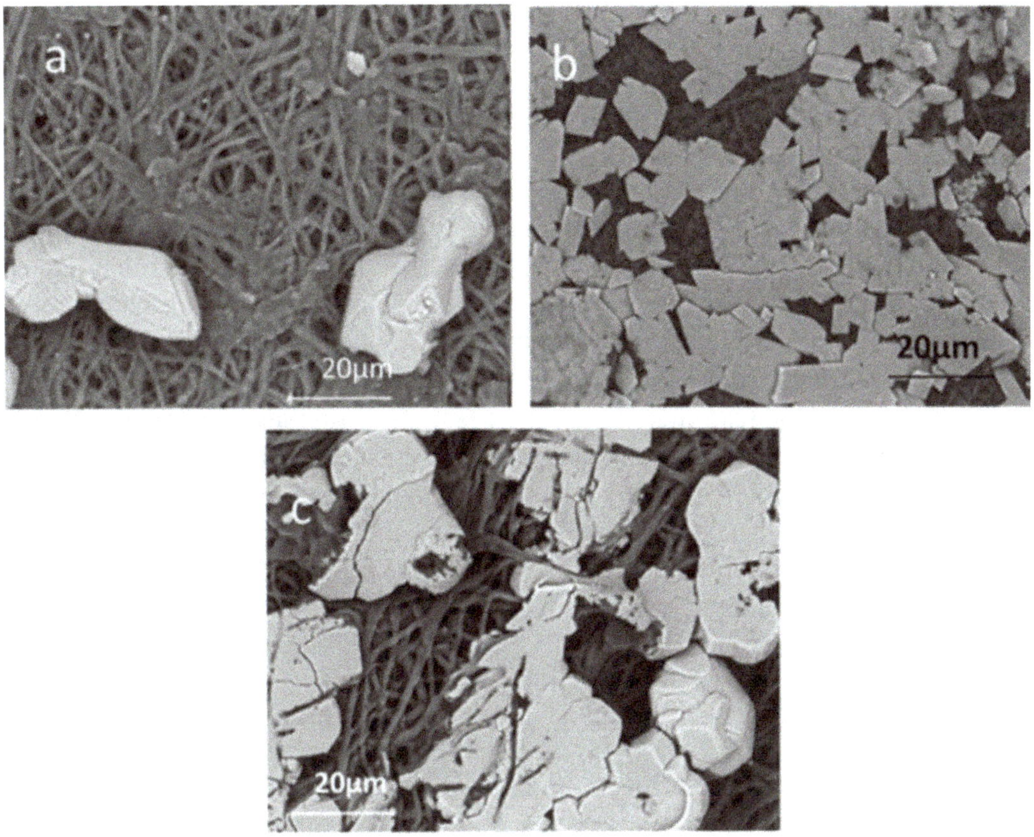

Fig. 4.3 Eggshell membrane (ESM) on top of the microbridge facing calcification medium after 24 h incubation: (**a**) ESM without treatment, 1000X; (**b**) ESM with immobilized CA, 1000X; (**c**) ESM with CA in solution in the calcification medium 1000X

rhombohedral calcite crystals (Fig. 4.2b), 31 ± 2.08 µm in average size were obtained (Table 4.1). When intact ESM was used in combination with CA dissolved in the calcification medium, rounded calcite crystals (Fig. 4.2c) with an average size of 20 ± 3.68 µm (Table 4.1), similar to those observed in the first condition were obtained.

4.3.2 ESM on Top of the Microbridge Facing the Calcification Medium After 24 H of Incubation

After 24 h incubation using ESM without treatment, polyhedral calcite crystals were obtained (Fig. 4.3a), with 22.1 ± 1.91 µm in average size (Table 4.1). But when ESM with immobilized CA was used, many polyhedral fused calcite crystals of 35.83 ± 3.13 µm in average size (Table 4.1) with symmetrical smooth edges (Fig. 4.3b) were observed. However, after using intact ESM with CA in solution, less polyhedral fused calcite crystals with curved edges (Fig. 4.3c) of 27.83 ± 2.47 µm in average size were observed (Table 4.1).

4.4 Discussion

When in vitro $CaCO_3$ crystallization experiments are done in a gas-liquid interface diffusion environment, the favorite place for crystal nucleation and growth must be considered. In fact, in this chamber-mediated experiment, CO_2 comes from the gas phase, while carbonate ions are in aqueous solution. If the reaction is done without any additional scaffold, such as the eggshell membrane, it is expected that nucleation of $CaCO_3$ crystals occurs close to the gas-liquid interface, and then, after a determined period of growth, crystals formed precipitate reaching the bottom of the reaction vessel (microbridge). However, here we showed that when an active heterogeneous nucleator scaffold, such as the eggshell membrane supplemented with immobilized or dissolved carbonic anhydrase, is located upside down at the gas-liquid interface for avoiding gravity effect, calcite nucleation and growth are sequestered by the scaffold from solution, thus affecting the morphology and size of the crystals formed. The morphology changes, including calcite aggregations occurs in a way that resembles the calcite column aggregation and fusion observed during natural eggshell formation.

Acknowledgment Work supported by Fondecyt project 1150681 from CONICYT.

References

Arias JL, Fernandez MS (2008) Polysaccharides and proteoglycans in calcium carbonate-based biomineralization. Chem Rev 108:4475–4482

Arias JL, Fernandez MS, Dennis JE, Caplan AI (1991) Collagens of the chicken eggshell membranes. Connect Tiss Res 26:37–45

Arias JI, Gonzalez A, Fernandez MS, Gonzalez C, Saez D, Arias JL (2008) Eggshell membrane as a biodegradable bone regeneration inhibitor. J Tiss Eng Regen Med 2:228–235

Dominguez-Vera JM, Gautron J, Garcia-Ruiz JM, Nys Y (2000) The effect of avian uterine fluid on the growth behavior of calcite crystals. Poult Sci 6:901–907

Fernandez MS, Moya A, Lopez L, Arias JL (2001) Secretion pattern, ultrastructural localization and function of extracellular matrix molecules involved in eggshell formation. Matrix Biol 19:793–803

Fernandez MS, Passalacqua K, Arias JI, Arias JL (2004) Partial biomimetic reconstitution of avian eggshell formation. J Struct Biol 148:1–10

Heuer AH, Fink DJ, Laraia VJ, Arias JL, Calvert PD, Kendall K, Messing GL, Rieke PC, Thompson DH, Wheeler AP, Veis A, Caplan AI (1992) Innovative materials processing strategies: a biomimetic approach. Science 255:1098–1105

Lowenstam HA, Weiner S (1989) On biomineralization. Oxford University Press, Oxford

Lu Y, Ye X, Zhang S (2013) Catalytic behavior of carbonic anhydrase enzyme immobilized onto nonporous silica nanoparticles for enhancing CO_2 absorption into a carbonate solution. Int J Greenh Gas Control 13:17–25

Mann S, Webb J, Williams RJP (1989) Biomineralization. VCH, Weinheim

Nys Y, Hincke M, Arias JL, Garcia-Ruiz JM, Solomon S (1999) Avian eggshell mineralization. Avian Poult Biol Rev 10:143–166

Panheleux M, Bain M, Fernandez MS, Morales I, Gautron J, Arias JL, Solomon S, Hincke M, Nys Y (1999) Organic matrix composition and ultrastructure of eggshell: a comparative study. Br Poult Sci 40:240–252

Rao A, Arias JL, Cölfen H (2017) On mineral retrosynthesis of a complex biogenic scaffold. Inorganics 5:16

Simkiss K, Wilbur KM (1989) Biomineralization. Academic, San Diego

Tembe S, Kubal BS, Karve M, D'Souza SF (2008) Glutaraldehyde activated eggshell membrane for immobilization of tyrosinase from *Amorphophallus companulatus*: application in construction of electrochemical biosensor for dopamine. Anal Chim Acta 612:212–217

Wanjari S, Labhsetwar N, Prabhu C, Rayalu S (2013) Biomimetic carbon dioxide sequestration using immobilized bio-composite materials. J Mol Catal B: Enzymatic 93:15–22

Chapter 5
Proteomic Analysis of Venomous Fang Matrix Proteins of *Protobothrops flavoviridis* (Habu) Snake

Tomohisa Ogawa, Asa Sekikawa, Hajime Sato, Koji Muramoto, Hiroki Shibata, and Shosaku Hattori

Abstract Venomous animals have specialized venom delivery apparatus such as nematocysts, stings, and fangs in addition to the poisonous organs consisting venom gland or sac, which produce and stock the venom. Snake is one of the major venomous animals, of which fangs are connected to the venom gland to inject the venom into prey. Snake's venomous fangs showed the unique characteristics including mechanical strength and chemical stability. Especially, *Protobothrops flavoviridis* (habu) snake fangs showed the resistance against its venom digestive proteases, whereas the bones and teeth of mouse were completely digested in the gastrointestinal tract, although habu fangs were also drawn into the body with the prey. These observations suggest that structural differences exist between venomous fangs and mammalian bones and teeth.

In this study, to reveal the molecular properties of venomous snake fangs, the matrix proteins of *P. flavoviridis* (habu) snake venom fang were analyzed by using proteomics experiments using 2D-PAGE and TOF MS/MS analyses. As a result, several biomineralization-related proteins such as vimentin, tectorin, adaptin, and collagen were identified in the venomous fang matrix proteins. Interestingly, the inhibitory proteins against venomous proteins such as metalloproteinase and PLA2 were also identified in fang's matrix proteins.

T. Ogawa (✉) · A. Sekikawa · H. Sato · K. Muramoto
Department of Biomolecular Sciences, Graduate School of Life Sciences, Tohoku University, Sendai, Japan
e-mail: tomohisa.ogawa.c3@tohoku.ac.jp; b1bm1012@s.tohoku.ac.jp; koji.muramoto.d5@tohoku.ac.jp

H. Shibata
Division of Genomics, Medical Institute of Bioregulation, Kyushu University, Fukuoka, Japan
e-mail: hshibata@gen.kyushu-u.ac.jp

S. Hattori
Amami Laboratory of Injurious Animals, The Institute of Medical Science, The University of Tokyo, Kagoshima, Japan
e-mail: shattori@ims.u-tokyo.ac.jp

K. Endo et al. (eds.), *Biomineralization*,
https://doi.org/10.1007/978-981-13-1002-7_5

Keywords Biomineralization · Matrix protein · Proteome · Snake · Venomous fang

5.1 Introduction

Venomous animals such as sea anemone, jellyfish, lizards, scorpion, fish, arachnids, bees, and snakes produce chemical weapon, toxic proteins, and peptides cocktail to kill and capture pray. They deliver the toxins as venom into prey through the sophisticated venom delivery systems consisting of an exocrine gland, a lumen, venom duct, and also injector such as nematocyst, sting, fangs, harpoon-like sting, and spine. These venomous apparatuses are thought to have evolved from the general biological organs, namely, an ovipositor, a tooth, radula, and dorsal fin, respectively. Snake is one of the major venomous animals, of which fangs are connected to the venom gland to inject the venom into prey. Venomous snakes can be classified into two groups according to the fang systems, front fanged (elapid and vipers) and rear fanged (grass snakes), and frontal fangs are further divided into two types, grooves and tubes (Kardong 1979; Savitzky 1980; Jackson 2002; Kuch et al. 2006). Vonk et al. (2008) reported the evolutionary origin and development of snake fangs, showing that front fangs develop from the posterior end of the upper jaw and are strikingly similar in morphogenesis to rear fangs. In the anterior part of the maxilla of front-fanged snakes, gene expression of sonic hedgehog, which is responsible among other things for the formation of the teeth, is suppressed. Despite such extensive studies and the recent genome sequence analyses for two venomous snakes, the king cobra (*Ophiophagus hannah*) (Vonk et al. 2013) and the five-pacer viper (*Deinagkistrodon acutus*) (Yin et al. 2016), the matrix proteins of venomous fangs, their evolutionary origins, and the biomineralization mechanisms of venomous fangs are still poorly understood.

Protobothrops flavoviridis (habu) snake that inhabits Ryukyu (Okinawa, Tokunoshima, and Amami) Islands are dangerous snakes having various toxic peptides and proteins (multiple protein families) as venom. Their venomous fangs are frequently lost and drawn into their own body with the prey after injection of the venom. Interestingly, venomous fangs are excreted with no change and no digestion, whereas the bones and teeth of the mouse (prey) are completely digested. These observations suggest that structural differences between venomous fangs and mammalian bones and teeth exist. In addition, it is conceivable that the adaptive evolution of the venomous organ and venomous fang bestowed them to have resistance to digestive juices. Thus, the snake fangs show the unique characteristics including mechanical strength and chemical stability.

In this study, to reveal the characteristics of habu snake fangs such as chemical stability, and their molecular evolution, proteomic analyses of fang matrix proteins were conducted by using 2D-PAGE and MALDI-TOF MS/MS.

5.2 Materials and Methods

5.2.1 Materials

The crude venomous fangs of *Protobothrops flavoviridis* (habu) snakes captured in Amami Island, Kagoshima Prefecture, Japan, were collected by dissection of the head from sacrifice. Subsequently, fangs and tissues were separately rinsed with phosphate-buffered saline and stored at −80 °C until use. Immobiline DryStrip for two-dimensional electrophoresis and the IPG buffer (pH 3–11) were obtained from GE Healthcare UK Ltd. (Buckinghamshire, England). Silver Stain MS kit was purchased from Wako Pure Chemical Industry, Ltd. (Osaka, Japan). *Achromobacter* protease I and *Staphylococcus aureus* V8 protease were obtained from Wako Pure Chemicals (Osaka, Japan) and Sigma-Aldrich Co. (St. Louis, MO, USA), respectively. ZipTip C18 was purchased from Millipore (Massachusetts, USA). All other reagents were of the best commercially available grade from Wako Pure Chemicals (Osaka, Japan) or Nacalai Tesque (Kyoto, Japan).

5.2.2 Isolation and Characterization of the Matrix Proteins from the Venomous Fang

Venomous fangs of habu snakes were decalcified with 50% formic acid at room temperature for 2 days. Then, the decalcified matrix proteins were dissolved in 6 M guanidinium hydrochloride in 50 mM Tris-HCl buffer (pH 8.8) containing 200 mM NaCl at 60 °C. After TCA-acetone precipitation, the pellet was dissolved in 8 M urea in 100 mM Tris-HCl buffer (pH 8.2) at 60 °C. For two-dimensional polyacrylamide gel electrophoresis (2D-PAGE), fang matrix proteins were directly dissolved in 400 μl of rehydration buffer (8 M urea, 4% CHAPS, 2% immobilized pH gradient (IPG) buffer (pH 3-11NL), DeStreak reagent (15 mg/ml), and 0.002% bromophenol blue) and were loaded onto IPG strips. After rehydration for 12 h, isoelectric focusing (IEF) was performed at 20 °C using the running conditions of the following focusing program: 500 V for 1 h, a gradient to 1000 V for 1 h, a gradient to 8000 V for 3 h, and 8000 V for 1.5 h (3225 V, 50 μA, 19,742 Vhs). After running IEF, IPG strips were equilibrated in a reducing equilibration buffer for 15 min and subsequently alkylated with iodoacetamide. Then, IPG strips were transferred onto 15% polyacrylamide gel (18 × 16 cm) and embedded with 0.5% agarose and electrophoresed. Gels were stained using Silver Stain MS kit or Coomassie Brilliant Blue.

5.2.3 *Proteome Analysis*

The spots on 2D gel were cut into pieces and washed with Milli-Q water. After the gels were dehydrated by acetonitrile with gentle agitation and completely dried in vacuo, gel samples were reduced by 10 mM DTT for 1 h at 56 °C. After cooling and washing by 25 mM ammonium bicarbonate buffer for 10 min, the gel samples were treated with 55 mM iodoacetamide in 25 mM ammonium bicarbonate solution in the dark. After removal of the solvent to be completely dried, gel particles were digested by *Achromobacter* protease I (Lys-C) or V8 protease at 37 °C for one night. After concentrating the digest in speed vacuum, samples were desalted on ZipTip C18 (Millipore). Samples were separated by using a DiNa Nano LC system equipped with a DiNa MALDI spotting device (KYA Technologies Co., Tokyo, Japan) and applied to MALDI-TOF MS and tandem MS/MS analysis using TOF/TOF™ 5800 Analyzer (AB SCIEX). Enzyme-digested matrix proteins without 2D-PAGE were also analyzed by nanoLC-MALDI-TOF MS/MS. Molecular masses were calibrated using the Sequazyme Peptide Mass Standards Kit (Applied Biosystems). Protein identification was performed by searching of each MS/MS spectrum against the protein sequence databases derived from the RNA-seq data of *P. flavoviridis* snake fang-forming tissues by using ProteinPilot software (version 3.0; AB Sciex) with the Paragon method.

5.3 Results and Discussion

5.3.1 *Isolation and Characterization of the Matrix Proteins from* **P. flavoviridis** *Venomous Fangs*

First, the decalcification conditions of venomous fangs were investigated by using hydrochloric acid and formic acid, respectively. The complete decalcification of the venomous fang without protein degradation was achieved by 50% formic acid at 30 °C for 2 days, resulting typical yield of 5.6 mg from 1.0 g of *P. flavoviridis* fangs, while the decalcification of fang by 10% HCl treatment caused the degradation of proteins (Fig. 5.1a). Then, the matrix proteins were subjected to the proteome analysis, *in-gel* enzymatic digestions for mass spectrometry characterization with 2D-PAGE and the shotgun proteomics of enzymatic digestions of total matrix proteins by nanoLC-MS/MS, respectively, after dissolved in 6 M guanidinium at 60 °C and concentrated by TCA-acetone precipitation.

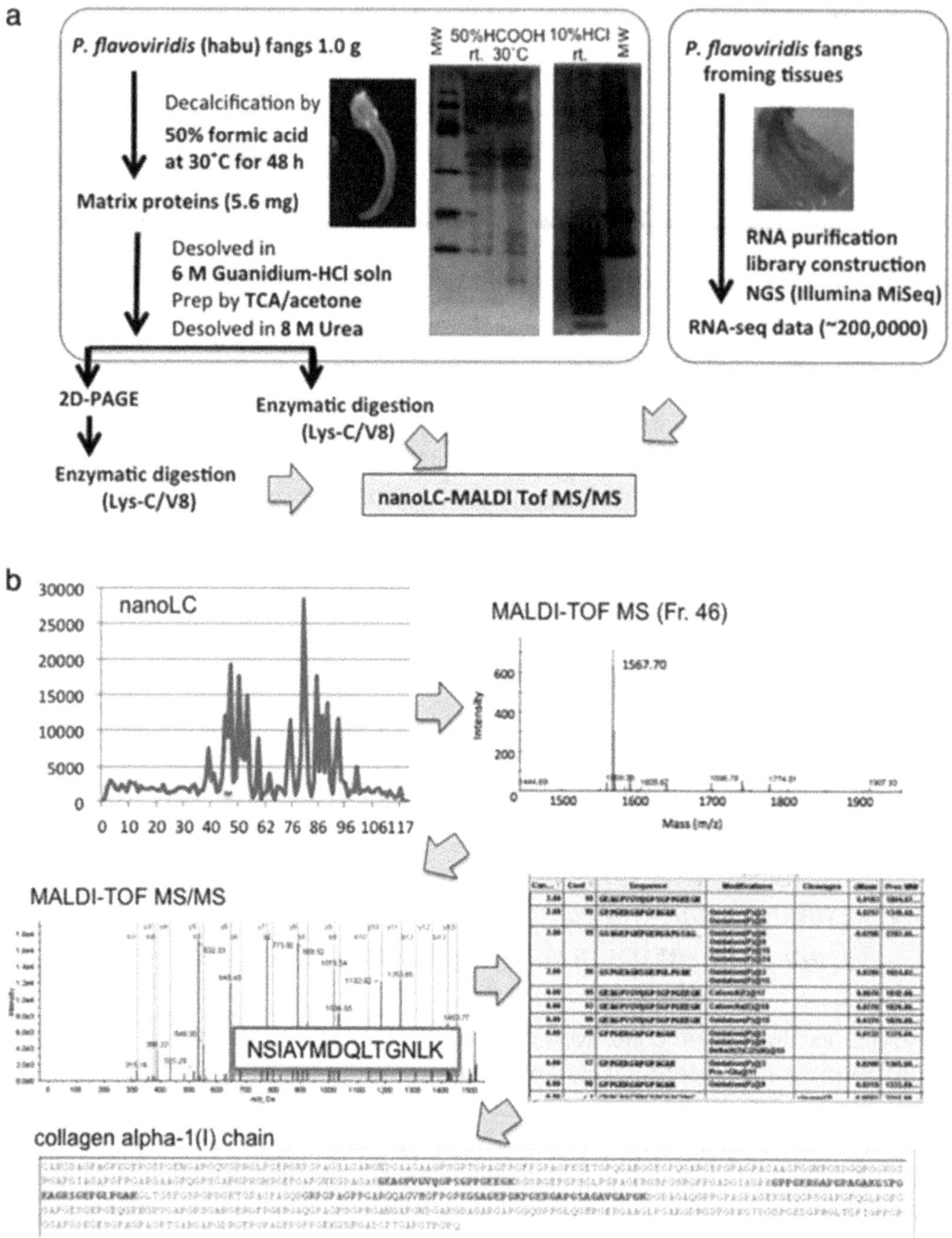

Fig. 5.1 Proteomic analysis of *P. flavoviridis* fang matrix proteins
Brief explanation of procedure through decalcification and mass spectrometry analysis (**a**) and typical profiles of digested matrix proteins on nanoLC-MALDI-TOF MS/MS (**b**)

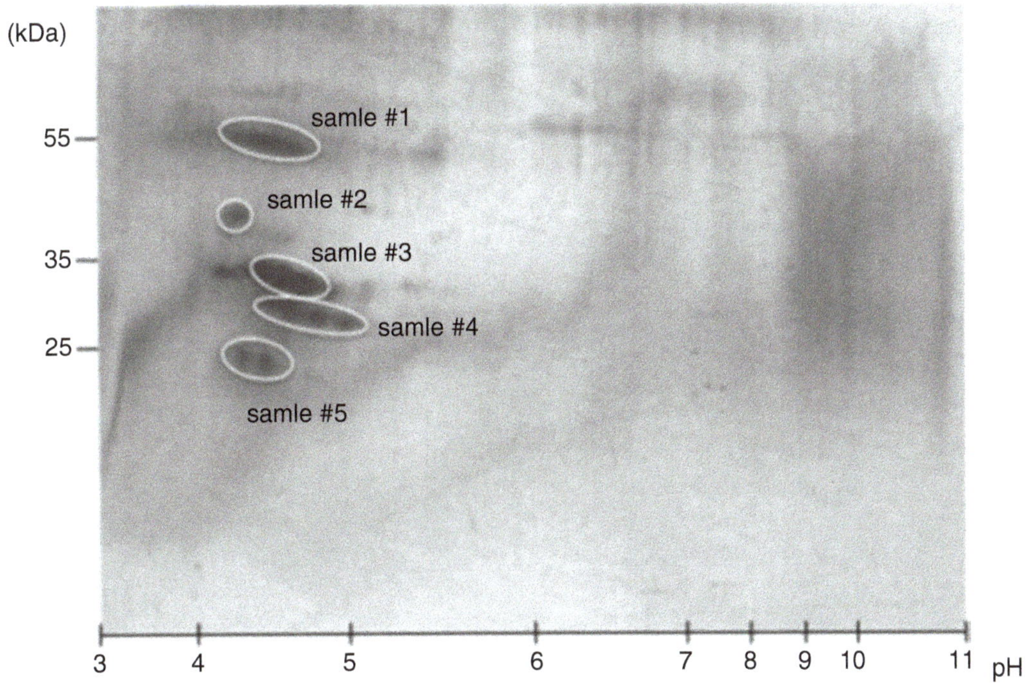

Fig. 5.2 2D-PAGE profile of *P. flavoviridis* venomous fang matrix proteins
Samples #1 to #5 were analyzed by nanoLC-MALDI-TOF MS/MS analysis after *in-gel* digestion, respectively

5.3.2 Proteome Analysis of the Fang Matrix Proteins

To identify the array of proteins in *P. flavoviridis* venomous fangs, the extracted matrix proteins were subjected to the 2D-PAGE (pH 3–11), resulting in identification in acidic region of around 20 appreciable major spots, of which pI values ranging from 4 to 6 (Fig. 5.2). These fang matrix proteins were roughly divided into five groups based on the molecular mass numbers: 55 kDa (sample #1), 40 kDa (#2), 35 kDa (#3), 30 kDa (#4), and 25 kDa (#5) proteins. Preliminary proteomic analyses of these protein spots allowed the identification of major components of fang matrix proteins including type I collagens alpha-1 and alpha-2 and UV excision repair protein RAD23-like protein (Table 5.1). Interestingly, antihemorrhagic factor HSF, which is a proteinaceous serum inhibitor against own venom metalloproteinases, was also detected as a matrix protein. However, these proteomic data from 2D-PAGE could not provide satisfactory results.

To improve the proteomic data of *P. flavoviridis* fang matrix proteins, a direct shotgun proteomic analysis was conducted. As a result of 4 independent experiments of shotgun proteomics, 36 proteins were identified as fang matrix proteins (Table 5.2). In addition to the type I collagen alpha1 (isoform X1 and X2) and alpha2 chains, the collagens type VI alpha2 and alpha3 chains and type XI alpha1 and alpha2 chains were identified. Because type I collagen has been reported to be related to the formation of dentin and enamel, contributing to the nanoscale architecture in the teeth (Wallace et al. 2010), type I collagen seems to be an important

Table 5.1 Proteomic data for 2D-PAGE analysis of *P. flavoviridis* fang matrix proteins

Sample[a]	Total	%Cov	Accession	Representative RNA-seq data	Peptides (95%)	Identified proteins
#2–1	2	7.390999794	m.3684	g.3684 ORF comp179282_c0_seq1:3–695(+)	1	Antihemorrhagic factor HSF
#3–1	4	7.451999933	m.304793	g.304793 ORF comp195637_c1_seq80:3108–4358(+)	2	Collagen alpha-1(I) chain isoform X1
#3–2	2	7.390999794	m.3684	g.3684 ORF comp179282_c0_seq1:3–695(+)	1	Antihemorrhagic factor HSF
#3–3	1.3	12.8700003	m.32414	g.32414 ORF comp189831_c0_seq6:1773–2078(+)	1	UV excision repair protein RAD23-like B
	2	12.8700003	m.32414	g.32414 ORF comp189831_c0_seq6:1773–2078(+)	1	
#4–1	2	12.30999976	m.228287	g.228287 ORF comp194729_c4_seq50:4684–5076(+)	1	Collagen alpha-2(I) chain isoform X1

[a]Sample numbers #2 to #4 correspond to the number of 2D-PAGE spots in Fig. 5.2

Table 5.2 *Protobothrops flavoviridis* fang matrix proteins identified by shotgun proteomic analyses

Trial/protein numbers	Total	% Cov	Accession	Representative RNA-seq data	Peptides (95%)	Identified proteins	Similarity (%) with mice homologs
1_1	8	9.855999798	m.304793	g.304793 ORF comp195637_c1_seq80:3108–4358(+)	4	Collagen alpha-1(I)	85
1_2	6	12.72999942	m.59430	g.59430 ORF comp191065_c4_seq27:514–1506(−)	3	Decorin	72
1_3	6	18.23000014	m.228281	g.228281 ORF comp194729_c4_seq49:3624–4235(+)	3	Collagen alpha-2(I)	75
1_4	4	3.852000087	m.380886	g.380886 ORF comp196768_c0_seq1:1–1872(+)	2	Serum albumin	32
1_5	4	10.79000011	m.280478	g.280478 ORF comp195368_c6_seq17:648–1679(−)	2	Osteonectin (SPARC)	83
1_6	2	4.098000005	m.229771	g.229771 ORF comp194758_c6_seq15:710–6349(+)	1	Collagen alpha-1(XI)	83
1_7	2	16.52999967	m.3685	g.3685 ORF comp179282_c1_seq1:1–366(+)	1	Antihemorrhagic factor HSF-like	–

1_8	2	3.260999918	m.380873	g.380873 ORF comp196660_c0_seq1:518–1624(+)	1	Biglycan	83
1_9	2	6.086999923	m.3684	g.3684 ORF comp179282_c0_seq1:3–695(+)	1	Antihemorrhagic factor HSF	–
1_10	1.7	12.8700003	m.32414	g.32414 ORF comp189831_c0_seq6:1773–2078(+)	1	UV excision repair protein RAD23-like B	73
1_11	0.4	8.122000098	m.15495	g.15495 ORF comp188251_c4_seq2:1–594(+)	0	Dual specificity protein phosphatase 3	79
1_12	0.17	2.26099994	m.302599	g.302599 ORF comp195617_c0_seq11:1965–3692(+)	0	Protein capicua homolog	66
1_13	0.14	8.653999865	m.361713	g.361713 ORF comp196120_c6_seq13:2390–3328(+)	0	L1-encoded reverse transcriptase-like protein	–
1_14	0.09	5.152000114	m.137751	g.137751 ORF comp193200_c4_seq25:1707–2699(+)	0	SLIT and NTRK-like protein 6/phospholipase A2 inhibitor-like	29
1_15	0.08	5.05400002	m.190269	g.190269 ORF comp194186_c4_seq5:195–1028(–)	0	Insulin-like growth factor binding protein 4	72
2_1	4	7.451999933	m.304793	g.304793 ORF comp195637_c1_seq80:3108–4358(+)	2	Collagen alpha-1(I)	85

(continued)

Table 5.2 (continued)

Trial/protein numbers	Total	% Cov	Accession	Representative RNA-seq data	Peptides (95%)	Identified proteins	Similarity (%) with mice homologs
2_2	2	7.390999794	m.3684	g.3684 ORF comp179282_c0_seq1:3–695(+)	1	Antihemorrhagic factor HSF	–
2_3	2	12.30999976	m.228287	g.228287 ORF comp194729_c4_seq50:4684–5076(+)	1	Collagen alpha-2(I)	75
2_4	1.4	8.147999644	m.4964	g.4964 ORF comp182948_c0_seq1:414–821(+)	1	Uncharacterized protein/ SOGA3-like	–
2_5	0.8	12.8700003	m.32414	g.32414 ORF comp189831_c0_seq6:1773–2078(+)	0	UV excision repair protein RAD23-like B	73
2_6	0.05	14.00000006	m.13350	g.13350 ORF comp187844_c0_seq6:399–701(+)	0	EF-hand domain-containing family member B	58
3_1	6	20.2000007	m.228281	g.228281 ORF comp194729_c4_seq49:3624–4235(+)	3	Collagen alpha-2(I)	75
3_2	4.11	14.35000002	m.3684	g.3684 ORF comp179282_c0_seq1:3–695(+)	2	Antihemorrhagic factor HSF	–
3_3	4	3.60600017	m.304793	g.304793 ORF comp195637_c1_seq80:3108–4358(+)	2	Collagen alpha-1(I)	85

3_4	2	7.97900036	m.59432	g.59432 ORF comp191065_c4_seq31:514–1080(−)	1	Decorin	72	
3_5	2	2.408000082	m.380886	g.380886 ORF comp196768_c0_seq1:1–1872(+)	1	Serum albumin	32	
3_6	2	12.3999998	m.3685	g.3685 ORF comp179282_c1_seq1:1–366(+)	1	Antihemorrhagic factor HSF-like	–	
3_7	2	0.585399987	m.229771	g.229771 ORF comp194758_c6_seq15:710–6349(+)	1	Collagen alpha-1(XI)	83	
3_8	0.8	3.78200002	m.2124	g.2124 ORF comp168486_c1_seq1:1–717(+)	0	Peroxisome proliferator-activated receptor gamma	92	
3_9	0.37	0.608900003	m.103143	g.103143 ORF comp192389_c5_seq5:3–4439(+)	0	Receptor-type tyrosine-protein phosphatase zeta isoform X2	70	
3_10	0.15	1.006999984	m.314611	g.314611 ORF comp195716_c7_seq95:1655–4339(−)	0	Probable methyltransferase TARBP1	60	
3_11	0.13	1.692000031	m.177447	g.177447 ORF comp193931_c1_seq1:2163–10,676(−)	0	Adenomatous polyposis coli protein	80	
3_12	0.09	1.070000045	m.56612	g.56612 ORF comp190997_c1_seq12:458–4387(+)	0	BAH and coiled-coil domain-containing protein 1	60	

(continued)

Table 5.2 (continued)

Trial/protein numbers	Total	% Cov	Accession	Representative RNA-seq data	Peptides (95%)	Identified proteins	Similarity (%) with mice homologs
3_13	0.09	2.153999917	m.41112	g.41112 ORF comp190336_c0_seq6:152–2104(−)	0	Leucine-rich repeat and fibronectin type III domain-containing protein 1	55
3_14	0.09	13.72999996	m.334963	g.334963 ORF comp195890_c6_seq76:1–309(+)	0	Unknown	–
3_15	0.07	7.086999714	m.14110	g.14110 ORF comp187994_c1_seq2:329–712(+)	0	39S ribosomal protein L55	43
4_1	10	11.0799998	m.380886	g.380886 ORF comp196768_c0_seq1:1–1872(+)	5	Serum albumin	32
4_2	10	25.65000057	m.3684	g.3684 ORF comp179282_c0_seq1:3–695(+)	5	Antihemorrhagic factor HSF	–
4_3	8	18.35999936	m.120416	g.120416 ORF comp192831_c6_seq13:1–1683(−)	9	Collagen alpha-1(I)X2	85
4_4	6	15.76000005	m.380873	g.380873 ORF comp196660_c0_seq1:518–1624(+)	3	Biglycan	83
4_5	6	11.77999973	m.304793	g.304793 ORF comp195637_c1_seq80:3108–4358(+)	5	Collagen alpha-1(I)X1	85

4_6	6	13.96999955	m.228235	g.228235 ORF comp194729_c4_seq37:1874–3379(+)	3	Collagen alpha-2(I)	75
4_7	4	13.84000033	m.68810	g.68810 ORF comp191390_c3_seq4:350–1024(+)	2	Transferrin-like	26
4_8	4	9.329000115	m.280478	g.280478 ORF comp195368_c6_seq17:648–1679(−)	2	Osteonectin (SPARC)	83
4_9	2	7.213000208	m.237824	g.237824 ORF comp194854_c3_seq3:504–3542(+)	1	Collagen alpha-2(VI)	55
4_10	2	2.072999999	m.85240	g.85240 ORF comp191877_c1_seq9:1401–8060(+)	1	Collagen alpha-3(VI)	55
4_11	2	1.752999984	m.164214	g.164214 ORF comp193681_c1_seq3:3–4967(+)	1	Venom factor	–
4_12	2	5.085000023	m.135289	g.135289 ORF comp193175_c0_seq8:3–1949(−)	1	Dentin matrix acidic phosphoprotein 1-like	36
4_13	2	7.97900036	m.59432	g.59432 ORF comp191065_c4_seq31:514–1080(−)	1	Decorin	72
4_14	2	12.8700003	m.32414	g.32414 ORF comp189831_c0_seq6:1773–2078(+)	1	UV excision repair protein RAD23-like B	73

(continued)

Table 5.2 (continued)

Trial/protein numbers	Total	% Cov	Accession	Representative RNA-seq data	Peptides (95%)	Identified proteins	Similarity (%) with mice homologs
4_15	2	6.25	m.209089	g.209089 ORF comp194475_c7_seq8:944–1474(+)	1	Galectin-9-like	61
4_16	1.7	13.0400002	m.1291	g.1291 ORF comp137400_c0_seq1:563–979(−)	1	Unconventional myosin-Ie	–
4_17	1.52	13.24999923	m.148536	g.148536 ORF comp193401_c3_seq19:317–1474(+)	1	Actin, cytoplasmic 1	99
4_18	0.64	2.26099994	m.302599	g.302599 ORF comp195617_c0_seq11:1965–3692(+)	0	Protein capicua homolog	66
4_19	0.47	0.630899984	m.259829	g.259829 ORF comp195117_c3_seq24:1–5709(+)	0	Collagen alpha-2(XI)	66
4_20	0.06	2.785000019	m.198369	g.198369 ORF comp194299_c9_seq1:2–2371(−)	0	Titin-like	31

component of venomous snake fang. Furthermore, the type VI collagen, which forms microfibrils and is primarily associated with the extracellular matrix of skeletal muscle and bone marrow, and type XI collagen, which is found in the cartilage of the nose and external ears in human, were also identified as matrix proteins in venomous fang, suggesting the unique distribution of type VI and type XI collagens as part of the fang matrix. On the other hand, noncollagenous dentin matrix proteins including proteoglycans (PGs), glycoproteins, serum proteins, enzymes, and growth factors are deemed to play structural, metabolic, and functional roles as key components in the mineralization process of dentin (Orsini et al. 2009). Shotgun proteomic analysis showed the fang noncollagenous dentin matrix proteins include proteoglycan such as decorin (1_2, 3_4, 4_13 in Table 5.2) and biglycan (1_8, 4_4), glycoproteins such as osteonectin (secreted protein acidic and rich in cysteine: SPARC) (1_5, 4_8), the SIBLING proteins such as dentin matrix acidic phosphoprotein 1 (4_12), and serum proteins such as albumin (1_4, 3_5, 4_1), phospholipase A_2 inhibitor (1_14) and antihemorrhagic factors, HSF (1_9, 2_2, 3_2, 4_2), and HSF-like protein (1_7, 3_6). The coexistence of these serum inhibitors as fang matrix proteins explains why venomous fang is stable against own venom enzymes compared with mouse-derived teeth and bones. Compared with the homologous proteins in mouse, several fang matrix proteins such as dentin matrix acidic phosphoprotein 1 (36%), titin-like protein (31%), transferrin-like protein (26%), and serum inhibitors including albumin (32%) and PLA2 inhibitor (29%) showed lower sequence similarities, suggesting that these differences in matrix proteins might be related to the functional differences and distinctive properties between venomous fang and mouse's teeth.

In this study, we identified 36 matrix proteins from *P. flavoviridis* snake fangs by proteomics analyses. They include proteinaceous inhibitor against own venom enzymes in addition to several types of collagens (types I, VI, and XI) and noncollagenous dentin matrix proteins. More recently, we have decoded the whole genome sequence of *P. flavoviridis* snakes (Shibata et al. 2018, in press). Further investigations are needed to elucidate the biomineralization mechanisms of venomous fang and their biological functions.

Acknowledgments The authors thank Prof. Noriyuki Satoh, Drs. Shinichi Yamasaki and Kanako Hisata, Okinawa Institute of Science and Technology Graduate University (OIST), Onna, Okinawa, for providing RNA-seq data from *P. flavoviridis* fang-forming tissues.

This study was partly supported by Grants-in-Aid of MEXT, Japan (#24651130 and #23107505 to TO). This study was also partly performed in the collaborative Research Project Program of the Medical Institute of Bioregulation, Kyushu University.

References

Jackson K (2002) How tubular venom-conducting fangs are formed. J Morphol 252:291–297

Kardong KV (1979) Protovipers and the evolution of snake fangs. Evolution 33:433–443

Kuch U, Müller J, Mödden C, Mebs D (2006) Snake fangs from the Lower Miocene of Germany: evolutionary stability of perfect weapons. Naturwissenschaften 93:84–87

Orsini G et al (2009) A review of the nature, role, and function of dentin non-collagenous proteins. Part 1: Proteoglycans Glycoproteins 21:1–18
Savitzky AH (1980) The role of venom delivery strategies in snake evolution. Evolution 34:1194–1204
Shibata H., Chijiwa T., Oda-Ueda N., Nakamura H., Yamaguchi K., Hattori S., Matsubara K., Matsuda Y., Yamashita A., Isomoto A., Mori K., Tashiro K., Kuhara S., Yamasaki S., Fujie M., Goto H., Koyanagi R., Takeuchi T., Fukumaki Y., Ohno M., Shoguchi E., Hisata K., Satoh N., and Ogawa T (2018) The habu genome reveals accelerated evolution of venom protein genes. Sci Rep (in press). https://doi.org/10.1038/s41598-018-28749-4
Vonk FJ, Admiraal JF, Jackson K, Reshef R, de Bakker MA, Vanderschoot K, van den Berge I, van Atten M, Burgerhout E, Beck A (2008) Evolutionary origin and development of snake fangs. Nature 454:630–633
Vonk FJ et al (2013) The king cobra genome reveals dynamic gene evolution and adaptation in the snake venom system. Proc Natl Acad Sci U S A 110:20651–20656
Wallace JM et al (2010) Type I collagen exists as a distribution of nanoscale morphologies in teeth, bones, and tendons. Langmuir 26:7349–7354
Yin W et al (2016) Evolutionary trajectories of snake genes and genomes revealed by comparative analyses of five-pacer viper. Nat Commun 7:13107. https://doi.org/10.1038/ncomms13107

Chapter 6
Characterization of Goldfish Scales by Vibrational Spectroscopic Analyses

Masayuki Nara, Yusuke Maruyama, and Atsuhiko Hattori

Abstract Scales of bony fishes are calcified tissues that contain osteoblasts, osteoclasts, and bone matrix, all of which are similar to those found in mammalian bone. The scales are composed of hydroxylapatite (HAP) and extracellular matrix which is mainly type I collagen fibers. We investigated the scales from goldfish by Fourier transform infrared (FTIR) and Raman spectroscopic analyses to characterize the components in the scales. The attenuated total reflection (ATR)-FTIR spectrum obtained from the surface coat of the normal goldfish scale was quite different from that of the backside coat of the same scale. The former showed a strong band at 1013 cm^{-1}, which was assignable to HAP, and weak bands at about 1643, 1415, and 870 cm^{-1}, whereas the latter showed a typical protein profile: strong bands at about 1631, 1550, and 1240 cm^{-1}, which were assignable to amide-I, amide-II, and amide-III of collagen, respectively. We also investigated the local structure of goldfish scales by using micro-Raman spectroscopy. The Raman spectrum of the normal scale showed the amide-I band at about 1640 cm^{-1} from the collagen and the PO_4^{3-} symmetric stretching band at about 961 cm^{-1} from the HAP. We discuss the implication of Raman and FTIR profiles for normal and regenerating goldfish scales.

Keywords Vibrational spectroscopy · Goldfish scale · Regeneration · Hydroxylapatite · Carbonate apatite

6.1 Introduction

Goldfish scale is a calcified tissue that contains osteoblasts, osteoclasts, and bone matrix, all of which are similar to those found in mammalian bone (Azuma et al. 2007). The scale is composed of hydroxyapatite (HAP) and extracellular matrix which is mainly type I collagen fibers, forming a highly ordered three-dimensional structure. It has been known that scales regenerate after being removed. Therefore,

M. Nara (✉) · Y. Maruyama · A. Hattori
College of Liberal Arts and Sciences, Tokyo Medical and Dental University (TMDU), Tokyo, Japan
e-mail: nara.las@tmd.ac.jp; ahattori.las@tmd.ac.jp

K. Endo et al. (eds.), *Biomineralization*,
https://doi.org/10.1007/978-981-13-1002-7_6

the goldfish scale is interesting from the viewpoint of the model system for the regeneration of mammalian bone.

Vibrational spectroscopy is useful for characterizing developmental changes in bone and other mineralized tissues. Infrared spectroscopy is used for examining the mineral properties and collagen maturity of bones (Boskey and Mendelsohn 2005; Paschalis et al. 2011) as well as protein structures such as collagen and osteocalcin (Jackson et al. 1995; Barth 2007; Mizuguchi et al. 2001). Raman spectroscopy is also available for bones and fish scales to provide information about protein and mineral components (Ikoma et al. 2003a, b).

In the present study, FTIR and Raman spectroscopic analyses were applied to scales from goldfish to characterize the components of the normal and regenerating ones. In particular, we focused on the pocket side of them, since the epidermal side of scales is more complicated because of the contribution of chromatophore.

6.2 Materials and Methods

We prepared normal scales and regenerating scales after 1 week and 2 weeks, extracted from goldfishes (*Carassius auratus*). As can be seen in Fig. 6.1, the picture of the regenerating scale after 2 weeks was morphologically different from that of the normal scale. There were about ten circular ridges for regenerated scales after 2 weeks, although a lot of circular ridges were observed for normal scales.

Attenuated total reflection (ATR)-Fourier transform infrared (FTIR) measurements were performed at 25 °C on a PerkinElmer Spectrum-One FTIR spectrometer equipped with a universal ATR unit and a liquid nitrogen-cooled MCT detector at resolution 2 cm^{-1}. A scale sample was placed on a diamond/ZnSe 1-reflection top-plate (PerkinElmer). The sampling depth of the ATR method was approximately 1–2 μm over the range of 2000–1000 cm^{-1}. We obtained the ATR-FTIR spectrum for the spot (about 1.5 mm in diameter) with the accumulations of 200 scans.

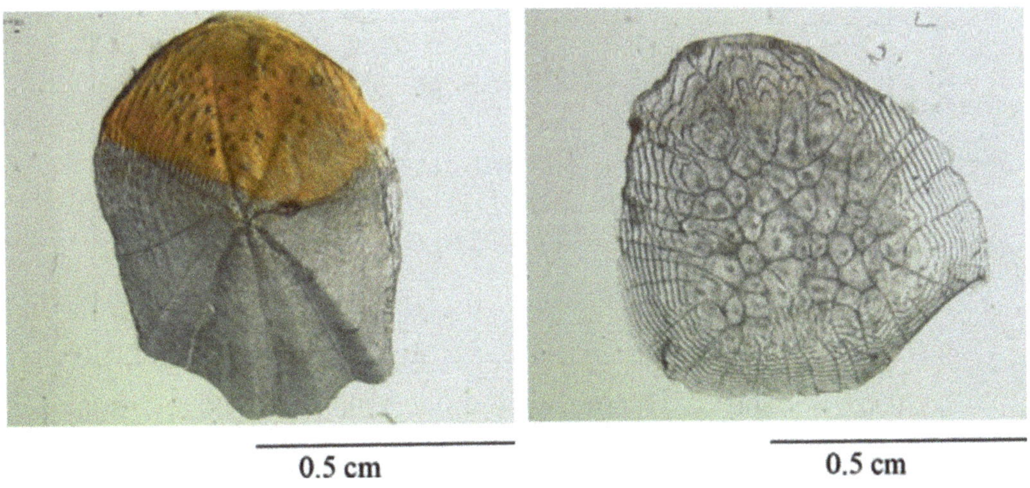

Fig. 6.1 Pictures of a normal scales (left) and a regenerating scale after 2 weeks (right) of goldfish (*Carassius auratus*)

Raman spectra were collected at room temperature (25 °C) with a Raman microscope (Kaiser HoloLab 5000 of Kaiser Optical System Inc.) using 532 nm Nd-YAG laser (2–5 mW at the sample surface), holographic transmission grating, and charge-coupled device (CCD). The spectral resolution in the present system is approximately 4.8 cm^{-1}. We obtained the Raman spectrum for a spot (about 2 μm in diameter) with two accumulations of 30 s each. The sampling depth of the Raman measurement was about 100 μm. A scale was set on a slide glass covered with aluminum foil, and the pocket sides of the surface were measured by Raman spectroscopy.

6.3 Results and Discussion

6.3.1 Characterization of a Normal Scale from Goldfish by FTIR Spectra

Figure 6.2 shows ATR-FTIR spectra of the surface and backside coats of a normal goldfish scale in the pocket side. Figure 6.2a showed a strong band at 1013 cm^{-1}, which was assignable to HAP, and weak bands at 1647, 1546, 1415, and 871 cm^{-1}. The bands at 1647 and 1546 cm^{-1} were probably assignable to proteins. The bands

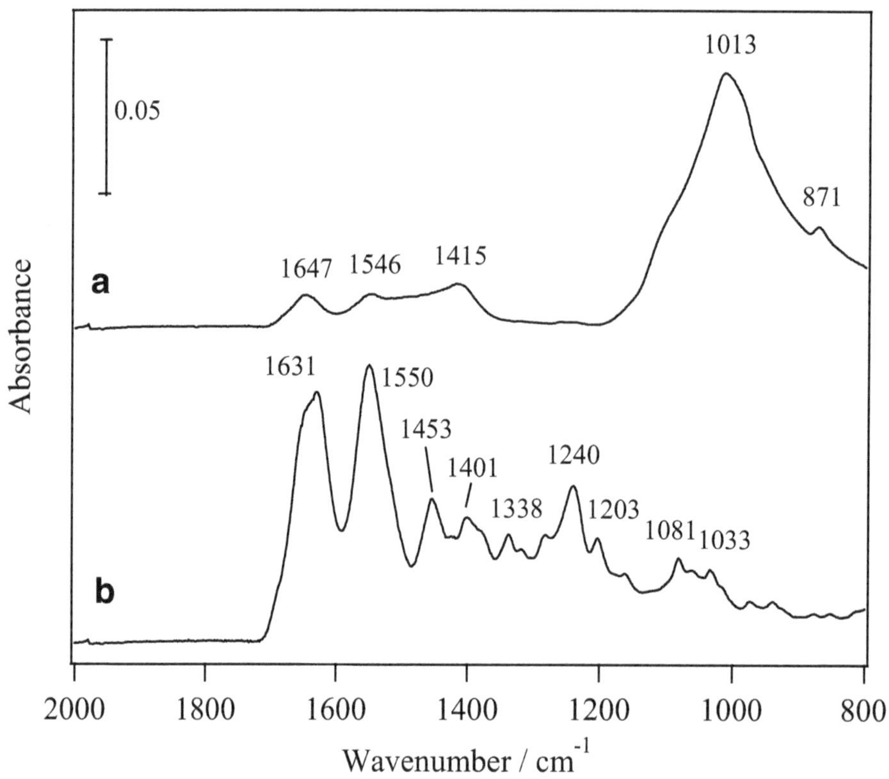

Fig. 6.2 ATR-FTIR spectra from (**a**) the surface coat and (**b**) the backside coat of the normal goldfish scale

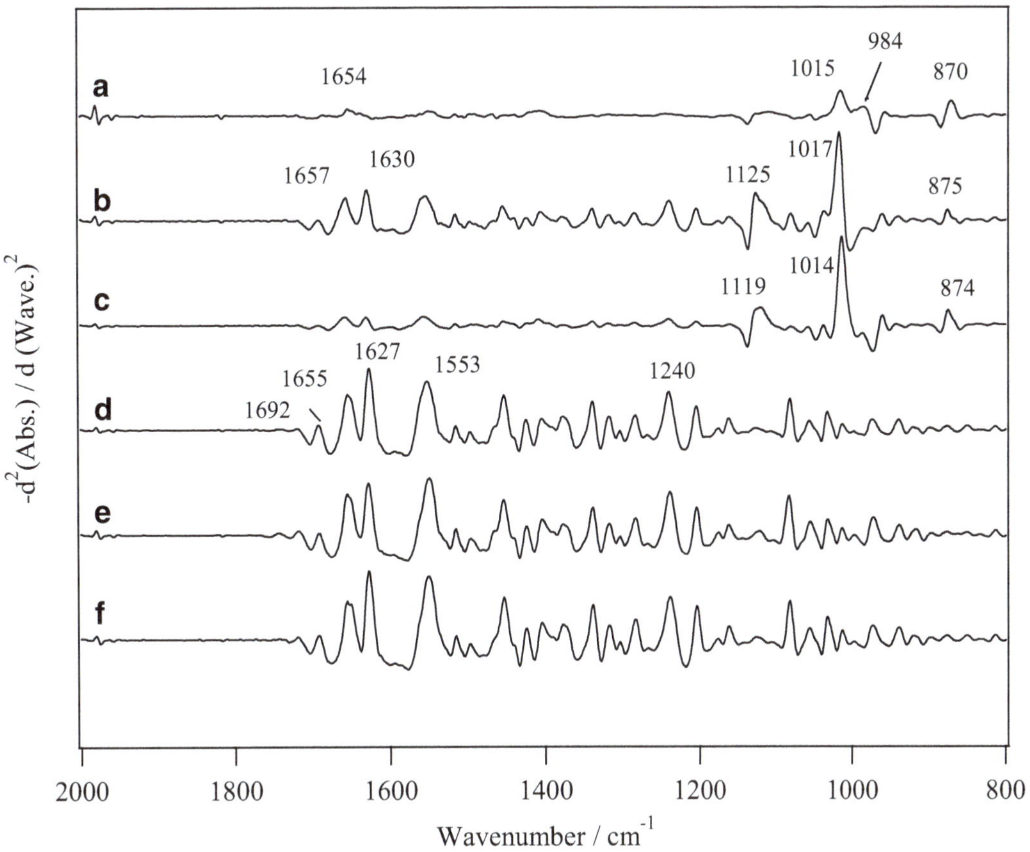

Fig. 6.3 ATR-FTIR second-derivative spectra of (**a–c**) the surface coat and (**d–f**) the back coat in the pocket side of three type of scales from goldfish: (**a**, **d**) a normal scale, (**b**, **e**) a regenerating scale after 1 week, and (**c**, **f**) a regenerating scale after 2 weeks. The second derivatives were multiplied by −1

at 1415 and 871 cm^{-1} were assigned to carbonate (CO_3^{2-}). Figure 6.2b showed a protein profile of collagen: strong bands at 1631, 1550, and 1240 cm^{-1}, which are undoubtedly assignable to amide-I, amide-II, and amide-III, respectively.

Figure 6.3a, d shows the ATR-FTIR second-derivative spectra of the corresponding spectra in Fig. 6.2. The second-derivative spectrum of surface coat showed the bands at 1654, 1015, 981, and 781 cm^{-1} in Fig. 6.3a, whereas that of the backside coat showed three bands at 1696, 1652, and 1625 cm^{-1} in the region of amide-I, one band at 1550 cm^{-1} in the region of amide-II, and one band at 1240 cm^{-1}. Obviously, the spectral profile for the surface coat reflected the HAP as the main component of the calcified layer, while the spectral profile for the back coat reflected the collagen as the main component of the fibrillary layer. The amide-I band observed from the surface coat may be due to proteins other than collagen, since the profile was different from that of collagen. The bands at 1415 and 871 cm^{-1} are probably originated from CO_3^{2-} (Ikoma et al. 2003b).

6.3.2 *Characterization of Regenerating Scales from Goldfish by FTIR Spectra*

Figure 6.3b, e shows the second-derivative spectra of the surface and back coats of the regenerating scale after 1 week in the pocket side, respectively. The band at 1017 cm^{-1} caused by HAP in Fig. 6.3b was quite sharper than the corresponding band of normal scale in Fig. 6.3a. The spectral profile of the amide-I region was similar to that of the back coat, which suggested that the ATR spectra reflected the fibrillary layer as well as the calcified layer, since the thickness of the calcified one was less than 2 μm. The spectral profile of the back coat of regenerating scales after 1 week (Fig. 6.3e) was almost the same as that of the back coat of a normal scale (Fig. 6.3d).

Figure 6.3c, f shows the second-derivative spectra of the surface and back coats of the regenerating scale after 2 weeks in the pocket side, respectively. The absorbance of amide-I band was weaker than that of Fig. 6.3b, which suggested that the calcified layer became thicker. The spectral profile of the back coat was almost the same as that of normal scale (Fig. 6.3d).

It was difficult to obtain an infrared spectrum of fish scale by using transmission mode, because the thickness of the normal scale is >100 μm and the absorbance of most interesting bands was saturated. ATR measurements have an advantage over transmission measurement, because ATR technique makes it possible to obtain not only the spectral profiles of fish scales but also the information about the surface and backside coats of the scales separately. Therefore, ATR-FTIR spectroscopy is promising for monitoring HAP and collagen components during the regeneration process of goldfish scale.

6.3.3 *Raman Spectra from Normal and Regenerating Scales of Goldfish*

Figure 6.4a, b shows Raman spectrum from the area between adjacent circular ridges in a normal scale. The bands at about 1669 cm^{-1} and 1242 cm^{-1} were assignable to collagen amide-I and amide-III, respectively, and the intense band at about 961 cm^{-1} was originated from the PO_4^{3-} symmetric stretching band for HAP (Penel et al. 1998). The intensity at 961 cm^{-1} was quite weak in the most outer part of the circular ridges, suggesting that HAP layer is not formed or thin on the collagen layers. The band at 1070 cm^{-1} was observed at the center of the scale, which was caused by type-B carbonate apatite (Awonusi et al. 2007). This interpretation was also confirmed by the FTIR bands at 1415 and 871 cm^{-1} (Fig. 6.2a). Furthermore, we found that the HAP layer became slightly thicker along the ridge line than the area between adjacent circular ridges (data not shown).

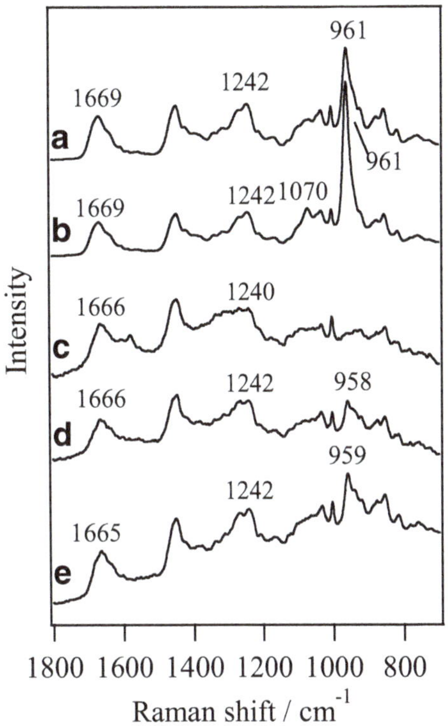

Fig. 6.4 Raman spectra from (**a**, **b**) the normal goldfish scale and from (**c**–**e**) the regenerating scale after 2 weeks. The spot position for (**a**, **c**) were on the outer part of the scale in the pocket side, and the spot positions for (**b**, **d**, **e**) were on the inner part of the scale in the pocket side. The spot position on (**d**) was in the middle of (**c**, **e**)

Figure 6.4c–e shows the Raman spectra from the area between adjacent circular ridges in regenerating scales after 2 weeks. The spectral profiles of the regenerating scales were similar to those of the normal ones except for the band at 961 cm^{-1}, which were weaker than that of normal scale (Fig. 6.4a, b). The intensities of the band at 961 cm^{-1} were the order (c) < (d) < (e). This result demonstrated that the HAP layers were formed from the center part to the outer part during the regeneration process of the scale.

Micro-Raman spectroscopy is a useful method for understanding the local components of goldfish scale because Raman spectroscopic method has higher resolution in the area compared with FTIR spectroscopic method. ATR-FTIR provides information regarding the surface component, because the sampling depth of Raman measurements was 100 μm. Therefore, Raman spectroscopy in combination with ATR-FTIR spectroscopy is powerful for analyzing HAP and carbonate apatite of the regenerating scales.

References

Awonusi A, Morris MD, Tecklenburg MMJ (2007) Carbonate assignment and calibration in the Raman spectrum of apatite. Calcif Tissue Int 81:46–52

Azuma K, Kobayashi M, Nakamura M, Suzuki N, Yashima S, Iwamuro S, Ikegame M, Yamamoto T, Hattori A (2007) Two osteoclastic markers expressed in multinucleate osteoclasts of goldfish scales. Biochem Biophys Res Commun 362:594–600

Barth A (2007) Infrared spectroscopy of proteins. Biochim Biophys Acta 1767:1073–1101

Boskey AL, Mendelsohn R (2005) Infrared spectroscopic characterization of mineralized tissues. Vib Spectrosc 38:107–114

Ikoma T, Kobayashi H, Tanaka J, Walsh D, Mann S (2003a) Microstructure, mechanical, and biomimetic properties of fish scales from *Pagrus major*. J Struct Biol 142:327–333

Ikoma T, Kobayashi H, Tanaka J, Walsh D, Mann S (2003b) Physical properties of type I collagen extracted from fish scales of *Pagrus major* and Oreochromis niloticus. Int J Biol Macromol 32:199–204

Jackson M, Choo LP, Watson PH, Halliday WC, Matsch HH (1995) Beware of connective tissue proteins: assignment and implications of collagen absorptions in infrared spectra of human tissues. Biochim Biophys Acta 1270:1–6

Mizuguchi M, Fujisawa R, Nara M, Kawano K, Nitta K (2001) Fourier-transform infrared spectroscopic study of Ca^{2+}-binding to osteocalcin. Calcif Tissue Int 69:337–342

Paschalis EP, Mendelsoln R, Boskey AL (2011) Infrared assessment of bone quality: a review. Clin Orthop Relat Res 469:2170–2178

Penel G, Leroy G, Rey C, Bres E (1998) Micro Raman spectral study of the PO_4 and CO_3 vibrational modes in synthetic and biological apatites. Calcif Tissue Int 63:475–481

Chapter 7
Relationship Between Bone Morphology and Bone Quality in Female Femurs: Implication for Additive Risk of Alternative Forced Molting

Natsuko Ishikawa, Chihiro Nishii, Koh-en Yamauchi, Hiroyuki Mishima, and Yoshiki Matsumoto

Abstract Calcium (Ca) storage in bone has a relationship with eggshell production. Forced molting by feeding restriction for older hens improves eggshell quality but leads to a decline in the bone quality. Dietary minerals improve the eggshell and bone quality; however, the effect on bone quality post-molting has not been clarified. This study evaluated the effects of dietary Ca and minerals on the eggshell and bone quality during both pre- and post-molting periods. The bone quality was evaluated by measurement of bone density and Fourier transform infrared spectroscopy (FT-IR) analysis. The eggshell quality was evaluated by morphological observation of the mammillary cores by scanning electron microscope and FT-IR analysis. The high Ca concentration feed group showed a low bone density post-molting and a high carbonate/phosphate ratio pre-molting. In high mineral concentration feed group, the eggshell strength, the thickness, and the proportion of large mammillary core areas were significantly higher ($p < 0.05$) than control group post-molting. These results suggest that the eggshell strength increases as the proportion of mammillary core areas increases. Furthermore, the high carbonate/phosphate ratio promoted a decrease in bone density. Therefore, the concentration of dietary mineral is strongly related with the maintenance of eggshells and bone quality post-molting.

Keyword Hens · Fourier transform infrared spectroscopy (FT-IR) · Scanning electron microscope (SEM) · Carbonate/phosphate ratio (C/P ratio) · Bone density · Mammillary cores · Calcium (Ca)

N. Ishikawa · C. Nishii · K.-e. Yamauchi · Y. Matsumoto (✉)
Faculty of Agriculture, Kagawa University, Miki, Japan
e-mail: myoshiki@ag.kagawa-u.ac.jp

H. Mishima
Department of Dental Engineering, Tsurumi University School of Dental Medicine, Yokohama, Japan

K. Endo et al. (eds.), *Biomineralization*,
https://doi.org/10.1007/978-981-13-1002-7_7

7.1 Introduction

A high egg laying ratio of laying hens is maintained by the metabolic mechanism of calcium (Ca) which is the main ingredient of eggshell. Approximately 70% of Ca derived from feed is accumulated in the marrow bones, a characteristic feature of birds, and approximately 68% of Ca in the bones is used for eggshell formation (Itoh 1971). Therefore, Ca storage in bones has a direct relationship with eggshell production. Consequently, the decline in Ca metabolism of the aging hens which leads to an increase in the number of broken eggs is a key issue in the poultry industry. In Japan, forced molting by feeding restriction of hens is applied in the latter stages of the laying period to improve the hen-day egg production and the eggshell quality and to extend the laying period (Roland and Bushong 1978). However a decrease in bone quality and bone density is caused by forced molting (Mazzuco and Hester 2005). Therefore, it is necessary to address the decline of bone quality in post-molting. Several studies have reported that dietary minerals and the particle size of Ca can lead to an improvement in the bone and eggshell quality (Calvo et al. 1982; Guinotte et al. 1991; Mekada et al. 1976). However, the effect on bone quality in post-molting has not yet been clarified. This study evaluated the effects of the particle size of Ca and the mineral components contained in feed on the eggshell and bone quality in fasting hens during pre- and post-molting periods.

7.2 Material and Method

7.2.1 *Breeding Test*

Sixteen egg-laying hens (Julia) were equally divided into four feeding groups, a control group (Group C) and three experimental groups (Group D, E, and F): Ca concentration ($CaCO_3$) was 3.8% $CaCO_3$ for Group C and 4.6% $CaCO_3$ for each experimental group by weight. $CaCO_3$ particle size was 40% $CaCO_3$ of 1–1.4 mm diameter for Groups C, D, and F. Group E was fed with powdered $CaCO_3$ less than 0.3 mm diameter. All groups, except Group F, received the same concentration of mineral additives, a mineral premix containing manganese sulfate, iron (III) sulfate, zinc sulfate, copper (II) sulfate, calcium iodate, and cobalt (II) sulfate. Group F received a richer mineral concentration.[1] The hens were fed from the age of 160 days old. Feed was given every day and there was no restriction on water intake by the hens. Forced molting by feeding restriction was applied for 8 days from the age of 503 days old to 510 days old. After forced molting, hens were refeed according to their group's respective feeding specification. All experiments were conducted in

[1]The amount of minerals added to feed is proprietary information and subject to a confidentiality agreement.

accordance with the regulations of the Kagawa University Animal Care and Use Committee.

7.2.2 *Sample Collection*

When the sample hens were 458 days old, two hens from each groups (a total of eight hens) were slaughtered, and femur samples were collected. The samples were regarded as pre-molting samples (PRE). When the hens were 512 days old, two hens from each groups (a total of eight hens) were slaughtered after 24 h of refeeding, and their femur samples were collected. These samples were regarded as post-molting samples (POST). The femur heads were fixed in 4% paraformaldehyde phosphate buffer solution (pH 7.4) and demineralized with 0.5 M EDTA (pH 8.0) for 3 weeks. Femur heads were embedded in paraffin and sectioned to obtain 10 μm sections.

7.2.3 *Bone Density*

The sections were stained by the Azan-Mallory method. The trabecular and bone marrow areas in femoral cancellous bone were observed at 10× magnification under a fluorescence microscope (Keyence Corp., Japan), and their central parts, 5500 μm away from periosteum, were analyzed using the software WinROOF version 7.4 (Mitani Corp., Japan). The area ratio of the trabecular to total area was determined as bone density.

7.2.4 *Fourier Transform Infrared Analysis of the Femoral Cortex*

The qualitative characteristics of the femoral cortex were determined using Fourier transform infrared spectroscopy (FT-IR) (Jasco Corp., Japan) analysis. The femoral cortex was powdered and mixed with potassium bromide (KBr). Spectroscopic analysis was based on two parameters: the calcification and the carbonate/phosphate ratio (C/P ratio) of the samples, both in PRE and POST. The calcification was calculated as the ratio of the area of the phosphate bands (900–1200 cm^{-1}) to the area of the amide I bands (1585–1720 cm^{-1}). The C/P ratio was calculated as the ratio of the area of the carbonate bands (850–890 cm^{-1}) to that of the phosphate bands (900–1200 cm^{-1}) (Boskey and Camacho 2007).

7.2.5 *Eggshell Quality Test*

The eggshell quality tests were performed twice in both PRE and POST. Eggshell thickness was determined three times on the eggshell equator for eight eggs per group. Eggshell strength was determined by an eggshell strength meter (Fujihira Industry Co., Ltd., Japan). The eggshells of 501 and 680 days old hens were used as morphological samples. The eggshells were cut into about 5 mm squares, and the eggshell membrane was dissolved with a mixture of 6% sodium hypochlorite, 4.12% sodium chloride, and 0.15% sodium hydroxide (Radwan et al. 2010). The mammillary cores were observed at 200× magnification under a scanning electron microscope (SEM) (JCM-6000: JEOL Ltd., Japan). The areas of approximately 100 mammillary cores were analyzed per piece, and 4 pieces per group were examined. Thereafter, the histogram of the areas of the mammillary cores was produced.

In the FT-IR analysis, the eggshells, including their membranes, were powdered and mixed with KBr. Spectroscopic analysis was calculated using the ratio of the peak at 873 cm^{-1} to the peak at 713 cm^{-1}, a parameter to evaluate the carbonate purity of the eggshells (Rodriguez-Navarro et al. 2015).

7.2.6 *Statistics*

Statistical processing was done using the IBM SPSS version 19 software (IBM Corp., USA). The significant differences among the groups were analyzed by the Tukey's HSD and Games-Howell post hoc tests. The level of significance was set at 5%, and the trend level was set at 10%.

7.3 Results

7.3.1 *Bone Density*

The trabecular areas in POST from all groups were significantly lower than those in PRE ($p < 0.05$). The area ratio of the trabecular to total area in PRE did not differ between any groups. However, the area ratio of the trabecular to total area in POST was significantly lower in Groups D and E than those in Groups C and F ($p < 0.05$) (Fig. 7.1a, b).

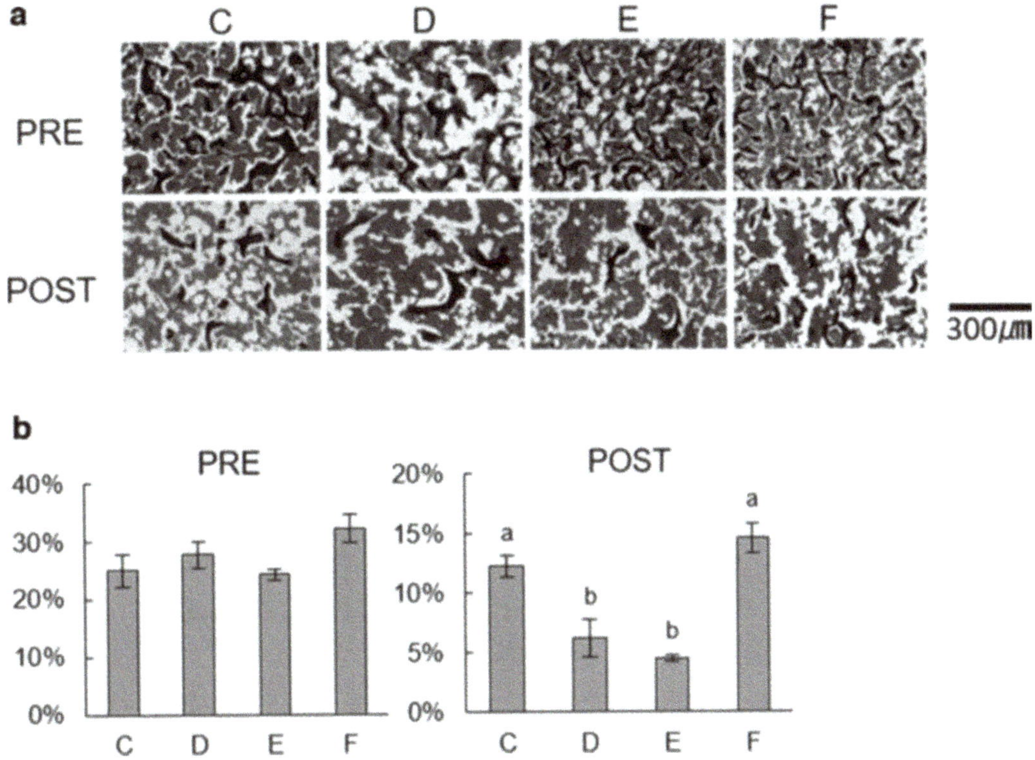

Fig. 7.1 (**a**) The trabecular and bone marrow areas in PRE and POST (black area, trabecular area; gray area, bone marrow area; white area, background). (**b**) The area ratio of the trabecular to total area in PRE and POST (a, b bars with different superscripts within a group are different at $p < 0.05$, $n = 4$)

7.3.2 Fourier Transform Infrared Analysis of Femoral Cortex

The calcification of the femoral cortex in Group F significantly decreased in POST ($p < 0.05$), whereas that in the other groups showed a decreasing trend ($p < 0.1$) (Fig. 7.2a). The C/P ratio of Groups D and E were significantly higher than Group F in PRE ($p < 0.05$) (Fig. 7.2b).

7.3.3 Egg Quality Test

Eggshell strength in Group F was significantly higher than those in Group C in POST ($p < 0.05$) (Fig. 7.3a). Eggshell thickness in Group F was significantly higher than those in Groups C and E in POST ($p < 0.05$) (Fig. 7.3b). The mammillary cores were observed as shown in Fig. 7.4a, and the proportions of the area of the eggshell mammillary cores did not differ in any group in PRE (Fig. 7.4b). There was a significant difference between Group C and Group F in POST with respect to their mammillary core areas larger than 6000 μm^2 ($p < 0.05$) (Fig. 7.4b). The ratio of the peak at 873 cm^{-1} to the peak at 713 cm^{-1} did not differ in any groups in PRE and POST (Fig. 7.5).

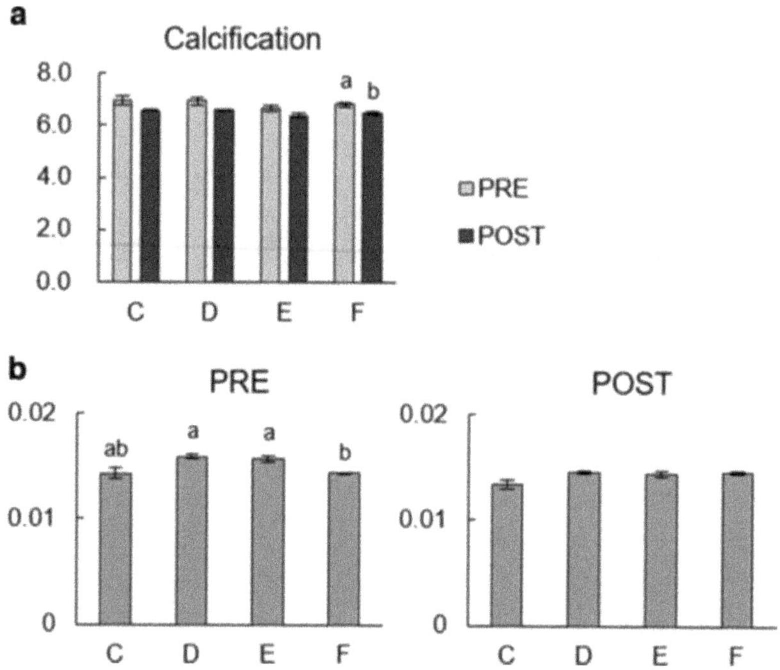

Fig. 7.2 (**a**) The calcification of the femoral cortex (a, b bars with different superscripts within a group are different at $p < 0.05$, $n = 6$). (**b**) The C/P ratio of the femoral cortex (a, b bars with different superscripts within a group are different at $p < 0.05$, $n = 6$)

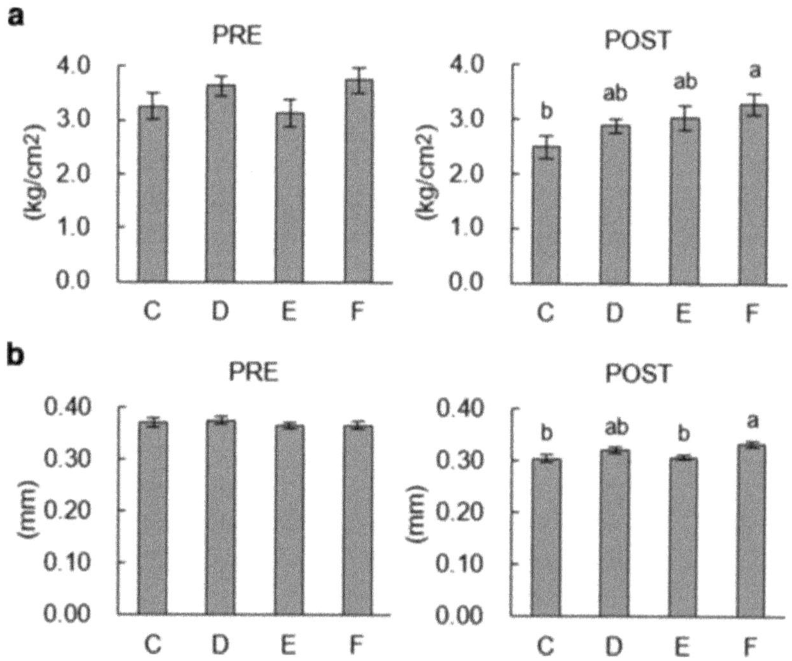

Fig. 7.3 (**a**) Eggshell strength in PRE and POST (a, b bars with different superscripts within a group are different at $p < 0.05$, $n = 16$). (**b**) Eggshell thickness in PRE and POST (a, b bars with different superscripts within a group are different at $p < 0.05$, $n = 16$)

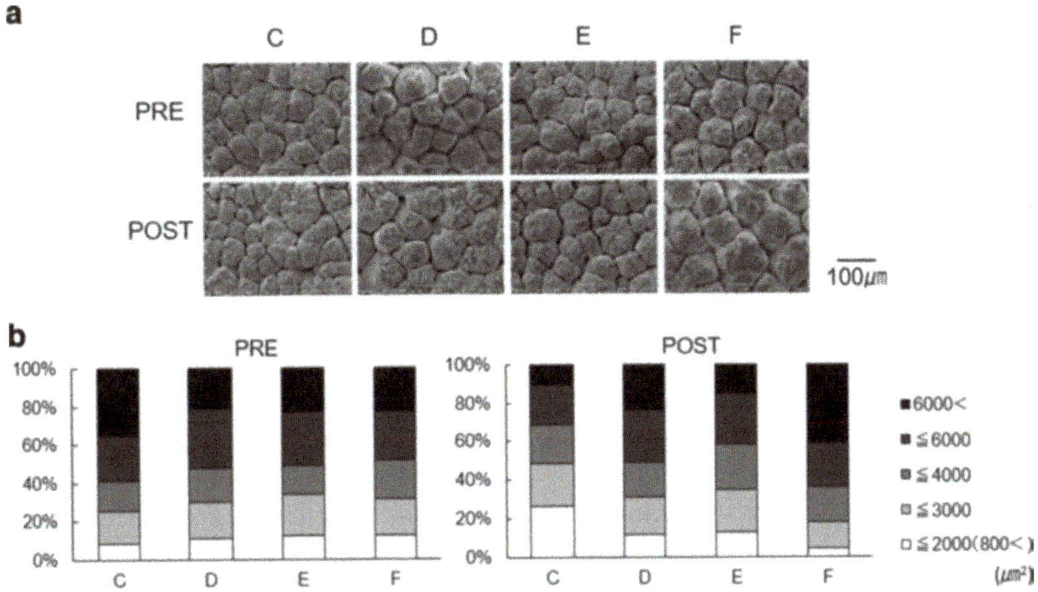

Fig. 7.4 (**a**) SEM microphotographs of eggshell mammillary core in PRE and POST. (**b**) Histogram of the areas of mammillary cores in PRE and POST ($n = 4$)

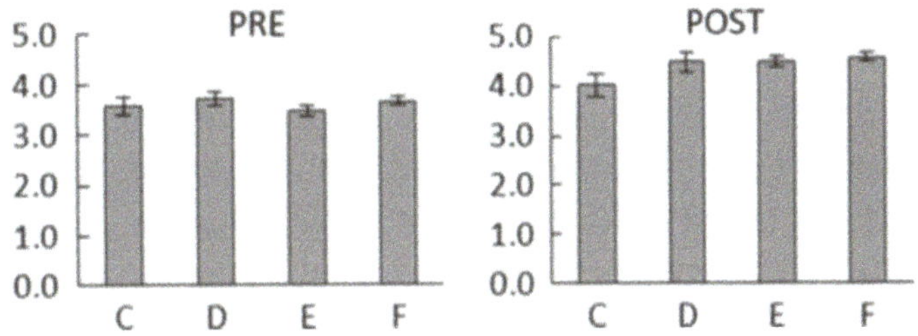

Fig. 7.5 The ratio of the peak at 873 cm^{-1} to the peak at 713 cm^{-1} (a parameter to evaluate the carbonate purity of the eggshell) in PRE and POST ($n = 6$)

7.4 Discussion

In this study, we focused on the effects of the mineral components and the particle size of $CaCO_3$ contained in feed and we investigated the morphology and quality of bone and eggshell in PRE and POST. The area ratio of the trabecular to total area is an index for evaluating bone density (Hagino, 2005). It was thought that a decrease in bone density of the femoral cancellous bone was due to the influence of forced molting because of the area ratio of the trabecular to total area diminished in all groups in POST (Fig. 7.1b). Thus, three experimental groups' feeds did not suppress the decline of the bone density.

Calcification is an index for evaluating bone strength, and high calcification indicates that the storage function of mineral in bone is high (Boskey and Camacho 2007). The decline of bone strength of the femoral cortex was also caused by the impact of forced molting because the calcification decreased in all groups in POST

(Fig. 7.2a). Furthermore, when the hardness of the part of the cortex of the femoral diaphysis was determined by Vickers hardness tester, the result of bone hardness and bone calcification were linked (data not shown), and further analysis is necessary about bone strength.

The C/P ratio is used as an index of the purity of bone minerals, and a low C/P ratio indicates a high degree of crystal purity (Malluche et al. 2012). The finding of this study suggested that crystal purity was low in PRE in Groups D and E (Fig. 7.2b). The main constituent of bone minerals are present in the bone as calcium phosphate and undergo a phase change to convert to stable apatite due to maturation. Apatite in bones replaces ions, such as carbonate ions(CO_3^{2-}) and phosphate ions, in the crystal lattice. Apatite containing a lot of CO_3^{2-} is reported to have high solubility and increase bone dissolution (Suetsugu 1996; Gourion-Arsiquaud et al. 2012). This suggested that the solubility of apatite was high in Groups D and E in PRE because a ratio of carbonate in Groups D and E were higher than Group F. Therefore, we think that the reduction of bone density was promoted further in Groups D and E in POST. These differences were thought to be due to the difference in the ratio of Ca and other mineral concentration in feed.

Eggshell strength and thickness in Group F were significantly higher than those in Group C in POST (Fig. 7.3a, b). Since zinc and manganese contained in mineral additives in feed have a relationship in eggshell formation, it was conclusive that the high mineral concentration feed improves eggshell quality and supports the previous research which mineral addition in feed improve eggshell quality (Mekada et al. 1976). Eggshell is formed by mammillary core formation on the eggshell membrane and deposition of Ca as a starting point from the mammillary cores. It was reported that as the number of large mammillary cores where several mammillary cores fused increases, the eggshell strength increases (Solomon 2010; Stefanello et al. 2014). As a result of the large number of mammillary core areas larger than 6000 μm^2 in POST, it was thought that the eggshell strength was linked the size of mammillary cores (Fig. 7.4b). Therefore, in addition to evaluating conventional eggshell strength, the morphological observation of the mammillary cores which is the microstructure of eggshell suggested that it is a new means to evaluate eggshell quality. The mechanism of action which mineral components in feed change the form of eggshell structure requires further investigation.

In the FT-IR analysis of eggshells, it was reported that the purity of carbonate changes during eggshell formation (Rodriguez-Navarro et al. 2015). We examined if the eggshell crystal quality could be evaluated after laying, however, the influence of feed on eggshell crystal quality was not detected.

The present result suggested that high mineral concentration feed improved eggshell quality, and high Ca concentration feed promoted the reduction of bone density in POST. In conclusion, the present study has demonstrated that the ratio of the minerals except Ca and the Ca concentration in the feed is important for maintenance of eggshell quality and bone quality in pre- and post-molting. It is necessary to analyze the bone metabolism in order to investigate the effect of feed in the future.

Acknowledgments This study was supported by Ise Foods, Inc., Japan, and Nichiwa Sangyo Co., Ltd., Japan, by providing hens and feeds.

References

Boskey A, Camacho NP (2007) FT-IR imaging of native and tissue-engineered bone and cartilage. Biomaterials 28(15):2465–2478

Calvo MS, Bell RR, Forbes RM (1982) Effect of protein-induced calciuria on calcium metabolism and bone status in adult rats. J Nutr 112(7):1401–1413

Gourion-Arsiquaud S, Lukashova L, Power J, Loveridge N, Reeve J, Boskey AL (2012) Fourier transform infrared imaging of femoral neck bone: reduced heterogeneity of mineral-to-matrix and carbonate-to-phosphate and more variable crystallinity in treatment-naive fracture cases compared with fracture-free controls. J Bone Miner Res 28(1):150–161

Guinotte F, Nys Y, De Monredon F (1991) The effects of particle size and origin of calcium carbonate on performance and ossification characteristics in broiler chicks. Poult Sci 70(9):1908–1920

Hagino H (2005) QUS no kijyunchi (Reference value of QUS). Osteoporosis Jpn 13(1):31–35

Itoh H (1971) Calcium metabolism in domestic fowl. Jpn Poult Sci 8(2):65–76

Malluche HH, Porter DS, Claude Monier-Faugere M, Mawad H, Pienkowski D (2012) Differences in bone quality in low- and high-turnover renal osteodystrophy. J Am Soc Nephrol 23:525–532

Mazzuco H, Hester PY (2005) The effect of an induced molt using a nonfasting program on bone mineralization of white leghorns. Poult Sci 84(9):1483–1490

Mekada H, Hayashi N, Okumura J, Yokota H (1976) Effect of dietary fossil shell on the quality of hen's egg shell in summer. Jpn Poult Sci 13(2):65–69

Radwan LM, Fathi MM, Galal A, Zein El-Dein A (2010) Mechanical and ultrastructural properties of eggshell in two Egyptian native breeds of chicken. Int J Poult Sci 9(1):77–81

Rodriguez-Navarro AB, Marie P, Nys Y, Hincke MT, Gautron JL (2015) Amorphous calcium carbonate controls avian eggshell mineralization: a new paradigm for understanding rapid eggshell calcification. J Struct Biol 190:291–303

Roland DA, Bushong RD (1978) The influence of force molting on the incidence of uncollectable eggs. Poult Sci 57(1):22–26

Solomon S (2010) The eggshell: strength, structure and function. Br Poult Sci 51(1):52–59

Stefanello C, Santos TC, Murakami AE, Martins EN, Carneiro TC (2014) Productive performance, eggshell quality, and eggshell ultrastructure of laying hens fed diets supplemented with organic trace minerals. Poult Sci 93:104–113

Suetsugu Y (1996) Carbonate ions in apatite structure. Inorg Mater 3:48–54

Chapter 8
Spectroscopic Investigation of Shell Pigments from the Family Neritidae (Mollusca: Gastropoda)

Toshiyuki Komura, Hiroyuki Kagi, Makiko Ishikawa, Mana Yasui, and Takenori Sasaki

Abstract Molluscan shells display a wide variety of pigmentation patterns. The diversity in molluscan shell color reflects the variety of different chemical species in the shell surface. Chemical characteristics of molluscan shell pigments have been extensively investigated, and compounds including porphyrins, polyenes, and melanins were identified as shell pigments. Here, we investigated shell pigments in 24 species in the family Neritidae using Raman spectroscopy. An excitation wavelength of 514.5 nm revealed two types of Raman spectra. One was characterized by two peaks ranging in wavenumber from 1100–1200 to 1500–1600 cm^{-1}, which indicate the presence of polyenes. Another type remained unassigned, implying the presence of other pigments such as porphyrins or melanins. The Raman spectra indicated a different distribution of the two types of pigments in shells. The patterns of the Raman spectra had no obvious relationship with taxonomical classification lower than the genus level and typical habitats. Measurement of the Raman spectrum at an excitation wavelength of 442 nm suggested that the wavelength can distinguish polyenes from other types of pigments.

T. Komura (✉) · H. Kagi
Graduate School of Science, The University of Tokyo, Bunkyo-ku, Tokyo, Japan
e-mail: komura@eqchem.s.u-tokyo.ac.jp; kagi@eqchem.s.u-tokyo.ac.jp

M. Ishikawa
Graduate School of Science, The University of Tokyo, Bunkyo-ku, Tokyo, Japan
Faculty of Animal Health Technology, Yamazaki Gakuen University, Hachioji, Tokyo, Japan
e-mail: maki.ishikawa.gm@gmail.com

M. Yasui
Department of Resources and Environmental Engineering, School of Creative Science and Engineering, Waseda University, Shinjuku-ku, Tokyo, Japan
e-mail: mana@aoni.waseda.jp

T. Sasaki
The University Museum, The University of Tokyo, Bunkyo-ku, Tokyo, Japan
e-mail: sasaki@um.u-tokyo.ac.jp

K. Endo et al. (eds.), *Biomineralization*,
https://doi.org/10.1007/978-981-13-1002-7_8

Keywords Mollusc · Neritidae · Shell pigment · Polyene · Porphyrin · Raman spectroscopy

8.1 Introduction

The phylum Mollusca is the second largest taxon in the animal kingdom. It is very diverse in size, shape, color, habitats, and other traits. The diverse pigmentation patterns on shells are a key trait. Diversity in molluscan shell color reflects the wide variety of chemical species included in the shell. Investigating the origin of shell pigmentation is very important to understand the evolutionary history of Mollusca (Williams 2017). Furthermore, chemical speciation of shell pigment molecules could provide insight into the interaction of pigment molecules with other shell components (Hedegaard et al. 2006), which is important for the better understanding of biomineralization during shell formation.

Shell pigments have been extensively investigated (Williams 2017; Ishikawa et al. 2013 and references therein). Comfort (1949a, b) reported the presence of porphyrin compounds in several groups of gastropods including the family Neritidae (described later) using ultraviolet fluorescence and absorption chromatography. Subsequently, the presence of polyene compounds was reported using Raman spectroscopy. For example, Hedegaard et al. (2006) estimated the chain length of conjugated polyenes and discussed the chemical modification of polyenes contained in the shell of the gastropod *Cypraea moneta* (Cypraeidae). Polyene pigments were observed in various taxa. However, the target samples used in previous studies were limited to common shells with strong colors. Here, we comprehensively studied the family Neritidae and conducted a preliminary study to detect porphyrin pigments using Raman spectroscopy. The family Neritidae comprises small- or medium-sized snails that inhabit a wide variety of shallow-water environments such as brackish areas and intertidal rocky zones. The family is characterized by clear and vivid color bands (Fig. 8.1), which make spectroscopic analysis easy to perform. Their various habitats are expected to have an effect on pigmentation because shell colors are affected by environmental factors (e.g., Sokolova and Berger 2000).

8.2 Materials and Methods

We investigated 24 species from 5 genera of the family Neritidae by using Raman spectroscopy (Table 8.1). Raman spectra were obtained from each differently colored area using an exposure time of 10 s for each measurement. Ten spectra were obtained for each area. Estimated energy resolution ranged from 1 to 2 cm^{-1}. Two Raman spectrometers with different excitation wavelengths (514.5 and 442 nm) were used (Table 8.2). The excitation wavelength of 514.5 nm has been previously demonstrated to detect polyenes. The excitation wavelength of 442 nm is near the Soret maxima of porphyrins and thus is expected to excite porphyrins that are

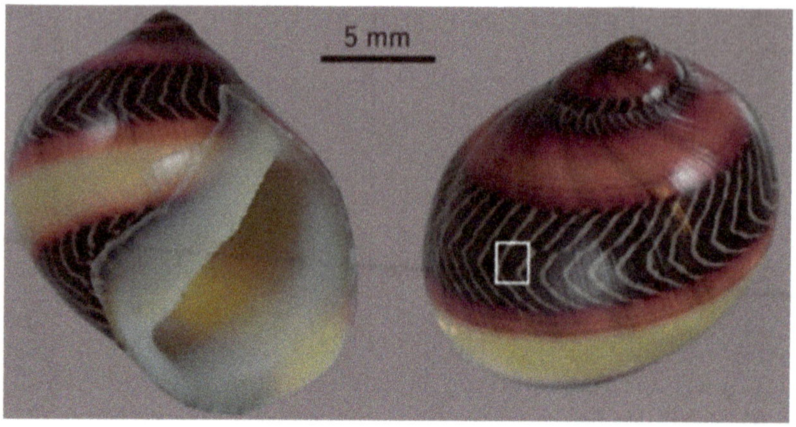

Fig. 8.1 *Neritina waigiensis* in the family Neritidae. A section of the shell denoted by the white square was used for Raman analysis (see Fig. 8.3)

Table 8.1 Collection numbers, species, locality, and typical habitats of the investigated samples

Coll. number	Species	Locality	Typical habitat
RM 32906	*Clithon oualaniense* (Lesson, 1831)	Bohol Island, Philippines	Brackish, on sandy or muddy substrate
RM 32907	*Clithon (Pictoneritina) chlorostoma* (Broderip, 1833)	Ishigaki Island, Japan	Under rocks, in estuaries
RM 32908	*Clithon cryptum* (Eichhorst, 2016)	Amami Island, Japan	Under rocks, in estuaries
RM 32909	*Nerita (Amphinerita) insculpta* (Récluz, 1841)	Okinawa Island, Japan	Intertidal, on rocks
RM 32910	*Nerita (Cymostyla) tristis* (Pilsbry, 1901)	Amami Oshima Island, Japan	Intertidal, on rocks
RM 32911	*Nerita (Cymostyla) striata* (Burrow, 1815)	Okinawa Island, Japan	Intertidal, on rocks
RM 32912	*Nerita (Ritena) plicata* (Linnaeus, 1758)	Ikema Island, Japan	Intertidal, on rocks
RM 32913	*Nerita (Ritena) costata* (Gmelin, 1791)	Amami Oshima Island, Japan	Intertidal, on rocks
RM 32914	*Nerita (Theliostyla) picea* (Récluz, 1841)	Australia	Uncertain
RM 32915	*Nerita (Theliostyla) exuvia* (Linnaeus, 1758)	Cebu Island, Philippines	Intertidal, on rocks
RM 32916	*Nerita (Theliostyls) albicala* (Linnaeus, 1758)	Amami Island, Japan	Intertidal, on rocks
RM 32917	*Nerita (Argonerita) signata* (Lamarck, 1822)	Bohol Island, Philippines	Intertidal, on rocks
RM 32918	*Nerita (Argonerita) chammaeleon* (Linnaeus, 1758)	Ishigaki Island, Japan	Intertidal, on rocks
RM 32919	*Nerita (Linnerita) incerta* (von dem Busch, 1844)	Zamami Island, Japan	Intertidal, on rocks

(continued)

Table 8.1 (continued)

Coll. number	Species	Locality	Typical habitat
RM 32920	*Neritina (Linnerita) rumphi* (Récluz, 1841)	Malakal Island, Palau	Intertidal, on rocks
RM 32921	*Neritina (Linnerita) polita* (Linnaeus, 1758)	Okinawa Island, Japan	Intertidal, on rocks near sand
RM 32922	*Neritina (Neritina) pulligera* (Linnaeus, 1767)	Okinawa Island, Japan	On rocks in rivers
RM 32923	*Neritina (Vittina) paralela* (Röding, 1798)	Cebu Island, Philippines	Brackish area
RM 32924	*Neritina (Vittina) waigiensis* (Lesson, 1831)	Cebu Island, Philippines	Mangrove swamp
RM 32925	*Neritina (Vittina) turritta* (Gmelin, 1791)	Cebu Island, Philippines	On mud in mangrove swamp
RM 32926	*Neripteron (Dostia) cornucopia* (Benson, 1836)	Cebu Island, Philippines	Brackish area and mangrove swamp
RM 32927	*Smaragdia rangiana* (Récluz, 1842)	Balicasag Island, Philippines	On seagrasses
RM 32928	*Neritodryas dubia* (Gmelin, 1791)	Cebu Island, Philippines	Intertidal, brackish area
RM 32929	*Neritodryas* sp.	Cebu Island, Philippines	Intertidal, brackish area

Scientific names and typical habitats follow the designation schemes of Tsuchiya and Kano (2017) and Eichhorst (2016)

Table 8.2 Excitation wavelength, laser source, laser power, calibration standard, and objective lens magnification data of the two Raman spectrometers

Excitation wavelength (nm)	Laser source	Laser power (mW)	Calibration standard	Objective lens magnification
514.5	Ar^+ laser	30	Naphthalene	×20
442	He-Cd laser	120	Silicon	×20

Laser power could be attenuated through the optical paths for both instruments

present in the mollusc shell (Comfort 1949a). We performed intact shell surface analysis without chemical treatments. The samples examined were registered in The University Museum, The University of Tokyo.

8.3 Results and Discussion

8.3.1 Raman Spectra at 514.5 nm

Figure 8.2 shows representative Raman spectra obtained from yellow, red, and black color bands of *N. waigiensis*. The Raman spectra of the black and red parts were similar, while the spectrum of the yellow part was markedly different from both. The spectrum obtained from the yellow part was characterized by two peaks with wavenumbers ranging from 1100–1200 cm^{-1} (ν_5) to 1500–1600 cm^{-1} (ν_1). These two peaks are assigned to polyene pigments contained in the shell (e.g., Bergamonti et al. 2013). These polyene-type spectra were obtained from the species listed in Table 8.3. While Raman shifts of ν_5 and ν_1 varied in all species, the observed values were within a certain range.

The spectra obtained from red and black parts of *N. waigiensis* had no obvious peaks that could be assigned to polyenes. This type of spectrum was also obtained from the species listed in Table 8.4. Similar spectra from the gastropod *Clunculus pharaonius* (Trochidae) were reported by Merlin and Delé-Dubois (1986) and Williams et al. (2016). The red and black pigments of *C. pharaonius* were identified as uroporphyrin and eumelanin, respectively, using high-performance liquid chromatography (Williams et al. 2016). However, the authors argued that the Raman spectra did not convey any definitive information concerning shell pigments, and it

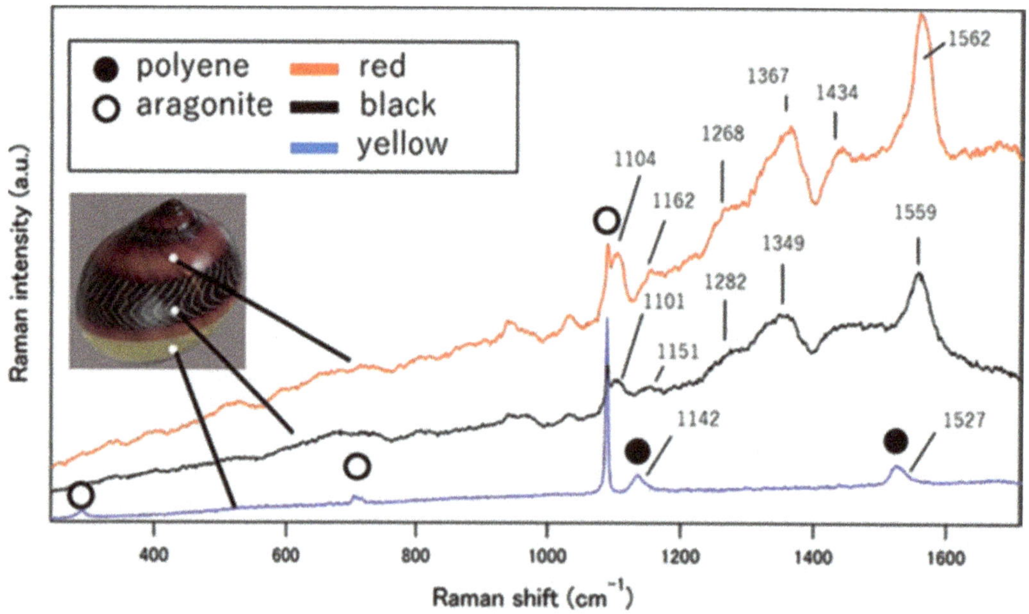

Fig. 8.2 Raman spectra obtained from each color band of *N. waigiensis* using 514.5 nm excitation. White circles in the figure indicate measurement points for Raman analysis

Table 8.3 Colors and wavenumbers of the ν_5 and ν_1 peaks using the 514.5 nm excitation from species containing polyenes

Species	Color	ν_5 (cm^{-1})	ν_1 (cm^{-1})
Clithonoualaniense (Lesson, 1831)	Pale yellow	1139	1532
Nerita (Amphinerita) insculpta (Récluz, 1841)	Black	1138	1528
Nerita (Linnerita) incerta (von dem Busch, 1844)	Green	1138	1526
Nerita (Cymostyla) tristis (Pilsbry, 1901)	Deep green	1138	1530
Nerita (Cymostyla) striata (Burrow, 1815)	Black	1135	1525
Nerita (Cymostyla) striata (Burrow, 1815)	Light green	1136	1527
Nerita (Ritena) plicata (Linnaeus, 1758)	Black	1135	1524
Nerita (Argonerita) signata (Lamarck, 1822)	Red	1133	1523
Nerita (Argonerita) chammaeleon (Linnaeus, 1758)	Black	1138	1524
Nerita (Theliostyls) albicilla (Linnaeus, 1758)	Deep green	1137	1527
Neritina (Linnerita) rumphii (Récluz, 1841)	Black	1136	1526
Neritina (Linnerita) rumphii (Récluz, 1841)	Green	1137	1525
Neritina (Linnerita) polita (Linnaeus, 1758)	Deep green	1135	1524
Neritina (Linnerita) polita (Linnaeus, 1758)	Green	1135	1524
Neritina (Neritina) pulligera (Linnaeus, 1767)	Deep green	1138	1528
Neritina (Neritina) pulligera (Linnaeus, 1767)	Orange	1139	1530
Neritina (Vittina) waigiensis (Lesson, 1831)	Yellow	1142	1527
Smaragdia rangiana (Récluz, 1842)	Green	1139	1534
Nerita (Ritena) costata (Gmelin, 1791)	Black (between spiral ribs)	1134	1524

was quite unclear whether the obtained spectra were assignable to uroporphyrin or eumelanin included in the shell. Presently, we also could not conclusively identify shell pigment from the Raman spectra. However, the difference in chemical origins of the black and red pigmentations of *N. waigiensis* from that of yellow pigmentation is a novel finding. It is worth noting that the Raman peaks obtained from red and black regions of *N. waigiensis* appeared at a similar frequency to those in the spectrum of eumelanin reported by Mbonyiryivuze et al. (2015). It is conceivable that the peaks we observed were due to background fluorescence.

Shell pigmentation may be relevant to taxonomical classification (Comfort 1949a, Williams 2017). However, the patterns and peak wavenumber of the Raman spectra (Tables 8.1, 8.2, and 8.3) had no obvious relationship with the taxonomical classification at the genus or lower level or with typical habitats. Different types of spectra could be observed even in the same individuals.

We fabricated the shell section perpendicular to the apertural margin of *N. waigiensis* (Fig. 8.3). The thickness of red- and black-colored layers was approximately 30 μm. The Raman spectra obtained from five points are shown in Fig. 8.4. No obvious peaks assignable to polyenes were observed from points 1 to 2. Two weak peaks assignable to polyenes were detected at point 3. The obtained spectra

Table 8.4 Colors and Raman shifts of representative peaks obtained at 514.5 nm excitation wavelength from species displaying other spectra

Species	Color	Raman shifts of representative peak (cm^{-1})
Clithon oualaniense (Lesson, 1831)	Black	1562
Clithon (Pictoneritina) chlorostoma (Broderip, 1833)	Black	1562
Clithon cryptum (Eichhorst, 2016)	Black	1566
Nerita (Linnerita) incerta (von dem Busch, 1844)	Deep green	1562
Nerita (Theliostyla) picea (Récluz, 1841)	Black	1560
Nerita (Theliostyla) exuvia (Linnaeus, 1758)	Black	1548
Neripteron (Dostia) cornucopia (Benson, 1836)	Deep green	1559
Neritina (Vittina) waigiensis (Lesson, 1831)	Red	1562
Neritina (Vittina) waigiensis (Lesson, 1831)	Black	1557
Neritina (Vittina) turritta (Gmelin, 1791)	Black	1566
Neritina (Vittina) parallella (Röding, 1798)	Black	1558
Neritodryas dubia (Gmelin, 1791)	Deep purple	1560
Neritodryas sp.	Red	1560
Neritodryas sp.	Black	1565
Nerita (Ritena) costata (Gmelin, 1791)	Black (on spiral ribs)	1554

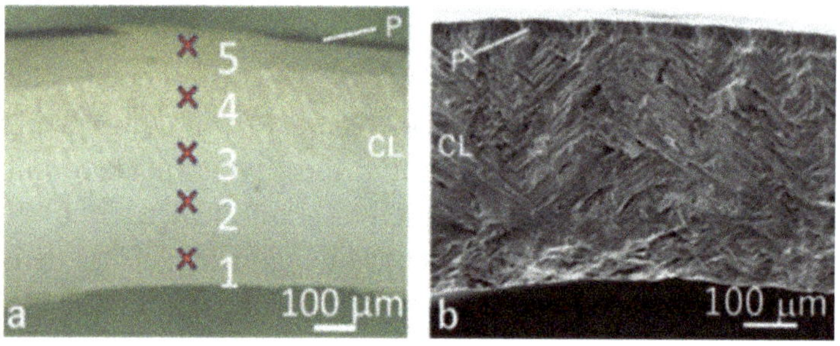

Fig. 8.3 (**a**) A section perpendicular to the apertural margin of *N. waigiensis*. The black and yellow patterns on the shell exterior are visible on the upper side of the figure. The numbers 1–5 indicate measured points. (**b**) Scanning electron microscopy image of the section of *N. waigiensis*. The multilayered structure of the shell is evident. The outermost region is a prismatic layer (P) that corresponds to the colored layer in (**a**). The inner layer has a crossed-lamellar structure (CL). These two figures were obtained from different individuals of *N. waigiensis*

raise the possibility that the concentration of polyenes increases continuously from the interior of the shell to the exterior surface. In contrast, black and red pigmentation appeared only in the narrow range on the surface, indicating that their distributions are quite different from the distribution of polyenes.

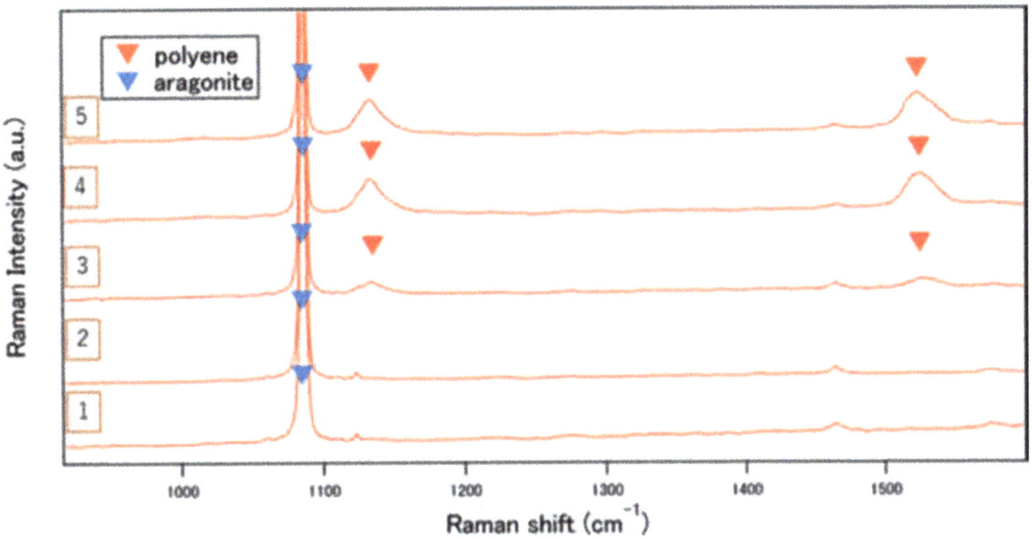

Fig. 8.4 Raman spectrum obtained from each measured point in Fig. 8.3

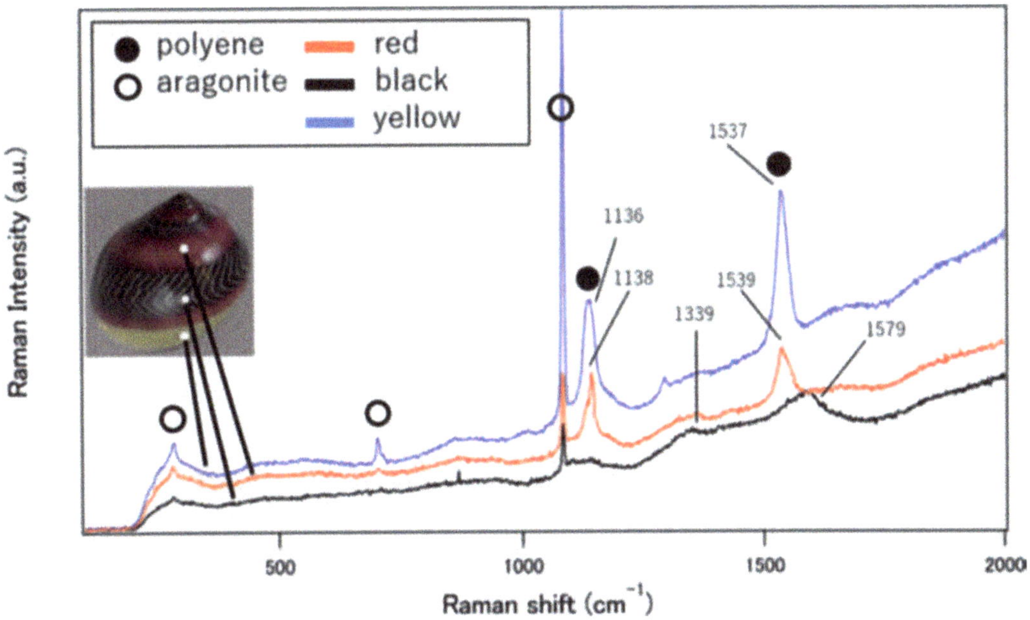

Fig. 8.5 Raman spectrum obtained from each color band of *N. waigiensis* using the 442 nm excitation wavelength. The white circles in the figure indicate the measurement points for Raman analysis

8.3.2 Raman Spectra at 442 nm Excitation

Figure 8.5 shows Raman spectra obtained from *N. waigiensis* using the 442 nm excitation wavelength. Clear peaks assignable to polyenes were observed from the yellow and red parts of the shell surface, but not from the black part. Polyene-type spectrum from the red part may be attributed to the polyenes of the yellow part existing just under the red color band on the surface. Williams et al. (2016) argued that it is difficult to distinguish polyenes from porphyrins only by the Raman spectra. However, our results suggest that polyenes can be distinguished from other pigments because the background fluorescence was relatively low compared to that for the peak heights at ν_5 and ν_1.

8.4 Conclusions

Analysis using the 514.5 nm excitation wavelength demonstrated that the pigmentation in the family Neritidae has at least two types of origins: polyenes and other unknown pigments such as porphyrins or melanins. The data from a shell section of *N. waigiensis* suggest that these two types of pigments are distributed in a different manner in the section. The patterns of the Raman spectra did not display obvious relationships with taxonomical classification and habitats. The Raman spectra obtained using the 442 nm excitation wavelength suggest that polyenes can be distinguished from other pigments by the presence of strong peaks of ν_5 and ν_1. However, definitive information on shell pigments was difficult using only Raman spectroscopy. Other analytical techniques such as high-performance liquid chromatography could be needed and will be studied.

Acknowledgment We thank Dr. Natsuhiko Sugimura from the Research Support Center at Waseda University for providing support for the measurement of the Raman spectra.

References

Bergamonti L, Bersani D, Mantovan S, Lottici PP (2013) Micro-Raman investigation of pigments and carbonate phases in corals and molluscan shells. Eur J Mineral 25:845–853

Comfort A (1949a) Acid-soluble pigments of shells. 1. The distribution of porphyrin fluorescence in molluscan shells. Biochem J 44:111–117

Comfort A (1949b) Acid-soluble pigments of shells. 4. Identification of shell porphyrins with particular reference to conchoporphyrin. Biochem J 45:208–210

Eichhorst TE (2016) Neritidae in the world. ConchBooks, Harxheim

Hedegaard C, Bardeau J-F, Chateigner D (2006) Molluscan shell pigments: an in situ resonance Raman study. J Molluscan Stud 72:157–162

Ishikawa M, Kagi H, Sasaki T, Endo K (2013) Current trend of research in molluscan shell pigments. Earth Mon 35(12):712–719 (In Japanese)

Mbonyiryivuze A, Omollo I, Ngom BD, Mwakikunga B, Dhlamini SM, Park E, Maaza M (2015) Natural dye sensitizer for Grätzel cells: Sepia Melanin. Phys Mater Chem 3(1):1–6

Merlin JC, Delé-Dubois ML (1986) Resonance Raman characterization of polyacetylenic pigments in the calcareous skeleton. Comp Biochem Physiol 84B(1):97–103

Sokolova IM, Berger VJ (2000) Physiological variation related to shell colour polymorphism in White Sea *Littorina saxatilis*. J Exp Mar Biol Ecol 245:1–23

Tsuchiya K, Kano Y (2017) Family Neritidae. In: Okutani T (ed) Marine Mollusks in Japan, 2nd edn. Tokai University Press, Tokyo

Williams ST (2017) Molluscan shell colour. Biol Rev 92:1039–1058

Williams ST, Ito S, Wakamatsu K, Goral T, Edwards NP, Wogelius RA et al (2016) Identification of shell colour pigments in marine snails *Clanculus pharaonius* and *C. margaritarius* (Trochoidea; Gastropoda). PLoSONE 11(7):e0156664

Chapter 9
3D Visualization of Calcified and Non-calcified Molluscan Tissues Using Computed Tomography

Takenori Sasaki, Yu Maekawa, Yusuke Takeda, Maki Atsushiba, Chong Chen, Koji Noshita, Kentaro Uesugi, and Masato Hoshino

Abstract Three-dimensional (3D) reconstruction is an essential approach in morphological studies in biology and paleontology. Seeking an optimized protocol for nondestructive observations, we attempted 3D visualization of various molluscan shells and animals with X-ray micro-computed tomography (micro-CT). Calcified parts of molluscs were easily visualized except for cases with marked differences in thickness heterogeneity. 3D imaging of shell microstructure was difficult. Visualization of soft tissue requires staining to enhance the image contrast. Especially for soft tissues, synchrotron X-ray microtomography is the most advanced method to generate clear 3D images. 3D data facilitates morphological quantification, enabling calculations of length and volume even for very complex forms. X-ray micro-CT is extremely useful in the morphologic examination of

T. Sasaki (✉) · Y. Maekawa · M. Atsushiba
The University Museum, The University of Tokyo, Bunkyo-ku, Tokyo, Japan
e-mail: atsushiba-7122@g.ecc.u-tokyo.ac.jp; yu.maekawa@um.u-tokyo.ac.jp; sasaki@um.u-tokyo.ac.jp

Y. Takeda
The University Museum, The University of Tokyo, Bunkyo-ku, Tokyo, Japan

Department of Earth and Planetary Science, Hokkaido University, Kita-ku, Sapporo, Hokkaido, Japan
e-mail: ytakeda@sci.hokudai.ac.jp

C. Chen
Japan Agency for Marine-Earth Science and Technology, Yokosuka, Kanagawa, Japan
e-mail: cchen@jamstec.go.jp

K. Noshita
Graduate School of Agricultural and Life Sciences, The University of Tokyo, Bunkyo-ku, Tokyo, Japan
e-mail: noshita@morphometrics.jp

K. Uesugi · M. Hoshino
Japan Synchrotron Radiation Research Institute, Sayo-gun, Hyogo, Japan
e-mail: hoshino@spring8.or.jp; ueken@spring8.or.jp

K. Endo et al. (eds.), *Biomineralization*,
https://doi.org/10.1007/978-981-13-1002-7_9

mineralized and soft tissues, although microstructural and histological details should be supplemented by other microscopic techniques.

Keywords Micro-CT · Synchrotron CT · Reconstruction · Anatomy

9.1 Introduction

The importance of computed tomography (CT) has been established in biology and paleontology. CT has also been used in examinations of vertebrate morphology (Gignac et al. 2016; du Plessis et al. 2017), and micro-CT has been used in invertebrate biology, mainly in entomology studies (Friedrich et al. 2014; Wipfler et al. 2016). The approach has been infrequently used for other animal groups. In malacology, the use of micro-CT is restricted to a small number of case studies involving anatomy (Golding and Jones 2007; Golding et al. 2009), ontogeny (Kerbl et al. 2013), paleontology (Takeda et al. 2016), and shell morphology (Monnet et al. 2009; Liew and Schilthuizen 2016; Noshita et al. 2016).

The application of CT is still in the testing and development stage. Having an optimized protocol for the nondestructive micro-CT analysis of various morphological characteristics would help expand the scope of CT applications and was the focus of the present study.

9.2 Material and Methods

The molluscan specimens used in this study are all registered and deposited in The University Museum, The University of Tokyo (UMUT). The abbreviations RM and CM in the registration numbers indicate recent and Cenozoic molluscs, respectively. Animals were fixed in 5% formaldehyde solution for several days, washed in tap water, and then preserved in 70% ethanol. Intact animals were extracted from shells by soaking the specimens in approximately 10% HCl to completely dissolve the shells. Most specimens were first digitally imaged (Fig. 9.1a–e) using a ScanXmate B100TSS110 industrial micro-CT device (Comscantecno Co., Ltd.) at UMUT. Scan parameters were adjusted according to samples and included source voltage (70–100 kV), source current (approximately 40–150 μA), and exposure time per frame (0.4–1.0 s). The total number of frames was 1200, the number of pixels of the detector was 1024 × 1012, and the highest resolution was approximately 2 μm. Samples larger than 3 cm were scanned in the laboratory of Comscantecno Co. Ltd. For scanning, embedding the sample in a heat-generated hole in Styrofoam on a rotating stage was the most effective method of sample fixation. For soft portions of samples, high-resolution X-ray CT was also performed (Fig. 9.1f–h) at the hutch 3 of the beamline BL20B2 in SPring-8 (Hyogo, Japan) with a resolution of 13.16 μm per pixel and an X-ray energy of 25 keV. Three-dimensional (3D) visualization was conducted using Molcer Plus (White Rabbit Corporation), OsiriX (OsiriX Foundation), and Amira 3.5.5 (Visage Imaging, Inc.) software.

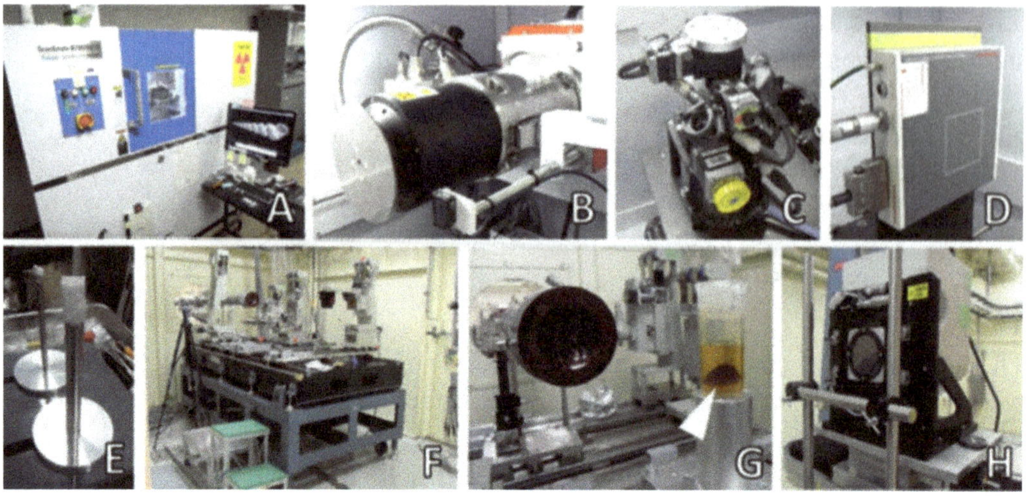

Fig. 9.1 CT facilities used in this study. (**a–e**) Industrial CT (UMUT). (**b**) X-ray tube. (**c**) Sample stage. (**d**) X-ray detector. (**e**) Sample holder. (**f–h**) Synchrotron CT (SPring-8 BL20B2). (**g**) Magnified view of sample stage. Arrowhead indicates sample. (**h**) X-ray detector

9.3 Results

9.3.1 Shells

Most samples of calcified shells were scanned without difficulty using conventional industrial micro-CT (Fig. 9.2). The internal structure of shells was also perfectly reconstructed from scan data. Exceptions included shells of specific groups of gastropods, with shells from different regions having extremely disparate thicknesses. For example, members of the families Ellobiidae (Figs. 9.2c, d), Olividae, and Conidae have shells in which the internal whorls are much thinner than the outer wall owing to the secondary resorption that occurs during growth. In such cases, the thinner inner whorls disappear or became patchy in distribution when the settings were optimized for the outer shell surface. Conversely, if contrast were enhanced to reveal the inner structures, outer surfaces were rendered unusable by the increased noise levels (the overexposure effect). So far, no viable solution to this problem has been identified in our current system.

Digitization using micro-CT is an excellent approach to display the overall 3D morphology and the internal structure of molluscan shells. Examples of specimens of small Cenozoic fossil gastropods are presented in Fig. 9.2e–j. Virtual slicing of type specimens along an arbitrary plane is possible only using micro-CT. Prominent columellar folds (Fig. 9.2f, h) or denticles in the outer lip (Fig. 9.2h) were important features to morphologically diagnose species. Construction of images from apical (Fig. 9.2i) and basal (Fig. 9.2j) views for fragile and minute specimens is easily acquired. However, imaging of the same specimens by photography with a digital camera and binocular microscope carries the risk of specimen loss or damage. Micro-CT allows the detailed nondestructive observation of the delicate structures of shells.

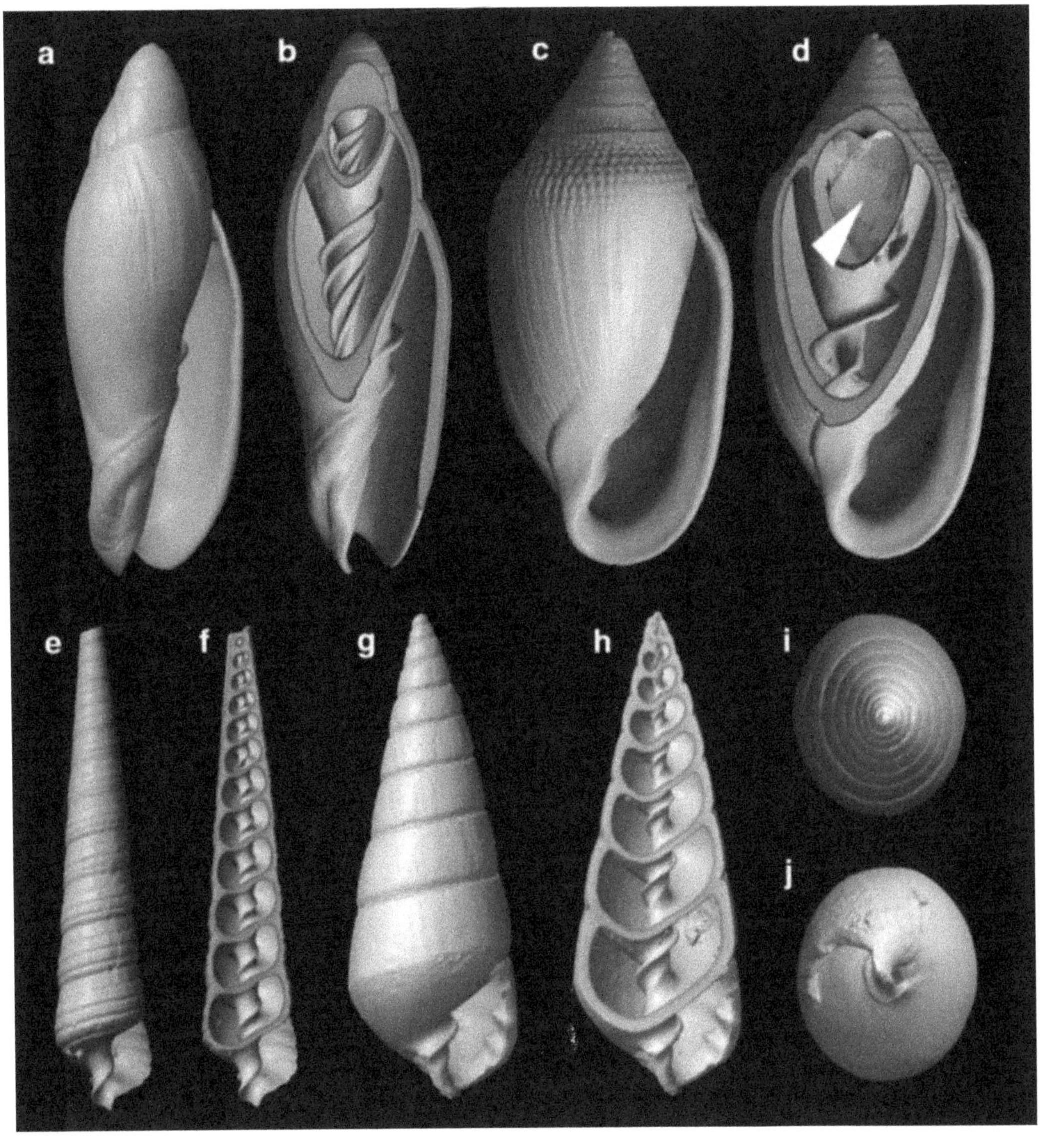

Fig. 9.2 Example of 3D reconstruction of calcified shells from industrial micro-CT data. (**a**, **b**) *Volutoconus bednalli* (Brazier, 1878) (Volutidae). UMUT RM32762. (**c**, **d**) *Ellobium aurismidae* (Linnaeus, 1758) (Ellobiidae). UMUT RM32763. Arrowhead indicates missing inner wall as artifact. (**e**, **f**) *Cerithiella trisulcata* (Yokoyama, 1922) (Newtoniellidae). UMUT CM20781. Holotype. (**g–i**) *Tiberia pseudopulchella* (Yokoyama, 1920) (Pyramidellidae). UMUT CM20242. Holotype. (**i**) Apical view. (**j**) Adapical view. Shell height: **a**, **b** = 90.6 mm; **c**, **d** 88.8 mm; **e**, **f** = 5.2 mm; **g**, **h** = 7.0 mm. Software: Molcer Plus

However, the use of micro-CT for shells is not entirely versatile. Most importantly, growth lines, shell layers, and shell microstructure cannot be observed. We were unable to detect any structure on sliced shell planes in the CT-derived 3D data. The observation of these fine structures still necessitates mechanical destruction or cutting of the actual shell samples.

Another issue is that high-resolution scanning of a specific part of a large shell is not possible. To achieve high-resolution scan data, it is necessary to place a sample

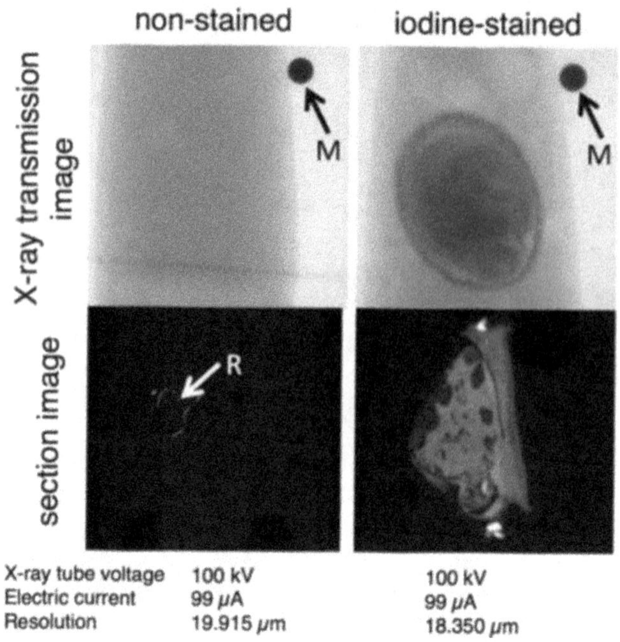

Fig. 9.3 Soft part of *Lottia dorsuosa* (Lottiidae). UMUT RM32764. Comparison of scanning results between iodine-free (left) and iodine-stained (right) samples with industrial micro-CT. *R* radular teeth, *M* metal ball for position correction. Body length = 22 mm

as close to the X-ray source as possible (for any given detector image size, the realized resolution depends on the field of view and, thus, the size of the specimen). In conventional micro-CT, it is necessary to rotate the specimen. Thus, if the sample is large, it must be placed further away from the X-ray source, which will decrease the resolution. This dilemma cannot be overcome at the present time.

9.3.2 *Soft Tissues*

Simultaneous visualization of both the shell and the soft regions from a single specimen could not be achieved with satisfactory results. If various parameters are optimized for shells, the settings are far from optimal for the soft regions, and vice versa. The only way to achieve high-quality scans for both features from a single individual is to obtain the shell scan first and to decalcify it to scan the soft regions. This destroys the shell. Therefore, development of a new algorithm or methodology is desired to enable the nondestructive scans of precious specimens (such as intact types) to reveal the anatomy of soft portions.

Applying CT to soft parts is more challenging than applying it to calcified parts. Animal tissues usually do not display any contrast in CT images without the aid of contrast-enhancing substances. Figure 9.3 shows an example of Patellogastropoda. In this organism, only iron-mineralized radular teeth are visible if the specimen is not treated with a contrast agent (e.g., iodine).

Installation of samples on the rotating stage is also an extremely sensitive part of the scanning process. If a wet sample is scanned while it is exposed to air, it quickly becomes dehydrated and deformed, which will result in a very blurred image that is

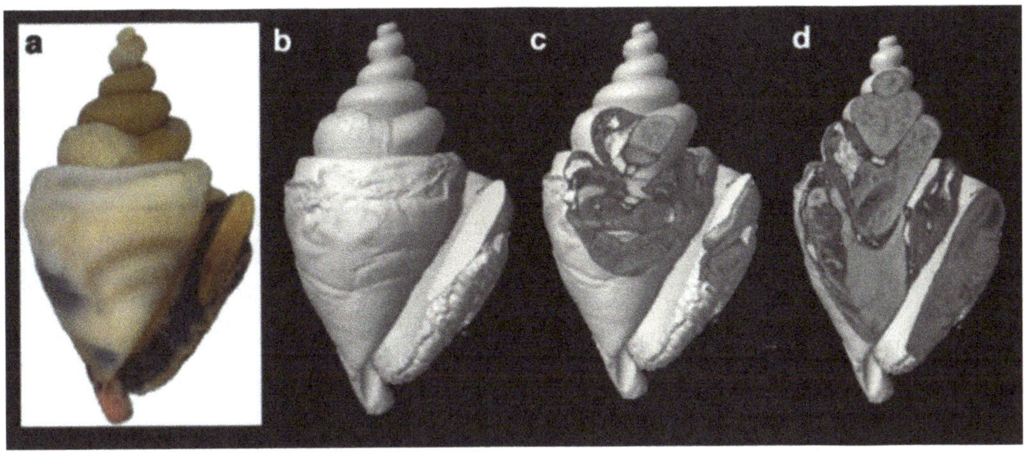

Fig. 9.4 Soft part of *Conus ebraeus* Linnaeus, 1758 (Conidae). UMUT RM32765. (**a**) Formalin-fixed animal with shell decalcified. (**b–d**) 3D reconstruction with software Molcer Plus from scan data of industrial CT. Body length = 19 mm

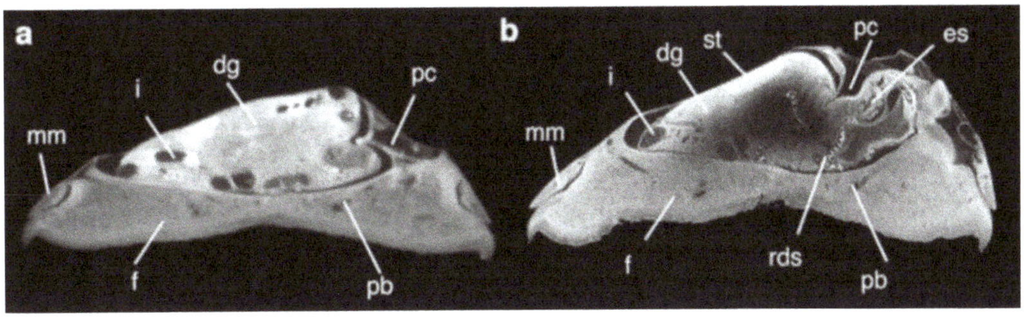

Fig. 9.5 Soft part of *Lottia dorsuosa* (Gould, 1859) (Lottiidae). UMUT RM32764. Comparison of scanning results between conventional industrial micro-CT (**a**) and synchrotron CT (**b** SPring-8 BL20B2). *dg* digestive gland, *es* esophagus, *f* foot, *i* intestine, *mm* mantle margin, *pb* pedal blood sinus, *pc* pallial cavity, *rds* radular sac, *st* stomach. Body length = 22 mm

unusable. Therefore, samples should be contained in a liquid medium such as ethanol, water, or physiological saline water in a (relatively) X-ray transparent container. Wrapping a sample with X-ray transparent film in a Styrofoam container can be an effective solution. Expelling air bubbles from the medium is essential because the bubbles can cause sample movement when they expand as they are subjected to heat generated during prolonged scanning.

In our experience, despite repeated experiments, scanning of soft parts with a conventional industrial micro-CT frequently resulted in insufficient contrast and clarity (Fig. 9.4). To explore other solutions, we attempted to use synchrotron CT instead of industrial CT (Fig. 9.1f–h). The results were clearly superior to the industrial CT data, as exemplified in an experiment in which the same specimen was used for both methods (Fig. 9.5). The synchrotron CT data were characterized by the clear edge of the outline and sharp boundaries of the internal organs. The configurations of internal organs were more reliably identified using this method.

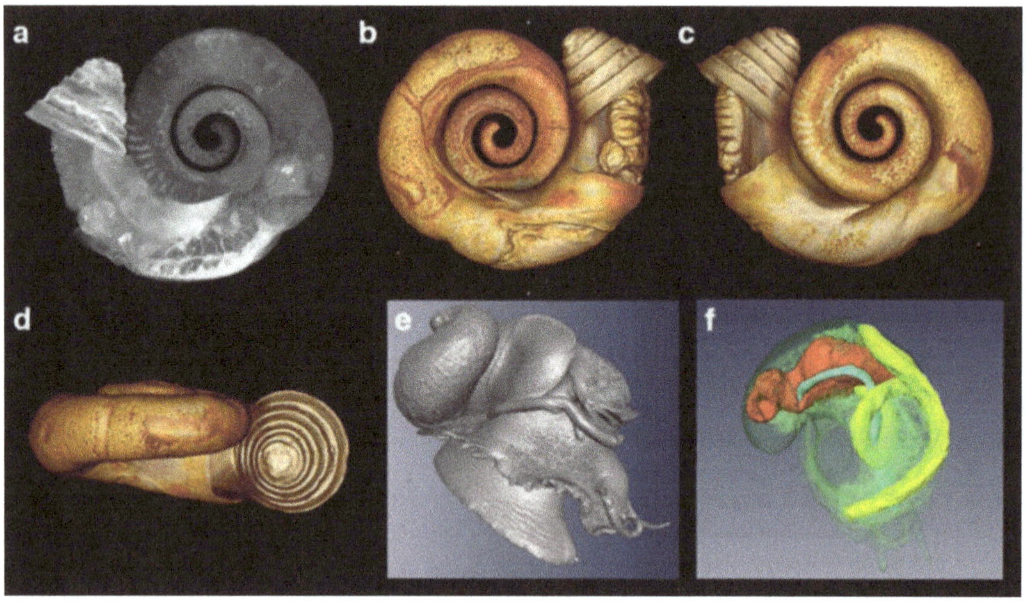

Fig. 9.6 Examples of 3D visualization of soft parts from synchrotron CT data. (**a–d**) *Spirostoma japonicum* (A. Adams, 1867) (Cyclophoridae). UMUT RM32766. Body length = 9.7 mm. (**a**) Transmission image. (**b**) Ventral view, (**c**) dorsal view, (**d**) frontal view. (**e**, **f**) *Granata lyrata* (Pilsbry, 1890) (Chilodontidae). UMUT RM32767. Body length = 9.9 mm. (**e**) Body surface. (**f**) Digestive tracts with translucent body surface. Software: (**a–d**) OsiriX. (**e**, **f**) Amira

A widely utilized method that was also used by us is to immerse samples in 1% iodine solution as the contrast agent for both laboratory and synchrotron CT scanning. This staining method is very handy and inexpensive. In our experiments, iodine rapidly penetrated into the samples, and immersion in iodine for 1 to several days was sufficient for samples smaller than 2 cm. However, slight shrinkage of the samples was unavoidable with iodine staining. This artifact was especially evident with the thin and membranous mantle tissue, which displayed numerous minute wrinkles after staining with iodine. In this study, we could not sufficiently test different contrast agents such as phosphomolybdic acid and osmium tetroxide. This will be the subject of a future study.

We tested Molcer Plus, OsiriX, and Amira software. Each has its own inherent advantages. Molcer Plus was the best software for visualizing calcified shells. OsiriX was able to create vivid 3D images of soft portions (Fig. 9.6b–d) with the most straightforward operation. Amira was superior in terms of results and operation for internal anatomy (Fig. 9.6e, f). By adjusting the threshold of brightness, the surface outline of a specimen could be automatically extracted (Figs. 9.6e and 9.7a–c). Different parts of internal organs could be illustrated in various colors after the segmentation procedure (Fig. 9.6f). Figure 9.7 is an example of the 3D visualization from three different angles, showing the animal's surface outline, digestive tracts with a translucent outline, and isolated digestive tracts only. This method allowed us to quantify the size and volume of various parts of the animal body.

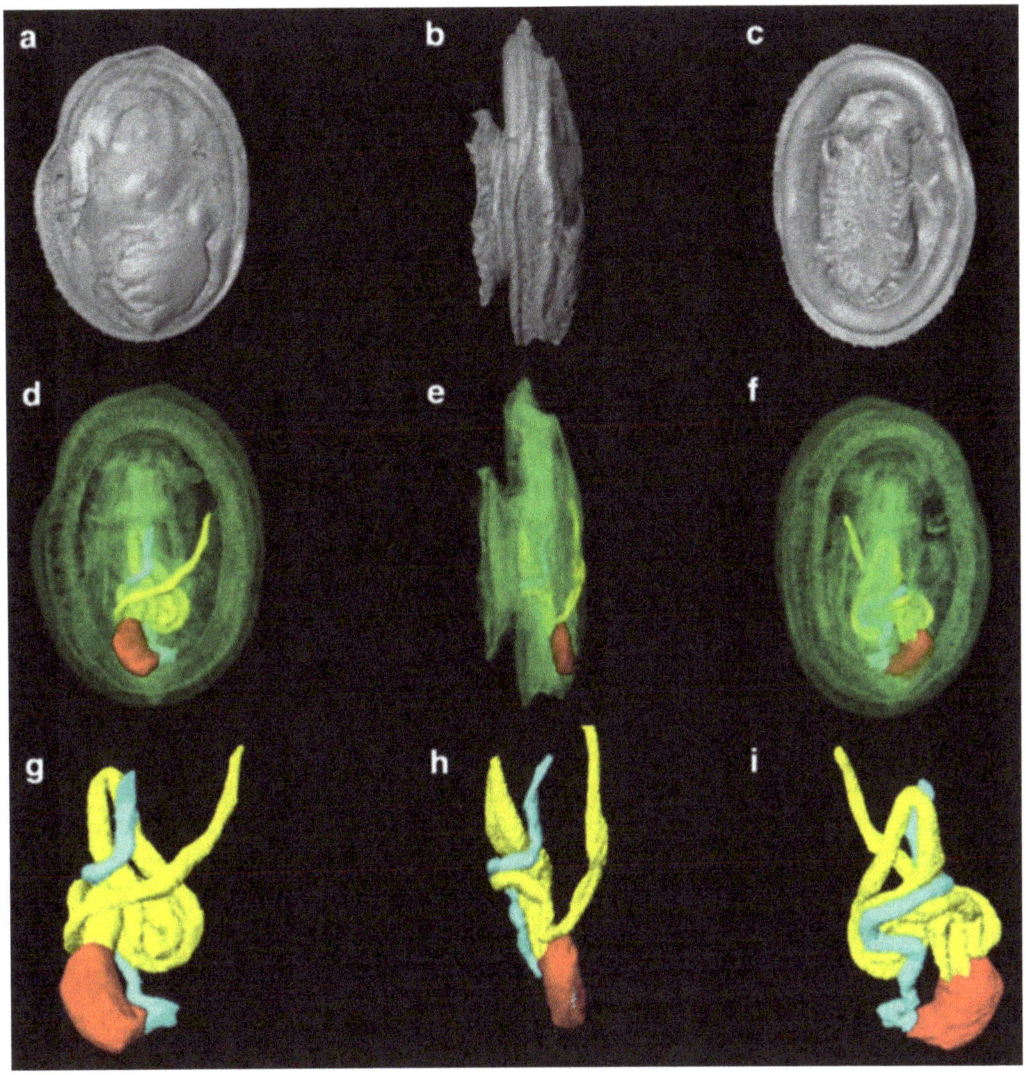

Fig. 9.7 Examples of 3D visualization of soft parts from synchrotron CT data (SPring-8 BL20B2). *Phenacolepas unguiformis* (Gould, 1859) (Phenacolepadidae). UMUT RM32768. (**a**–**c**) Exterior. (**d**–**f**) Digestive tracts with translucent outline. (**g**–**i**) Extracted digestive tracts. (**a**, **d**, **g**) Dorsal view. (**b**, **e**, **h**) Left lateral view. (**c**, **f**, **i**) Ventral view. Esophagus (blue), stomach (red), and intestine (yellow) are indicated in different colors. Body length = 6.0 mm. Software: Amira

9.4 Discussion

Through this experimental study, we confirmed that micro-CT is a very useful method for 3D presentation of various hard and soft features of molluscs. CT scanning has three important advantages. First, observations of internal shell structures are possible without having to cut the shells. Second, acquisition of a complete series of serially sectioned images without damaging soft portions is feasible. Third, the use of synchrotron CT allows 3D reconstruction of soft parts in much less time.

Scanning calcium carbonate shells is relatively easily performed and should be applied widely to other biominerals of invertebrates such as corals, barnacles, and echinoderms (Okanishi et al. 2017). The most comprehensive method for understanding shell morphology is achieved by the combination of micro-CT and scanning electron microscopy (SEM). Micro-CT has the advantages of 3D digitization and nondestructive internal observation. For example, it is possible to reveal internal morphological characteristics of specimens without cutting through them (Fig. 9.2) and can be achieved from any direction and for specimens of any size. On the other hand, SEM has a much higher resolution, which enables the observation of microscopic sculptures at higher magnification. Therefore, SEM is still necessary for characterizing micromolluscs (Sasaki 2008). In addition, shell microstructure and shell layer structure are most reliably observed with SEM (Nishida et al. 2012; Sato and Sasaki 2015).

We confirmed that micro-CT is also extremely effective for the study of soft parts. In particular, this method has a tremendous benefit for samples that are difficult to section with a microtome. For example, the digestive tracts of deposit feeders such as infaunal bivalves are often filled with many sediment grains, which easily damage knives during histological sectioning. In patellogastropod limpets (Fig. 9.3) and chitons, the radular teeth are heavily mineralized and also cause serious knife damage. Using micro-CT avoids these problems.

Before the introduction of micro-CT, serial histological sectioning was the only method available for 3D reconstruction (Chen et al. 2015; see Ruthensteiner 2008 for detailed methodology). However, with micro-CT, we are liberated from the difficult and time-consuming demand of making a complete series of serial sections of whole animals. For 3D reconstruction from serial sections, considerable time is spent aligning the stacks. This issue does not exist in micro-CT because the image stack generated is completely aligned without skew. In addition, complete anatomical reconstruction of large specimens becomes possible (the realistic upper size limit of resin-embedded serial sectioning is approximately 5 mm wide, and paraffin sections are too skewed to be useful for 3D visualization). Therefore, CT presents a high-throughput, highly efficient approach compared to sectioning, as has previously been pointed out by Golding and Jones (2007) and Kerbl et al. (2013).

Generating 3D data from a 2D image stack is still a time-consuming process with regard to internal anatomy. At present, we do not have a practical algorithm for automatic segmentation of the various internal organs. This continues to hinder advances in 3D morphological analysis.

The resolution of CT data is still much lower than that of histological sectioning. In addition, we cannot distinguish different organs using distinctive staining, as is used for paraffin-embedded sectioning or immunohistochemistry. For example, muscle and connective tissue can be vividly distinguished by trichrome staining (Katsuno and Sasaki 2008), but such a distinction is not possible with CT data. Therefore, it is advisable to reconstruct various 3D morphologies from CT data and supplement the details from histological sections. In this approach, much less histology data are needed for an overall understanding of the specimen. In this way, we can greatly improve the efficiency of morphological studies with CT.

3D data with segmentation may be exploited for various morphological analyses, especially quantitative analysis. For example, we can calculate the length and volume of various structures that are difficult to measure in actual specimens. Quantification of shape and its applications are topics for the future.

In conclusion, X-ray micro-CT is extremely useful in the morphological characterization of both mineralized and non-mineralized tissues of molluscs. Although this method has the potential to greatly improve the efficiency of morphological studies, it does not entirely replace conventional approaches and should be supplemented by data from other destructive microscopic methods.

Acknowledgments Dr. Osamu Sasaki (The Tohoku University Museum) and Dr. Akiteru Maeno (National Institute of Genetics) kindly provided technical advice when we introduced the Comscantechno CT scanner to The University Museum, The University of Tokyo. This study was funded by a JSPS Kakenhi Grant, number 15K14589 and JP16J06269. The synchrotron radiation experiments were performed at the BL20B2 of SPring-8 with the approval of the Japan Synchrotron Radiation Research Institute (JASRI) (Proposal Nos. 2015B1833, 2016A1706, 2017A1720, 2017B1767).

References

Chen C, Copley JT, Linse K, Rogers AD, Sigwart JD (2015) The heart of a dragon: 3D anatomical reconstruction of the 'scaly-foot gastropod' (Mollusca: Gastropoda: Neomphalina) reveals its extraordinary circulatory system. Front Zool 12(13):1–16

du Plessis A, Broeckhoven C, Guelpa A, le Roux SG (2017) Laboratory x-ray micro-computed tomography: a user guideline for biological samples. Gigascience 6:1–11

Friedrich F, Matsumura Y, Pohl H, Bai M, Hoernschemeyer T, Beutel RG (2014) Insect morphology in the age of phylogenomics: innovative techniques and its future role in systematics. Entomol Sci 17:1–24

Gignac PM, Kley NJ, Clarke JA, Colbert MW, Morhardt AC, Cerio D, Cost IN, Cox PG, Daza JD, Early CM, Echols MS, Henkelman RM, Herdina AN, Holliday CM, Li Z, Mahlow K, Merchant S, Mueller J, Orsbon CP, Paluh DJ, Thies ML, Tsai HP, Witmer LM (2016) Diffusible iodine-based contrast-enhanced computed tomography (diceCT): an emerging tool for rapid, high-resolution, 3-D imaging of metazoan soft tissues. J Anat 228:889–909

Golding RE, Jones AS (2007) Micro-CT as a novel technique for 3D reconstruction of molluscan anatomy. Molluscan Res 27:123–128

Golding RE, Ponder WF, Byrne M (2009) Three dimensional reconstruction of the odontophoral cartilages of Caenogastropoda (Mollusca: Gastropoda) using micro-CT: morphology and phylogenetic significance. J Morphol 270:558–587

Katsuno S, Sasaki T (2008) Comparative histology of radula-supporting structures in Gastropoda. Malacologia 50:13–56

Kerbl A, Handschuh S, Noedl M-T, Metscher B, Walzl M, Wanninger A (2013) Micro-CT in cephalopod research: investigating the internal anatomy of a sepiolid squid using a non-destructive technique with special focus on the ganglionic system. J Exp Mar Biol Ecol 447:140–148

Liew TS, Schilthuizen M (2016) A method for quantifying, visualising, and analysing gastropod shell form. PLoS One 11:e0157069

Monnet C, Zollikofer C, Bucher H, Goudemand N (2009) Three-dimensional morphometric ontogeny of mollusc shells by micro-computed tomography and geometric analysis. Palaeontol Electron 12.3(12A):1–13

Nishida K, Ishimura T, Suzuki A, Sasaki T (2012) Seasonal changes in the shell microstructures of the bloody clam, Scapharca broughtonii (Mollusca: Bivalvia: Arcidae). Palaeogeogr Palaeoclimatol Palaeoecol 363–364:99–108

Noshita K, Shimizu K, Sasaki T (2016) Geometric analysis and estimation of the growth rate gradient on gastropod shells. J Theor Biol 389:11–19

Okanishi M, Fujita T, Maekawa Y, Sasaki T (2017) Non-destructive morphological observations of the fleshy brittle star, *Asteronyx loveni* using micro-computed tomography (Echinodermata, Ophiuroidea, Euryalida). ZooKeys 663:1–19

Ruthensteiner B (2008) Soft part 3D visualization by serial sectioning and computer reconstruction. Zoosymposia 1:63–100

Sasaki T (2008) Micromolluscs in Japan: taxonomic composition, habitats, and future topics. In: Geiger DL, Ruthensteiner B (eds) Micromollsucs: methodological challenges – exciting results. Zoosymposia 1:147–232

Sato K, Sasaki T (2015) Shell microstructure of Protobranchia (Mollusa: Bivalvia): diversity, new microstructures and systematic implications. Malacologia 59(1):45–103

Takeda Y, Tanabe K, Sasaki T, Uesugi K, Hoshino M (2016) Non-destructive analysis of in situ ammonoid jaws by synchrotron radiation X-ray micro-computed tomography. Palaeontol Electron 19.3(46A):1–13

Wipfler B, Pohl H, Yavorskaya MI, Beutel RG (2016) A review of methods for analysing insect structures – the role of morphology in the age of phylogenomics. Curr Opin Insect Sci 18:60–68

Part II
Molecular and Cellular Regulation of Biomineralization

Chapter 10
Calcium Ion and Mineral Pathways in Biomineralization: A Perspective

Gal Mor Khalifa, Keren Kahil, Lia Addadi, and Steve Weiner

Abstract Calcium transport from the environment to the final site of mineral deposition involves uptake from the water or the food into cells. Within the cells calcium ions are translocated to various organelles and vesicles where they accumulate, in such a way as to not raise the very low calcium concentrations in the cytosol. In various biomineralizing systems, the calcium is stored in vesicles as a highly disordered hence relatively soluble solid phase. The concentrated calcium phase is then translocated out of the cell to the site of mineralization. Additional pathways may involve transport through the vasculature as ions and possibly mineral from distant sites. Understanding calcium pathways is the foundation for not only better understanding biomineralization processes but also for better understanding calcium and its fundamental role in cell signaling.

Keywords Calcium uptake and transport · Seawater vacuoles · Calcium signaling · Mineral-containing vesicles

10.1 Introduction

One common attribute of all biologically mineralizing processes is that huge amounts of ions must be acquired from the environment, and transported to the site of mineralization, where they are deposited. In many mineralizing processes, the ions are temporarily stored in the form of highly unstable and disordered membrane-bound mineral phases inside the cells (Weiner and Addadi 2011). Furthermore, in many cases the mineral first deposited at the site of mineralized tissue formation is also an unstable disordered mineral ("precursor phase") that subsequently crystallizes into the mature phase (Beniash et al. 1997; Crane et al. 2006; Mahamid et al. 2010; Weiss et al. 2002).

G. M. Khalifa · K. Kahil · L. Addadi · S. Weiner (✉)
Department of Structural Biology, Weizmann Institute of Science, Rehovot, Israel
e-mail: Gal.Mor@weizmann.ac.il; keren.kahil@weizmann.ac.il; lia.addadi@weizmann.ac.il; steve.weiner@weizmann.ac.il

K. Endo et al. (eds.), *Biomineralization*,
https://doi.org/10.1007/978-981-13-1002-7_10

Ion uptake and transport into cells and its temporary storage in cells are by no means confined to mineralization processes. In fact all cells need a suite of ions in order to function. Probably the best-studied ion in this respect is calcium. Calcium is used by all cells for signaling (Altin and Bygrave 1988; Carafoli 2005). For this to work, the cell needs to maintain a very low concentration of calcium in its cytosol – about 100–200 nM (Carafoli 2005), which is at least 10,000 times less concentrated than calcium in seawater (about 10 mmol) (Pietrobon et al. 1990). This signaling role of calcium requires the cell to take up calcium and store it in locations that do not contaminate the cytosol. This requirement must be even more stringent for cells that are involved in the calcium mineralization process, as they need to transport large amounts of calcium but also must have a functioning calcium signaling system.

Although a lot is known about the functions of calcium in cell metabolism, the actual distributions and concentrations of calcium ions in cells (not only in the cytosol) are not well documented. The main reasons for this are probably technical, as such mapping and measurements cannot be carried out on fixed and dehydrated specimens but require either in vivo measurements or a suitable fixation method. In vivo options for identifying ion concentrations are fluorescent probes which are sensitive to nanomolar concentrations (Rudolf et al. 2003) but not to the much higher concentrations that are relevant for the different stages in biomineralization. Identification of minerals in vivo is at present limited to micro-Raman spectroscopy, although the laser could conceivably induce amorphous minerals to crystallize. A most suitable fixation method for preserving ion concentrations and stabilizing unstable mineral phases is cryo-fixation. Cryo-fixation is the very rapid freezing of water such that ice crystals do not form, but the water is essentially frozen into a glassy or vitrified state. This method was developed by Dubochet (Dubochet et al. 1988). Mapping and measuring calcium concentrations in vivo or after cryo-fixation are, however, still technically very challenging. One promising option is cryo-soft X-ray tomography (Pereiro and Chichón 2014; Sviben et al. 2016).

10.2 Calcium Uptake and Transport

The ultimate source of ions is from the environment in which the organism lives. The ions can be extracted directly from the aqueous medium (seawater or freshwater) and/or from the food. Active ion-by-ion uptake takes place through ion-specific channels and pumps located in the cell membranes. Many proteins that bind one or several ions are known, and many are thought to be involved in ion transport (Pietrobon et al. 1990). These ion uptake and transport processes also occur in cells that are responsible for depositing mineral. Even if sufficient ions can be transported in these ways during rapid mineralization, or even during normal mineralization, are these the only pathways used? Much still remains to be learned about ion and mineral pathways in biology.

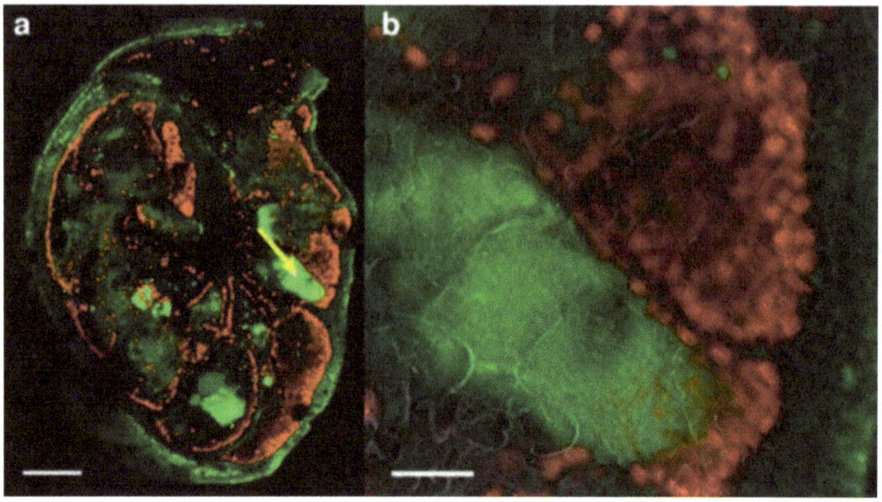

Fig. 10.1 Cryo-fluorescence images superimposed on a micrograph of high-pressure frozen and freeze-fractured *Amphistegina lessonii*. (**a**) A cryo-fluorescent image of a whole *A. lessonii* specimen superimposed on a freeze-fractured surface showing symbiont autofluorescence (red) and calcein labeling (green). The white arrow shows the location of one large seawater vacuole. Scale bar = 100 μm. (**b**) Magnified correlative cryo-SEM- fluorescence image of the seawater vacuole identified in image **a**. Scale bar = 20 μm

One approach is to use fluorescent molecules that are not able to pass through membranes: such as calcein and large fluorescently labeled polymers such as dextran (e.g., Butko et al. 1996). Organisms are grown in a medium in which one or both of these molecules are dissolved. If the fluorescent label enters the cell, then the marker molecules must have entered without passing through the membrane. One such process is endocytosis. As calcein is also a calcium-binding molecule, this is of particular relevance to tracking calcium in biomineralization. Bentov et al. (2009) monitored both these molecules in rapidly re-mineralizing benthic foraminifera whose shells had been previously dissolved so that the fluorescent signal could be imaged. These re-mineralizing foraminifera do indeed take up the fluorescent molecules, and these fluorescent molecules end up in the shell itself (Bentov et al. 2009). In this way Bentov et al. (2009) demonstrated that these organisms must be incorporating seawater droplets and at least some of the components of these droplets could be incorporated in the shell. Seawater droplet uptake was subsequently confirmed for intact foraminifera by imaging cryo-fixed fracture surfaces onto which fluorescent maps of the same cryo-fracture surface were superimposed (Khalifa et al. 2016). The calcein distribution in the foraminifer cytoplasm, investigated using this technique, shows that the foraminifer cell incorporates seawater droplets in a variety of sizes, starting from small micron-sized vesicles up to vacuoles tens of microns in size (Fig. 10.1). Seawater uptake was subsequently shown to occur in sea urchin larvae also using fluorescent dextran and calcein (Vidavsky et al. 2016). Surprisingly, the fluorescent markers labeled many sea urchin larval cells, in addition to the primary mesenchymal cells (PMCs) that are responsible for calcite spicule formation. Here the fluorescent calcein, but not the dextran, ends up in the calcitic spicule (Vidavsky et al. 2016). As seawater endocytosis is now known from

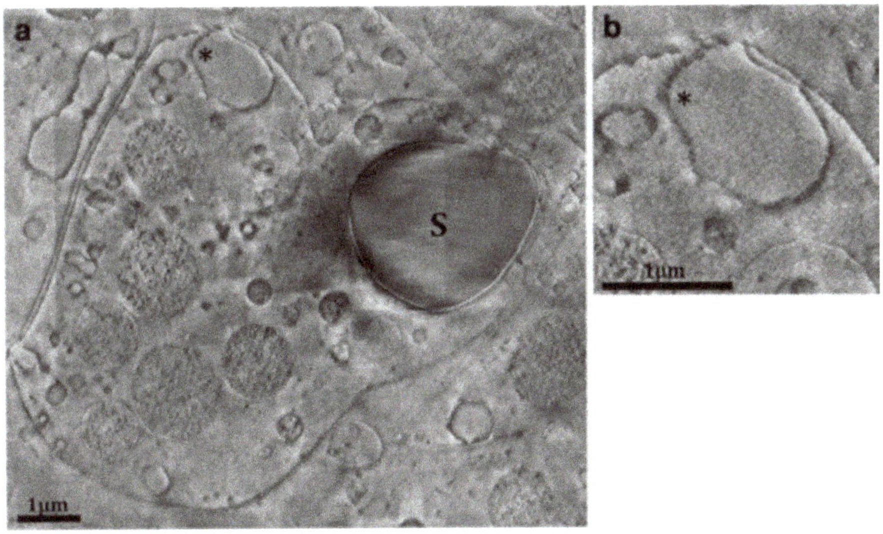

Fig. 10.2 Cryo-FIB-SEM micrograph of a single section of a high-pressure frozen sea urchin larva at the prism stage. (**a**) A primary mesenchyme cell attached to the spicule (S). A vesicle containing a uniform content similar in texture and gray levels to the cytoplasm and extracellular fluids is marked by an asterisk. This vesicle is close to the plasma membrane and has an opening to the extracellular fluids. (**b**) Higher magnification of the vesicle in **a**

two very different organisms, we suspect that the seawater occlusion uptake pathway may be widespread. This in turn opens up a fascinating question of how seawater can be manipulated chemically and/or biologically to enable specific ions, such as calcium, to be extracted without extracting all the other ions such as magnesium or strontium that are also present in seawater, in some cases in greater abundance than calcium.

In sea urchin larvae, seawater is incorporated into the body cavity (blastocoel). Many filopodia traverse the blastocoel, and it has been observed that the cells concentrate the calcein label into intracellular vesicles, and these vesicles move along the filopodia. They are transporting calcium in the form of a mineral, as shown by Raman spectroscopy, to the epithelial and mesenchymal cells (Vidavsky et al. 2015). Another possible mode of seawater uptake from the blastocoel was observed using cryo-FIB SEM to reconstruct the 3D organization of the constituents of the primary mesenchyme cells (PMCs) of sea urchin larvae – the cells responsible for calcite spicule formation. These cells contain vesicles, some of which have openings to the seawater-containing blastocoel (Fig. 10.2). In one case it was shown that such a vesicle is connected to other vesicles and/or vacuoles to form a large membrane-bound intracellular network (Vidavsky et al. 2016). It is conceivable, but not proven, that such a conduit might allow seawater with its calcium ions to move through the cell without contaminating the cytosol. Another option is to transport ions and/or minerals outside cells – either between cells as has been observed in coral epithelia responsible for skeletal mineralization (Gattuso et al. 1999) or as mineral-containing vesicles that have been observed in blood vessels of vertebrates (Kerschnitzki et al. 2016) and mollusks (Mount et al. 2004) and in the vertebrate extracellular matrix (so-called matrix vesicles) (Anderson 1995).

10.3 Temporary Calcium Storage in Cells

Intracellular calcium is known to be stored in the sarcoplasmic reticulum, the endoplasmic reticulum, mitochondria, and various vesicles including the acidosomes (Docampo et al. 2005; García et al. 2006; Pezzati et al. 1997). Apparently what is not known is how the calcium is transported to these organelles or vesicles without contaminating the cytosol. It is also not known in which forms the calcium is stored at these locations. It is however known that in some sea urchin larval cells, calcium is stored in vesicles in the form of a highly disordered mineral phase, amorphous calcium carbonate (Beniash et al. 1999; Weiner and Addadi 2011). A particularly interesting mineral storage vesicle is present in Coccolithophoridae. This vesicle stores a calcium polyphosphate mineral (Sviben et al. 2016). This is surprising as Coccolithophoridae produce calcitic bodies (coccoliths). Intracellular mineral storage vesicles are also known in cells that are involved in bone formation (Akiva et al. 2015; Mahamid et al. 2011).

10.4 Many Open Questions and Challenges Remain

Many mineralization processes take place either in the extracellular environment or in relatively large vacuoles within the cell. The first formed mineral phase, however, is often found in membrane-bound vesicles within the cell (Weiner and Addadi 2011). Almost nothing is known about whether the temporarily stored calcium in the membrane-bound vesicles is transferred to the extracellular or intracellular sites of mineralized skeletal formation, and if so how is the calcium transferred out of the cell. In one case mineral-containing vesicles were observed to be exocytosed into the extracellular environment during bone formation (Boonrungsiman et al. 2012).

Foraminifera and sea urchin larvae are now known to take up ions by introducing seawater into the intracellular environment (Bentov et al. 2009; Vidavsky et al. 2016). This in turn raises the question of how this seawater is manipulated chemically and/or biologically to extract the calcium ions. One interesting observation is the presence of mineral bodies rich in magnesium in the seawater vesicles of foraminifera (Khalifa et al. 2016). How the Mg-rich mineral forms and for what purpose are as yet unanswered questions.

It was reported that the vasculature in developing chick bones contains membrane-bound mineral particles (Kerschnitzki et al. 2016). These vesicles must have formed at some other location and were introduced into the blood system. It is not known where these mineral particles form, but the implication is that bone formation involves many different cells, some of which may be located at considerable distances from the site of bone mineralization.

A 3D map of the distributions of ions in a cell would contribute significantly to our understanding of how all cells translocate and store large concentrations of ions without contaminating the cytosol. We still however do not have appropriate techniques to map the full range of ion concentrations in cells.

10.5 Concluding Comment

Biologically mineralizing processes involve the uptake, transport, and deposition of large amounts of ions, often within a relatively short time. These systems are therefore advantageous for elucidating ion and mineral pathways in biology. Some of these pathways may be confined to mineralizing systems, but other pathways may also operate in all cells, as all cells require calcium and many other ions for performing basic functions. Thus elucidating these ion and mineral pathways in biomineralization may well contribute to our understanding of a fundamental biological process.

Acknowledgments LA and SW are the incumbents of the Dorothy and Patrick Gorman Professorial Chair of Biological Ultrastructure and the Dr. Trude Burchardt Professorial Chair of Structural Biology, respectively.

References

Akiva A, Malkinson G, Masic A, Kerschnitzki M, Bennet M, Fratzl P, Addadi L, Weiner S, Yaniv K (2015) On the pathway of mineral deposition in larval zebrafish caudal fin bone. Bone 75:192–200

Altin JG, Bygrave FL (1988) Second messengers and regulation of Ca2+ fluxes by Ca2+-modulating agonists in rat liver. Biol Rev 63:551–611

Anderson HC (1995) Molecular biology of matrix vesicles. Clin Orthop 314:266–280

Beniash E, Aizenberg J, Addadi L, Weiner S (1997) Amorphous calcium carbonate transforms into calcite during sea-urchin larval spicule growth. Proc R Soc Lond B Ser 264:461–465

Beniash E, Addadi L, Weiner S (1999) Cellular control over spicule formation in sea urchin embryos: a structural approach. J Struct Biol 125:50–62

Bentov S, Brownlee C, Erez J (2009) The role of seawater endocytosis in the biomineralization process in calcareous foraminifera. Proc Natl Acad Sci U S A 106:21500–21504

Boonrungsiman S, Gentleman E, Carzaniga R, Evans ND, McComb DW, Porter AE, Stevens MM (2012) The role of intracellular calcium phosphate in osteoblast-mediated bone apatite formation. Proc Natl Acad Sci 109:14170–14175

Butko P, Huang F, Pusztai-Carey M, Surewicz WK (1996) Membrane permeabilization induced by cytolytic δ-endotoxin CytA from Bacillus thuringiensis var. israelensis. Biochemistry 35:11355–11360

Carafoli E (2005) Calcium – a universal carrier of biological signals. FEBS J 272:1073–1089

Crane NJ, Popescu V, Morris MD, Steenhuis P, Ignelzi MA (2006) Raman spectroscopic evidence for octacalcium phosphate and other mineral species deposited during intramembraneous mineralization. Bone 39:431–433

Docampo R, de Souza W, Miranda K, Rohloff P, Moreno SNJ (2005) Acidocalcisomes – conserved from bacteria to man. Nat Rev 3:251–261

Dubochet J, Adrian M, Chang J-J, Homo J-C, Lepault J, McDowall AW, Schultz P (1988) Cryo-electron microscopy of vitrified specimens. Q Rev Biophys 21:129–228

García AG, García-De-Diego AM, Gandía L, Borges R, García-Sancho J (2006) Calcium signaling and exocytosis in adrenal chromaffin cells. Physiol Rev 86:1093–1131. https://doi.org/10.1152/physrev.00039.02005

Gattuso JP, Allemand D, Frankignoulle M (1999) Photosynthesis and calcification at cellular, organismal and community levels in coral reefs: a review on interactions and control by carbonate chemistry. Am Zool 39:160–183

Kerschnitzki M, Akiva A, Ben Shoham A, Koifman N, Shimoni E, Rechav K, Arraf AA, Schultheiss TM, Talmon Y, Zelzer E, Weiner S, Addadi L (2016) Transport of membrane-bound mineral particles in blood vessels during chicken embryonic bone development. Bone 83:65–72

Khalifa MG, Kirchenbuechler D, Koifman N, Kleinerman O, Talmon Y, Elbaum M, Addadi L, Weiner S, Erez J (2016) Biomineralization pathways in a foraminifer revealed using a novel correlative cryo-fluorescence-SEM-EDS technique. J Struct Biol 196:155–163

Mahamid J, Aichmayer B, Shimoni E, Ziblat R, Li C, Siegel S, Paris O, Fratzl P, Weiner S, Addadi L (2010) Amorphous calcium phosphate transformation into crystalline mineral in zebrafish fin bones: mapping the mineral from the cell to the bone. Proc Natl Acad Sci U S A 107:6316–6321

Mahamid J, Sharir A, Gur D, Zelzer E, Addadi L, Weiner S (2011) Bone mineralization proceeds through intracellular calcium phosphate loaded vesicles: a cryo-electron microscopy study. J Struct Biol 174:527–535

Mount AS, Wheeler AP, Paradkar RP, Snider D (2004) Hemocyte-mediated shell mineralization in the Eastern oyster. Science 304:297–300

Pereiro E, Chichon FJ (2014) Cryo-soft X-ray tomography of the cell. eLS. Wiley, Chichester

Pezzati R, Bossi M, Podini P, Meldolesi J, Grohovaz F (1997) High-resolution calcium mapping of the endoplasmic reticulum-golgi-exocytic membrane system. Mol Biol Cell 8:1501–1512

Pietrobon D, Di Virgilio F, Pozzan T (1990) Structural and functional aspects of calcium homeostasis in eukaryotic cells. Eur J Biochem 193:599–622

Rudolf R, Mongillo M, Rizzuto R, Pozzan T (2003) Looking forward to seeing calcium. Nat Rev 4:579–586

Sviben S, Gal A, Hood MA, Bertinetti L, Politi Y, Bennet M, Krishnamoorthy P, Schertel A, Wirth R, Sorrentino A, Pereiro E, Faivre D, Scheffel A (2016) A vacuole-like compartment concentrates a disordered calcium phase in a key coccolithophorid alga. Nat Commun. https://doi.org/10.1038/ncomms11228

Vidavsky N, Masic A, Schertel A, Weiner S, Addadi L (2015) Mineral-bearing vesicle transport in sea urchin embryos. J Struct Biol 192:358–365

Vidavsky N, Addadi S, Schertel A, ben-Ezra D, Shpigel M, Addadi L Weiner S (2016) Calcium transport into the cells of the sea urchin embryo: implications for spicule formation. Proc Natl Acad Sci U S A 113:12637–12642

Weiner S, Addadi L (2011) Crystallization pathways in biomineralization. Annu Rev Mater Res 41:21–40

Weiss IM, Tuross N, Addadi L, Weiner S (2002) Mollusk larval shell formation: amorphous calcium carbonate is a precursor for aragonite. J Exp Zool 293:478–491

Chapter 11
Identification of Barnacle Shell Proteins by Transcriptome and Proteomic Approaches

Yue Him Wong, Noriaki Ozaki, Wei-Pang Zhang, Jin Sun, Erina Yoshimura, Mieko Oguro-Okano, Yasuyuki Nogata, Hsiu-Chin Lin, Benny K. K. Chan, Pei-Yuan Qian, and Keiju Okano

Abstract In barnacle shell, the calcified shell layer is laid on top of the epicuticle. Here, we report our strategy and some preliminary results on the identification of potential shell proteins of the barnacle *Megabalanus rosa*. At first, *M. rosa* proteins from acid-soluble and acid-insoluble shell extracts were subjected to proteomic analysis and searched against *M. rosa* complete transcriptome. Then using the information that the calcified shell is formed just after the larval-adult molt, juvenile

Y. H. Wong · N. Ozaki · K. Okano (✉)
Department of Biotechnology, Faculty of Bioresource Sciences, Akita Prefectural University, Akita, Japan
e-mail: timwong@akita-pu.ac.jp; ozanor@akita-pu.ac.jp; keijuo@akita-pu.ac.jp

W.-P. Zhang · J. Sun · P.-Y. Qian
Division of Life Science, School of Science, The Hong Kong University of Science and Technology, Hong Kong, China
e-mail: wzhangae@connect.ust.hk; boqianpy@ust.hk

E. Yoshimura · Y. Nogata
Environmental Science Research Laboratory, Central Research Institute of Electric Power Industry, Chiba, Japan
e-mail: yoshimura@ceresco.jp; noga@criepi.denken.or.jp

M. Oguro-Okano
Department of Biotechnology, Faculty of Bioresource Sciences, Akita Prefectural University, Akita, Japan

Department of Animal, Health Technology, Yamazaki Gakuen University, Tokyo, Japan
e-mail: m-oguro@yamazaki.ac.jp

H.-C. Lin
Department of Marine Biotechnology and Resources, National Sun Yat-sen University, Kaohsiung, Taiwan
e-mail: hsiuchinlin@mail.nsysu.edu.tw

B. K. K. Chan
Biodiversity Research Center, Academia Sinica, Taipei, Taiwan
e-mail: chankk@gate.sinica.edu.tw

K. Endo et al. (eds.), *Biomineralization*,
https://doi.org/10.1007/978-981-13-1002-7_11

differentially expressed genes against larval stages were screened. Sixty secretory protein sequences were identified as primary candidates of *M. rosa* shell proteins, among which 37 are novel proteins.

Keywords Barnacle · Shell formation · Transcriptome · Proteomics

11.1 Introduction

Thoracican barnacles produce a heavily calcified shell that, unlike their crustacean relatives, does not shed away (Walley 1969). The calcified shell offers physical protection against predators and wave actions (Astachov et al. 2011). The shell also enables barnacles to prevent desiccation in the intertidal region.

The calcified shell plates produced by the subtidal thoracican barnacle *Megabalanus rosa* are composed of the operculum plates (OPs), the lateral wall plates (WPs), and the basal shell plate (BP) (Fig. 11.1). OPs consist of two pairs of shell plates, namely, terga and scuta. These are movable plates that serve as the shutter of the soft body. *M. rosa* produces four pairs of WPs, which are the major shell plates that protect the interior soft body from mechanical impact. BP is the calcified shell plate at the bottom of the barnacle, separating the barnacle soft body from the rock substratum surface. Hence, each of these plates has different functions. Details of barnacle shell anatomy can be found in Chan et al. (2009).

Obviously, it is important to understand what molecules are involved in the formation of these shell structures. Matsubara et al. (2008) isolated two C-type lectin proteins BRA-2 and BRA-3 from the regenerating *M. rosa* shell. Zhang et al. (2015) reported a list of acid-soluble shell proteins, including carbonic anhydrase and an aspartic acid-rich partial protein sequence from the intertidal barnacle *Amphibalanus amphitrite*. The aspartic acid-rich partial protein, however, has shown no sequence homology to the molluscan Asprich shell protein family (Gotliv et al. 2005),

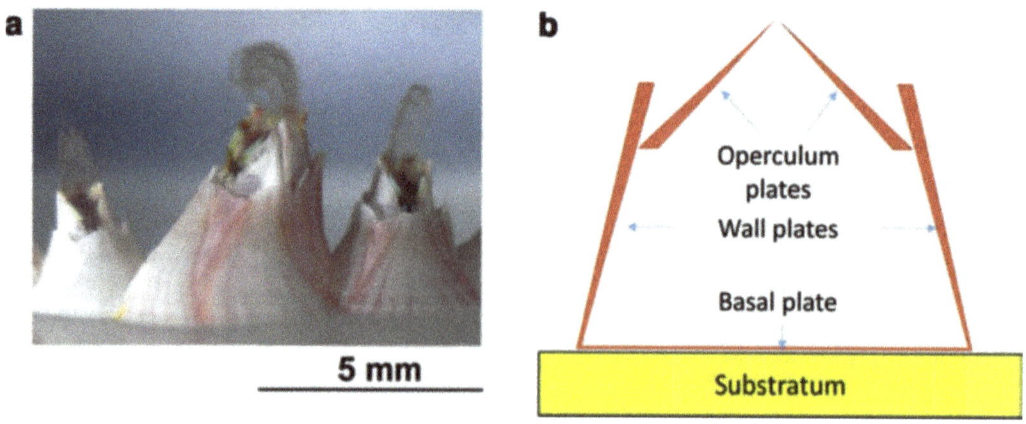

Fig. 11.1 The thoracican barnacle *Megabalanus rosa* and a schemetic drawing of the adult shell structure. (**a**) 2-month *M. rosa* juvenile, with cirri reaching out from its calcified shell for feeding on planktons. (**b**) A schemetic drawing of *M. rosa* shell structure. *M. rosa* shell composes of the operculum plates (OPs), the wall plates (WPs), and a basal plate (BP)

suggesting that aspartic acid-rich proteins in barnacles and mollusks have independently evolved.

In this study, we used *M. rosa* as the study model for barnacle shell formation. We present an integrated transcriptomic and proteomic approach for the identification of barnacle shell protein candidates.

11.2 Material and Methods

11.2.1 M. rosa *and Its Larval Culture Construction*

Adult individuals of *M. rosa* were obtained in the Oga Peninsula, Akita, Japan, from the bouy deployed by local fishermen. Upon arriving the lab, the *M. rosa* individuals were maintained in a 20 °C aquarium until being sampled. Larval samples were prepared at Central Research Institute of Electric Power Industry, according to Yoshimura et al. (2006a, b).

11.2.2 Transcriptome Data Analysis

The details of the preparation of *M. rosa* Illumina transcriptome will be reported elsewhere. The *M. rosa* transcriptome assembly covered various larval stages, attached larvae, metamorphosing larvae, 1-day and 3-day-old juveniles, and adult tissues. The transcriptome data were mainly assembled using Trinity v2.3.2 (Grabherr et al. 2011). But we soon discovered that Trinity failed to resolve highly repetitive tandem repeat structures often found among potential shell protein transcripts, owing to the use of fixed short kmer length (kmer = 25 bp). Therefore, we switched to a multiple kmer strategy, in which the Illumina read data were assembled using Transabyss v1.6.3 (Robertson et al. 2010) with kmer size ranging from 21 to 161 bp, for every 10 bp. These assemblies were then merged using the script Transabyss-merge. Transcript abundance estimation was performed using the software RSEM (Li and Dewey 2011). The levels of transcript expression were normalized according to coverage and then converted to the relative expression levels in FPKM values. Differential expression analysis was performed using the software edgeR (Robinson et al. 2010).

11.2.3 Preparation of Shell-Soluble and Shell-Insoluble Fractions

To extract shell proteins, the mineralized shell plates, namely, OPs, WPs, and BP as described above, were subjected to acid decalcification. After removing the promosa (all soft body parts) from the shell, OPs, WPs, and BP were then cleaned by

10% bleach solution (household bleach) for 3 days, with daily exchange of the bleach solution. After bleaching, the shell plates were washed with distilled water extensively and then dried in freeze drier for 1 day. The dried shell plates were then crushed into fine powder smaller than 110 μm (filtered by a mesh filter). Altogether, 20 *M. rosa* specimens (integument diameter ranging from 2 to 5 cm) were being sacrificed. Then, around 12 g of OP powder, 20 g of WP powder, and 20 g of BP powder were independently decalcified by 10% acetic acid overnight in 4 °C. By 4000 × g centrifugation, the supernatants, which represent the acid-soluble fractions (ASF), and the pellets, which represent the acid-insoluble fractions (AIF) of OP, WP, and BP, were separated. Acetic acid in the ASF of OP, WP, and BP was exchanged with Milli-Q water by dialysis (6–8 kDa dialysis membrane). Proteins in the ASFs were then concentrated by 3 kDa cutoff centrifugal filtering device (Amicon Ultra, Millipore). After removal of lipids by methanol-chloroform precipitation, purified ASF protein samples were redissolved in 40 μl 2 M thiourea. To extract proteins from AIF, Milli-Q water-washed insoluble pellets from OP, WP, and BP were treated with 1 ml of 8 M urea for 1 h at room temperature. The retrieved solubilized AIFs were then subjected to methanol-chloroform precipitation. The purified AIF proteins were redissolved in 40 μl 2 M thiourea. ASF and AIF protein samples were then loaded onto a 4–20% SDS-PAGE gradient gel. The gel was subsequently stained with Coomassie Brilliant Blue G-250.

11.2.4 In-Gel Digestion, LC-MS/MS Analysis, and Protein Identification

The AIF and ASF samples from OPs, WPs, and BP were divided into nine size fractions and independently retrieved for in-gel digestion. Destaining, reduction, alkylation, in-gel digestion, and the final peptide digest retrieval were performed as in Sun et al. (2012), except that 1 μg of trypsin (sequencing grade) dissolved in 100 μl of 10 mM of triethylammonium bicarbonate was applied to the gel pieces from each sample; standard shotgun proteomics techniques were used to analyze the samples on a Thermo Scientific LTQ VelosTM platform (Thermo Fisher Scientific, Bremen, Germany). Operation details of the LC-MS/MS can refer to Zhang et al. (2014). Identification of protein was performed using MASCOT search engine (v2.3.02), with the parameter setting the same as in Zhang et al. (2014). The transcriptome data generated from *M. rosa* (method and sample details mentioned above) were *in silico* translated to a protein database using Transdecoder v.3.0.3 (Haas and Papanicolaou 2016), with minimum length of the open reading frame set at 100 amino acid. Decoy sequences consisting of shuffled protein sequences for each of the proteins were concatenated to the original protein database to generate a target-decoy database for protein identification.

11.2.5 Analysis of M. rosa *Shell Protein Candidates*

The identified protein sequences were analyzed for the presence of N-terminal signal sequence using SignalP server 4.1 (Nielsen 2017), followed by manual correction. The identified proteins with N-terminal signal peptide were then selected and categorized based on their annotation status.

11.3 Results and Discussion

11.3.1 Development of Shell Formation in M. rosa *Juvenile*

Figure 11.2a shows the life cycle of thoracican barnacles including *M. rosa*. *M. rosa* larvae are in general encased in chitinous cuticles. They do not produce any calcified shell structure at any larval stage. Formation of calcium carbonate shell occurs only after post-settlement metamorphosis, that is, the transition of a cypris larva into a juvenile barnacle. This means that the genes responsible for barnacle shell formation start to be expressed during metamorphosis and in the early juvenile stage. As shown in Fig. 11.2b, in *M. rosa*, the progression of calcification was the most obvious at the first 5 days of juvenile development. At 5 days after metamorphosis, all shell plates are completely nontransparent, indicating these shell plates are all mineralized.

11.3.2 Identification of Proteins in M. rosa *Shell Extract*

In total, 431 translated protein sequences (Fig. 11.3a) from all the 6 samples, that is, the AIF and ASF of BP/OPs/WPs, were identified using the translated protein database generated from the multiple kmer Transabyss pipeline (contains 35,998 translated nonredundant protein sequences).

11.3.3 Filtering Shell Proteome Data with Transcriptome Analysis

We noticed that, among the 431 identified translated protein sequences identified from all the shell samples, ovary proteins such as vitellogenin were detected (Fig. 11.3a), indicating that the shell plate samples were contaminated by ovary tissue, and bleaching obviously was not effective in removing all of these ovary

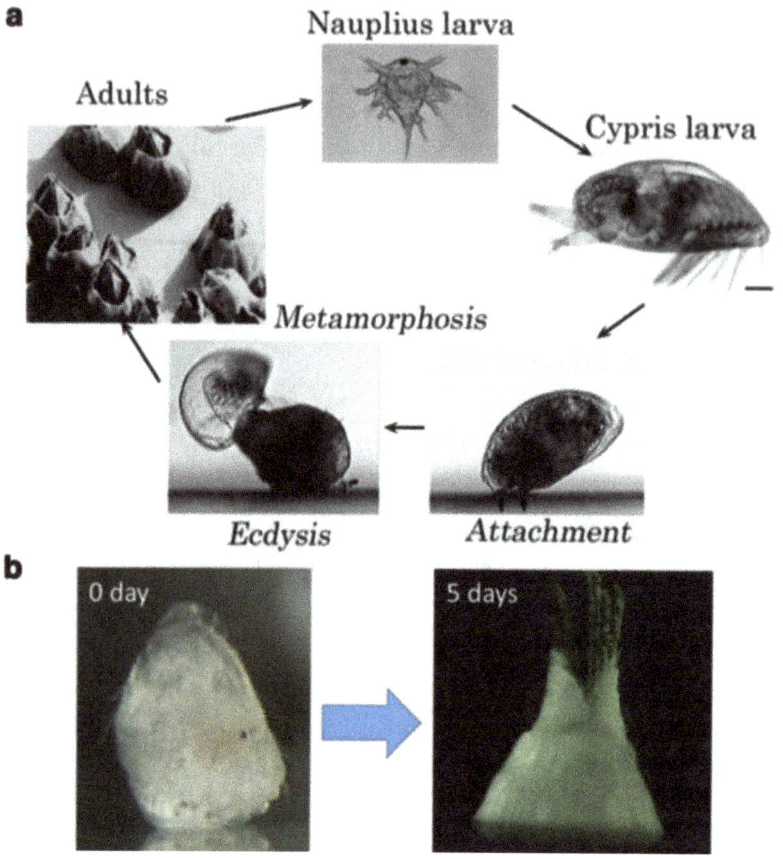

Fig. 11.2 Life cycle of *M. rosa* and the development of young juvenile. (**a**) The barnacle spawned as nauplius larva, which undergoes four successive molts and then transforms into a cypris larva. The cypris larva actively searches for an appropriate substratum and will then fully commit to settlement, which involves attachment of the larval body onto the substratum by cement secretion, and metamorphosis, which involves ecdysis of the cyprid body molt. The soft newly metamorphosed juvenile soon begins to feed on planktons using the cirri and develops into an adult barnacle, protected by calcified shells. (**b**) Development of young juvenile. The 0 day juvenile, that is, the stage when ecdysis was just completed. Five days after completion of metamorphosis, the juvenile has developed mineralized shell plates

proteins stuck to the shell during sampling. From our preliminary SEM and EDX analyses, we have observed that at the juvenile stage, shell material is being actively synthesized. We therefore selected the identified proteins whose transcripts were four-folds (16 times) more highly expressed in the juvenile stages than in the larval stages (FDR <0.001). This criterion filtered out 349 proteins, leaving 82 relevant shell proteins, among which 60 contain a signal peptide (Fig. 11.3b). With the juvenile-specific expression pattern and the presence of signal peptide as the criteria, the list of identified shell protein candidates became much smaller yet specific. Among the 60 shell protein candidates, some of them were implicated in shell formation in other systems, including carbonic anhydrase, C-type lectin domain protein, and chitin-binding domain proteins (Miyamoto et al. 1996; Suzuki et al. 2007; Joubert et al. 2010). In addition, 37 unknown/novel proteins were also discovered, and these proteins are now under our major investigation. Our results clearly

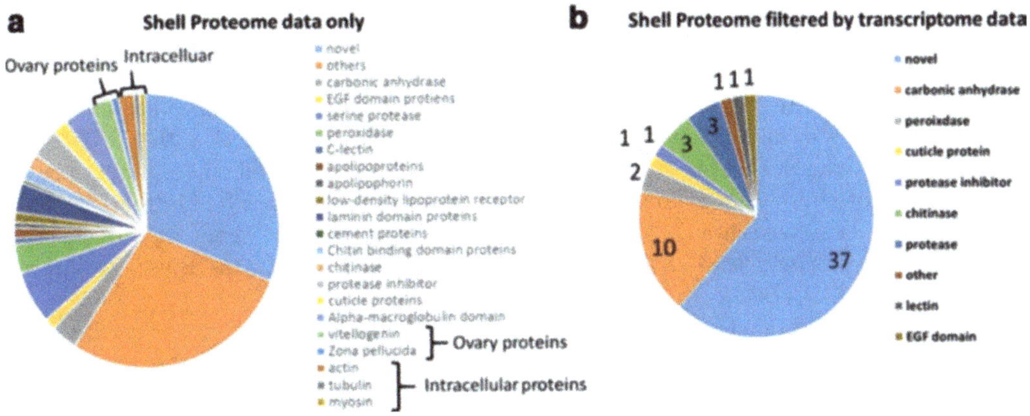

Fig. 11.3 Proteins identified from the acid-soluble and acid-insoluble extract of all the shell parts of *M. rosa*. (**a**) The whole shell proteome as identified in this study. Four hundred and thirty-one translated protein sequence identified by Mascot protein identification pipeline. (**b**) Shell proteome filtered by transcriptome data. Sixty translated proteins with a predicted N-terminal signal peptide and whose transcripts were 16 times upregulated during metamorphosis and the juvenile stages

indicate that our transcriptome-based filtering method, that is, to filter the shell proteome data with the corresponding transcript expression patterns, is an excellent pipeline for the purpose of relevant shell protein identification.

References

Astachov L, Nevo Z, Brosh T, Vago R (2011) The structural, compositional and mechanical features of the calcite shell of the barnacle *Tetraclita rufotincta*. J Struct Biol 175:311–318

Chan BKK, Prabowo RE, Lee KS (2009) Crustacean fauna of Taiwan: barnacles, volume I-Cirripedia: thoracica excluding the Pyrgomatidae and Acastinae. National Taiwan Ocean University, Keelung

Gotliv BA, Kessler N, Sumerel JL, Morse DE, Tuross N, Addadi L, Weiner S (2005) Asprich: a novel aspartic acid-rich protein family from the prismatic shell matrix of the bivalve *Atrina rigida*. ChemBioChem 6:304–314

Grabherr MG, Haas BJ, Yassour M, Levin JZ, Thompson DA, Amit I, Adiconis X, Fan L, Raychowdhury R, Zeng Q, Chen Z (2011) Full-length transcriptome assembly from RNA-Seq data without a reference genome. Nat Biotechnol 29:644–652

Haas BJ, Papanicolaou A (2016) TransDecoder (finding coding regions within transcripts)

Joubert C, Piquemal D, Marie B, Manchon L, Pierrat F, Zanella-Cléon I, Cochennec-Laureau N, Gueguen Y, Montagnani C (2010) Transcriptome and proteome analysis of *Pinctada margaritifera* calcifying mantle and shell: focus on biomineralization. BMC Genomics 11:613

Li B, Dewey CN (2011) RSEM: accurate transcript quantification from RNA-Seq data with or without a reference genome. BMC Bioinformatics 12:323

Matsubara H, Hayashi T, Ogawa T, Muramoto K, Jimbo M, Kamiya H (2008) Modulating effect of acorn barnacle C-type lectins on the crystallization of calcium carbonate. Fish Sci 74:418–424

Miyamoto H, Miyashita T, Okushima M, Nakano S, Morita T, Matsushiro A (1996) A carbonic anhydrase from the nacreous layer in oyster pearls. Proc Natl Acad Sci U S A 93:9657–9660

Nielsen H (2017) Predicting secretory proteins with SignalP. In: Protein function prediction: methods and protocols. Springer, New York, pp 59–73

Robertson G, Schein J, Chiu R, Corbett R, Field M, Jackman SD, Mungall K, Lee S, Okada HM, Qian JQ, Griffith M (2010) De novo assembly and analysis of RNA-seq data. Nat Methods 7:909–912

Robinson MD, McCarthy DJ, Smyth GK (2010) edgeR: a bioconductor package for differential expression analysis of digital gene expression data. Bioinformatics 26:139–140

Sun J, Zhang H, Wang H, Heras H, Dreon MS, Ituarte S et al (2012) First proteome of the egg perivitelline fluid of a freshwater gastropod with aerial oviposition. J Proteome Res 11(8):4240–4248

Suzuki M, Sakuda S, Nagasawa H (2007) Identification of chitin in the prismatic layer of the shell and a chitin synthase gene from the Japanese pearl oyster, *Pinctada fucata*. Biosci Biotechnol Biochem 71:1735–1744

Walley LJ (1969) Studies on the larval structure and metamorphosis of *Balanus balanoides* (L.). Philos Trans R Soc B 256:237–280

Yoshimura E, Nogata Y, Sakaguchi I (2006a) Experiments on rearing the barnacle *Megabalanus rosa* to the cyprid stage in the laboratory. Sessile Organisms 23(2):33–37

Yoshimura E, Nogata Y, Sakaguchi I (2006b) Simple methods for mass culture of barnacle larvae. Sessile Org 23:39–42

Zhang Y, Sun J, Mu H, Li J, Zhang Y, Xu F et al (2014) Proteomic basis of stress responses in the gills of the pacific oyster *Crassostrea gigas*. J Proteome Res 14(1):304–317

Zhang G, He LS, Wong YH, Xu Y, Zhang Y, Qian PY (2015) Chemical component and proteomic study of the *Amphibalanus (= Balanus) amphitrite* shell. PLoS One 10(7):e0133866

Chapter 12
The Optical Characteristics of Cultured Akoya Pearl Are Influenced by Both Donor and Recipient Oysters

Toshiharu Iwai, Masaharu Takahashi, Chiemi Miura, and Takeshi Miura

Abstract The characteristics of a cultured pearl are influenced by two kinds of pearl oysters. One is the donor pearl oyster, which provides a small piece of mantle to be transplanted, and the other is the recipient pearl oyster, in which the pearl nucleus and a small piece of mantle are transplanted. Generally, the brightness, luster, and color of pearls are affected by the donor oyster, while the thickness of nacre is affected by the recipient oyster. Previously, we have indicated that the sex of recipient pearl oyster directly affects the quality of pearl, and the optical characteristics measured by FT-IR (Fourier transform infrared spectroscopy) of pearl produced from male and female pearl oysters significantly differ (Iwai et al. Aquaculture 437:333–338, 2015). Moreover, using the various strains of Akoya pearl oyster as recipient and the same donor oyster, the produced Akoya pearl had different spectra for each strain. Also, besides the culture of the Akoya pearl oyster, the transplantation also produced different optically characterized pearls by breeding them in various environments. These results suggested that the optical characteristics underlying pearl quality are not only the influence by donor oyster but also the sex, the strain, and the breeding conditions of recipient oyster.

Keywords Cultured pearl · Optic characteristic · FT-IR

T. Iwai · T. Miura (✉)
Graduate School of Agriculture, University of Ehime, Matsuyama, Ehime, Japan
e-mail: t-iwai@agr.ehime-u.ac.jp; miutake@agr.ehime-u.ac.jp

M. Takahashi
Pearl Oyster Research Laboratory, Shimonada Fisheries Cooperative, Uwajima, Japan
e-mail: simonada-jf-t-i@md.pikara.ne.jp

C. Miura
Graduate School of Agriculture, University of Ehime, Matsuyama, Ehime, Japan

Department of Global Environment Studies, Faculty of Environmental Studies, Hiroshima Institute of Technology, Hiroshima, Japan
e-mail: chiemi8@agr.ehime-u.ac.jp

K. Endo et al. (eds.), *Biomineralization*,
https://doi.org/10.1007/978-981-13-1002-7_12

12.1 Introduction

The technique of producing pearls in the body of Akoya pearl oyster by transplantation is a biotechnology developed in Japan that skillfully utilized the biomineralization ability of oysters (Southgate and Lucas 2008; Wada 1999). The characteristics of a cultured pearl are influenced by two kinds of pearl oysters. One is the donor pearl oyster, which provides a small piece of mantle to be transplanted; the other is the recipient pearl oyster, in which the pearl nucleus and a small piece of mantle are transplanted to produce a pearl. Generally, the brightness, luster, and color of pearls are affected by the donor oyster, while the thickness of nacre is affected by the recipient oyster (Wada and Komaru 1996). Only the recipient oyster is required to have good growth rate and disease-resistance trait; hence, the effect of recipient oysters on the quality of produced pearls has been underestimated.

In transplantation, the pearl nucleus and a small piece of mantle were transplanted into the gonads of recipient pearl oyster. The sex and state of gonads affect the characteristics and quality of cultured pearl. In our previous study, we have clearly indicated that the sex of recipient pearl oyster directly affects the quality of pearl, and the optical characteristics measured by FT-IR of pearl produced from male and female pearl oysters significantly differed (Iwai et al. 2015). These results showed that the optical characteristics and quality of pearls have strong influence not only by donor oysters but also by recipient oysters. Moreover, it is also known that the characteristics and quality of pearls are affected by the difference of pearl cultivation area in general. In this study, we measured the FT-IR spectra of the pearls produced with various recipient and donor strain combinations and pearls cultured in various culture area and, then based on these characteristics, clustered and investigated what kind of factors influence the quality of pearls.

12.2 Materials and Methods

12.2.1 Akoya Pearl Oysters

Akoya pearl oysters, *Pinctada fucata*, were obtained from K, S, U, and M pearl farmers. The strains “U-H” and “U-T” were two types of Akoya pearl oyster strains produced by U pearl farmer. The strain “M-H” was one of several strains produced by M pearl farmer.

12.2.2 Pearl Culture

Various conditions, such as transplantation date and harvest date, in pearl culture used in each test are described in each figure legend. The method of pearl culture used for this study was generally in accordance with the method that the pearl farmer carried out.

12.2.3 *Fourier Transform Infrared Spectroscopy and Data Analysis*

The methods in this study were described previously (Iwai et al. 2015). Briefly, a Fourier transform infrared (FT-IR) ALPHA Platinum ATR spectrometer (Bruker Optics, Germany) was used to acquire spectral data of the pearl surface. A spectral resolution of 4 cm^{-1} was applied, and 64 scans were co-added and averaged for each spectrum. Transmission/absorption FT-IR spectra were collected, and data from 400 to 4000 wavenumbers were stored on a computer while purging the instrument continuously with dry air to reduce water vapor absorption. Ward's algorithm was used for hierarchical clustering as described previously (Helm et al. 1991). The hierarchical clustering was performed with the cluster analysis module of OPUS 7.2 software (Bruker Optics, Germany). Hierarchical cluster analysis was used to objectively assess clustering of the FT-IR vector-normalized spectra obtained from the different culture site or recipient and donor combination.

12.3 Results

12.3.1 *The Cultured Pearls from Various Culture Sites*

In order to evaluate the characteristics of cultured pearls, ten culture areas mainly carrying pearl culture in Uwa Sea, Ehime Prefecture, Japan, were selected (Fig. 12.1a). Nine months after transplantation at various culture areas, the pearls were collected and analyzed by FT-IR spectrometry (Fig. 12.1b, c). However, visual evaluation of the quality of these pearls was difficult. Accordingly, we examined the differences between the pearls from various culture area based on the optical properties of the pearl surface using the FT-IR spectrometer (Fig. 12.1c). By performing hierarchical cluster analysis with FT-IR spectrometry, these pearls were classified into two clusters. When comparing this result with the actual culture area, the culture pearls were separated into a north area and a south area. These results indicated that the optical characteristics of pearls from various culture areas were significantly different. Furthermore, the optical characteristics of each pearl were determined according to the culture area of Akoya pearl oyster.

12.3.2 *The Cultured Pearls from Combination of Donor and Recipient Pearl Oysters*

In order to investigate how the characteristics of pearls change by combination of donor and recipient oysters, pearls were produced using three kinds of Akoya pearl oyster strains as donors and two kinds as recipients (Fig. 12.2a). Unlike pearls produced by various culture area, pearls differed greatly in appearance. Pearls using

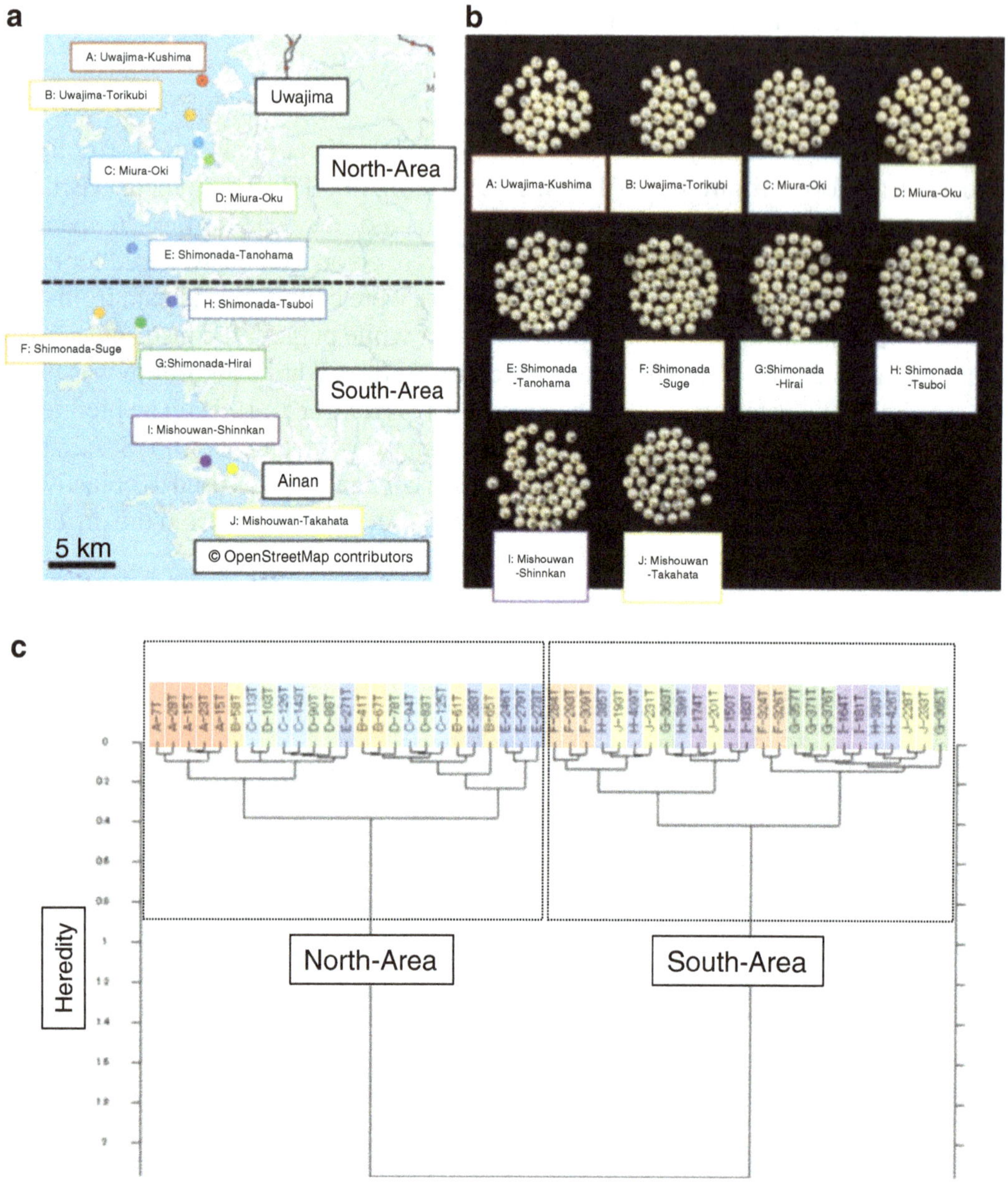

Fig. 12.1 The cultured pearls from various culture sites. The pearls were cultured by the following conditions: transplantation date, July 20, 2014; harvest date, Feb 23, 2015–Mar 6, 2015; pearl nucleus size, 6.67 mm at single transplantation; donor oyster, Akoya pearl oyster strain-K; recipient oyster, Akoya pearl oyster strain-S; transplantation was operated by single pearl farmer. (**a**) A map showing the point where pearls were cultivated. (**b**) A picture of the cultured pearls. (**c**) Dendrogram of a hierarchical cluster analysis showing objective spectral diversity in pearls from vrious culture sites. Cluster analysis was performed with vector-normalized spectra. The spectral distances were calculated with Pearson's correlation coefficient, and Ward's algorithm was used for hierarchical clustering. Hierarchical clustering is a statistical data analysis procedure for the classification of similar objects into North-Area and South-Area groups. The name of each sample is as follows: taking "A-7T," for example, "A" indicates the cultured area shown in (**a**, **b**), "7" means a serial number of the obtained pearl, and "T" is the initial of *Tounen* in Japanese and means that the cultivated period is within 1 year

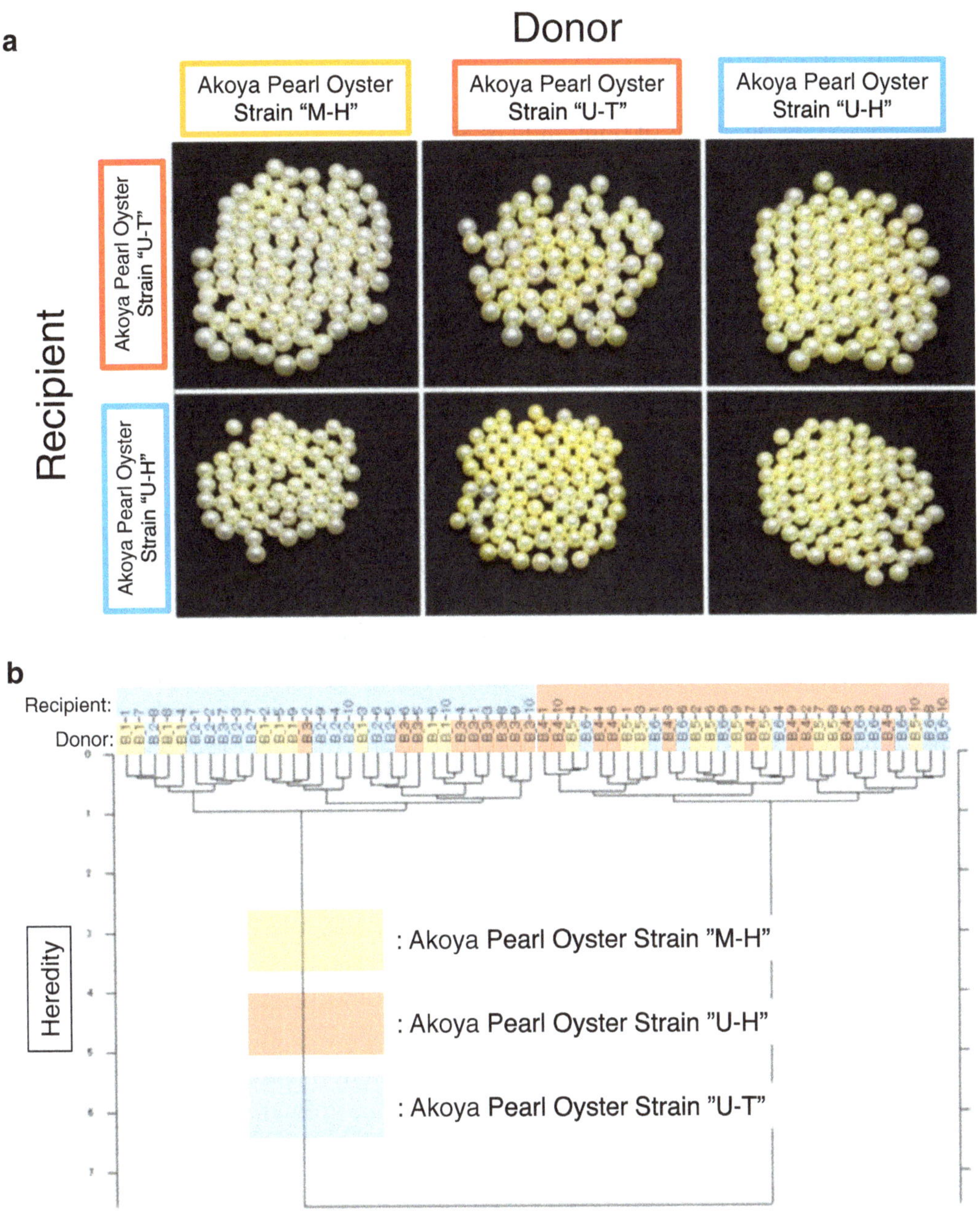

Fig. 12.2 The cultured pearls from combination of donor and recipient pearl oyster. The pearls were cultured by the following conditions: transplantation date, July 2–3, 2015; harvest date, Jan 19, 2016; pearl nucleus size, 6.67 mm at single transplantation were operated by single pearl farmer. (**a**) A picture of the cultured pearl. (**b**) Dendrogram of a hierarchical cluster analysis showing objective spectral diversity in pearls from combination of donor and recipient pearl oyster. Cluster analysis was performed with vector-normalized spectra. The spectral distances were calculated with Pearson's correlation coefficient, and Ward's algorithm was used for hierarchical clustering. Hierarchical clustering is a statistical data analysis procedure for the classification of similar objects into strain "U-T" and "U-H" as recipient pearl oyster groups

Akoya pearl oyster strain “M-H” as a donor clearly produced white pearls compared to the other four pearls, irrespective of using the Akoya pearl oyster strain “U-H” or “U-T” as recipient. Accordingly, we examined the differences between the pearls from various combinations of donor and recipient oysters based on the optical properties of the pearl surface using the FT-IR spectrometer (Fig. 12.2b). By performing hierarchical cluster analysis with FT-IR spectrometry, these pearls were classified into two clusters. These two clusters were highly dependent on the recipient strain. These results suggested that the effect on the optical characteristics of pearls was stronger in recipients than in donor.

12.4 Discussion

What is the factor that affects the quality of pearls which has been the great attention of pearl culture farmers and researchers since the beginning of pearl culture? From various experiments and experience of pearl farmers, it was known that the donor’s characteristics have a great influence on the quality of pearls, and research on donors has been actively conducted in recent research (Fujimura and Komaru 2017; Odawara et al. 2017). However, the recipient oysters that actually produce the pearl were considered to affect only the size of the pearl, such as the thickness of the nacre, and attention has not been paid to recipient oysters. Our study revealed that the sex of the recipient oysters affects not only the thickness of the pearl nacre but also the optical characteristics and quality of the pearl (Iwai et al. 2015). Therefore, in this study, we investigated the influence of donor and recipient on pearls, which is a factor influencing the optical characteristics of pearls. As a result, it was revealed that the influence of the recipient on the optical characteristics of the pearl surface by the FT-IR is larger than that of the donor which has been conventionally mentioned. It was suggested that in order to further improve quality in the future pearl culture, it was necessary to carry out seedling production and selective breeding of pearl oyster as a recipient with consideration of the influence on the quality of pearls. Moreover, the quality of pearls was also known to be strongly influenced by the pearl culture area. However, there were not many cases comparing pearls with different pearl culture environments. In this study, comparison of produced pearls was possible according to Akoya pearl oysters, which was transplanted under the same condition and was bred in each culture area, and the optical characteristics of pearls using FT-IR could be evaluated objectively. As a result of the comparison, the pearls produced in each culture area of Uwa Sea had two different optical characteristics, and it was able to distinguish from the north area and the south area clearly. These results are consistent with the actual impression of the pearl culture farmer, and it became clear that the method of distinguishing pearls by FT-IR is useful. It is necessary to investigate in detail what kind of environmental factors in breeding culture areas are affecting the optical characteristics of pearls. We investigate various factors on the quality and optical characteristics of culture pearls, and we could contribute to the improvement of pearl quality by investigating the influence.

Acknowledgments This study was supported by a grant-in-aid from the Science and Technology Research Promotion Program for Agriculture, Forestry, Fisheries, and Food Industry (26019A). This research was supported by grants from the Project of the NARO Bio-oriented Technology Research Advancement Institution (The Special Scheme to Create Dynamism in Agriculture, Forestry, and Fisheries Through Deploying Highly Advanced Technology). This research was supported by grants from the Project of the NARO Bio-oriented Technology Research Advancement Institution (The Special Scheme Project on Regional Developing Strategy).

References

Fujimura T, Komaru A (2017) The influence of nacreous crystal thickness of donor oysters on interference color appearance and crystal thickness of pearls in Pinctada fucata (Japanese pearl oyster). Nippon Suisan Gakkaishi 83:971–980 (in Japanese with English abstract)

Helm D, Labischinski H, Schallehn G, Naumann D (1991) Classification and identification of bacteria by Fourier-transform infrared spectroscopy. J Gen Microbiol 137:69–79

Iwai T, Takahashi M, Ido A, Miura C, Miura T (2015) Effect of gender on Akoya pearl quality. Aquaculture 437:333–338

Odawara K, Ozaki R, Takagi M (2017) Influence of the thickness of the nacreous elemental lamina of the pearl oyster Pinctada fucata used as donor oysters on the pearls. Nippon Suisan Gakkaishi 83:981–995 (in Japanese with English abstract)

Southgate PC, Lucas JS (2008) The pearl oyster. Elsevier, Oxford

Wada KT (1999) Science of the pearl oyster. Shinju Shinbunsha, Tokyo (in Japanese)

Wada KT, Komaru A (1996) Color and weight of pearls produced by grafting the mantle tissue from a selected population for white shell color of the Japanese pearl oyster *Pinctada fucata*. Aquaculture 142:25–32

Chapter 13
Influence of B Vitamins on Proliferation and Differentiation of Osteoblastic Bovine Cell Cultures: An In Vitro Study

Kent Urban, Julia Auer, Sebastian Bürklein, and Ulrich Plate

Abstract Minerals and vitamins affect bone formation, genetics, nutrition, and hormones. Studies mainly focus on the elucidation of the metabolic pathways during biomineralization to get an idea of how to promote the process of biomineralization in vivo and in vitro. One qualified approach to reach this is to investigate the influence of different substances on the proliferation and differentiation of osteoblastic cell cultures in vitro. The aim of this study was to investigate the effects of different types of single B vitamins (B_6, B_9, and B_{12}) and a vitamin B complex (B_1, B_2, B_3, B_5, B_6, B_9, and B_{12}) on proliferation and differentiation of primary bovine osteoblastic cells in vitro. The proliferation of osteoblastic cells during the experiments was evaluated by cell number analysis while cultivating. The expression of marking proteins of the osteogenic differentiation was evaluated by immunohistochemistry. Previous experiments with seven different B vitamins in different concentrations revealed a positive effect on cell proliferation with increasing concentration caused by three B vitamins: pyridoxal (B_6), folic acid (B_9), and cobalamine (B_{12}). The use of vitamin B_6, B_9, and B_{12} in different concentrations resulted in a significant increase of cell proliferation *($p < 0.05$)*. But neither the B vitamins nor the B vitamin complexes stimulated the expression of the typical bone cell proteins.

Keywords Vitamins · Vitamin B · Bone formation · Bone regeneration · Bone metabolism · In vitro biomineralization

---

K. Urban
Department of Periodontology and Operative Dentistry in the School of Dentistry, University of Münster, Münster, Germany
e-mail: Kent.Urban@ukmuenster.de

J. Auer · U. Plate (✉)
Department of Maxillofacial Surgery, VABOS, University of Münster, Münster, Germany
e-mail: plateu@uni-muenster.de

S. Bürklein
Central Interdisciplinary Ambulance in the School of Dentistry, University of Münster, Münster, Germany
e-mail: Sebastian.Buerklein@ukmuenster.de

K. Endo et al. (eds.), *Biomineralization*,
https://doi.org/10.1007/978-981-13-1002-7_13

13.1 Introduction

Focussing on the rapid development of implant- and bone-substitute materials as well as their integration in autologous tissue and optimized wound healing processes, it gets more and more important to give well-known therapies new perspectives. For a better adaption of implants in surrounding tissue, not only material's biocompatibility but also bone regeneration as a part of wound healing becomes subject of scientific research. Many existing therapies on bone regeneration dealing with vitamin D and calcium supplementation are well established (Avenell et al. 2014; Javed et al. 2016; Vandenbroucke et al. 2017). The effect of some other single vitamins or vitamin complexes is already investigated (Masse et al. 2010; Elste et al. 2017). Nevertheless, the effects in direct supplementation with vitamins in bone defects on bone regeneration are not completely understood yet (Owen et al. 1990; Herrmann et al. 2013).

13.2 Materials and Methods

For the experiments, two different cell culture mediums were used:

(a) Medium MP (High Growth Enhancement Medium without L-glutamine, MP Biomedicals GmbH, Eschwege, Germany) and
(b) Medium PAN (High Growth Enhancement Medium without L-glutamine and without B vitamins; PAN Bio-Tek, Bad Frierdrichshall, Germany).

Both mediums were supplemented with 4% FCS (fetal calf serum) (Biochrom, Berlin, Germany), 10.000 IU/ml penicillin, 10.000 μg/ml streptomycin, 250 μg/ml amphotericin B, and 200 mM L-glutamine (Biochrom KG Seromed, Berlin, Germany). Primary bovine osteoblast-like cells were used in this study. The cells were derived from the periosteum of calf metacarpus according to the instructions of Jones and Boyde (1977). Tissue explants were cultured for 4 weeks in medium MP supplemented with 10% FCS, 10.000 IU/ml penicillin, 10.000 μg/ml streptomycin, 250 μg/ml amphotericin B, 10 mM ß-glycerophosphate, and 200 mM L-glutamine (Biochrom KG Seromed, Berlin, Germany), at 37 °C and 5% CO_2 in humidified air. The medium was replaced once a week. When cells reached confluence, they were harvested (20 min incubation at 37 °C with 0.4 g collagenase, 98.8 mg nutrient mixture (HAM's F – 10) in 10 ml HEPES (2-[4-(2-hydroxyethyl)-1-piperazinyl] ethane sulfonic acid), repeatedly washed with phosphate-buffered saline (PBS), subsequently incubated for 15 min, and centrifuged. Pellets were resuspended in PBS and the cell number was determined in a cell counter (CASYWI Modell TT, Schärfe System, Reutlingen, Germany). Osteoblasts (10.000/cm^2) were seeded on 24-well plate plastic petri dishes (Nunc TFS, Roskilde, Denmark) with different mediums and B vitamin concentrations. Cell proliferation was determined after 1, 3, and 5 days, respectively. Cell morphology evaluation was performed by means of light microscopy. To determine the cell number, digital photos were taken under standardized conditions and cells were counted using the software program ImageJ with the plug-in Cell Counter. The experiments were repeated six times and all data were analyzed using one-way analysis of variance and post hoc Scheffé Test. As basic level of vitamin complex, the standard concentration of included B vitamins in medium MP was used (4 mg/l thiamine, 0, 4 mg/l riboflavin, 4 mg/l niacin, 4 mg/l pantothenic acid, 4 mg/l pyridoxal, and 4 mg/l folic acid). This concentration was called medium MP_0 and served as negative control for each group. Vitamin concentration was increased to achieve different concentrations (from basic level up to fourfold concentration) and called MP_1–MP_3 (Table 13.1). Vitamin B_{12} was not included and only solely added to medium MP. Based on medium PAN without B vitamins, single B vitamins were also added in different concentrations (from 4 to 12 μg/ml) (Table 13.1). Medium PAN without any B vitamins was called PAN_0 and was used as negative control for all experiments with medium PAN. An increase in cell number after 3 and 5 days was observed in all test groups (Figs. 13.1 and 13.2). For cell differentiation, collagen I, osteonectin, and osteocalcin were assessed by immunohistochemistry (Dako EnVision System, Dako, Hamburg, Germany) under standardized conditions with fluorescence microscopy

Table 13.1 Different B-vitamin concentrations in μg/ml for (a) medium MP, MP_0 = standard B vitamin concentration (negative control), MP_1 = double concentration of vitamin, MP_2 = triple concentration of vitamin, MP_3 = fourfold concentration of vitamin and (b) medium PAN, PAN_0 = without vitamin (negative control), PAN_1 = 4 μg/ml, PAN_2 = 8 μg/ml, and PAN_3 = 12 μg/ml vitamin

Medium/vitamin	B1	B2	B3	B5	B6	B9	B12
MP_0	4	0,4	4	4	4	4	0
PAN_0	0	0	0	0	0	0	0
MP_1 B6	4	0,4	4	4	8	4	0
MP_2 B6	4	0,4	4	4	12	4	0
MP_3 B6	4	0,4	4	4	16	4	0
MP_1 B9	4	0,4	4	4	4	8	0
MP_2 B9	4	0,4	4	4	4	12	0
MP_3 B9	4	0,4	4	4	4	16	0
MP_1 B12	4	0,4	4	4	4	4	8
MP_2 B12	4	0,4	4	4	4	4	12
MP_3 B12	4	0,4	4	4	4	4	16
PAN_1 B6	0	0	0	0	4	0	0
PAN_2 B6	0	0	0	0	8	0	0
PAN_3 B6	0	0	0	0	12	0	0
PAN_1 B9	0	0	0	0	0	4	0
PAN_2 B9	0	0	0	0	0	8	0
PAN_3 B9	0	0	0	0	0	12	0
PAN_1 B12	0	0	0	0	0	0	4
PAN_2 B12	0	0	0	0	0	0	8
PAN_3 B12	0	0	0	0	0	0	12

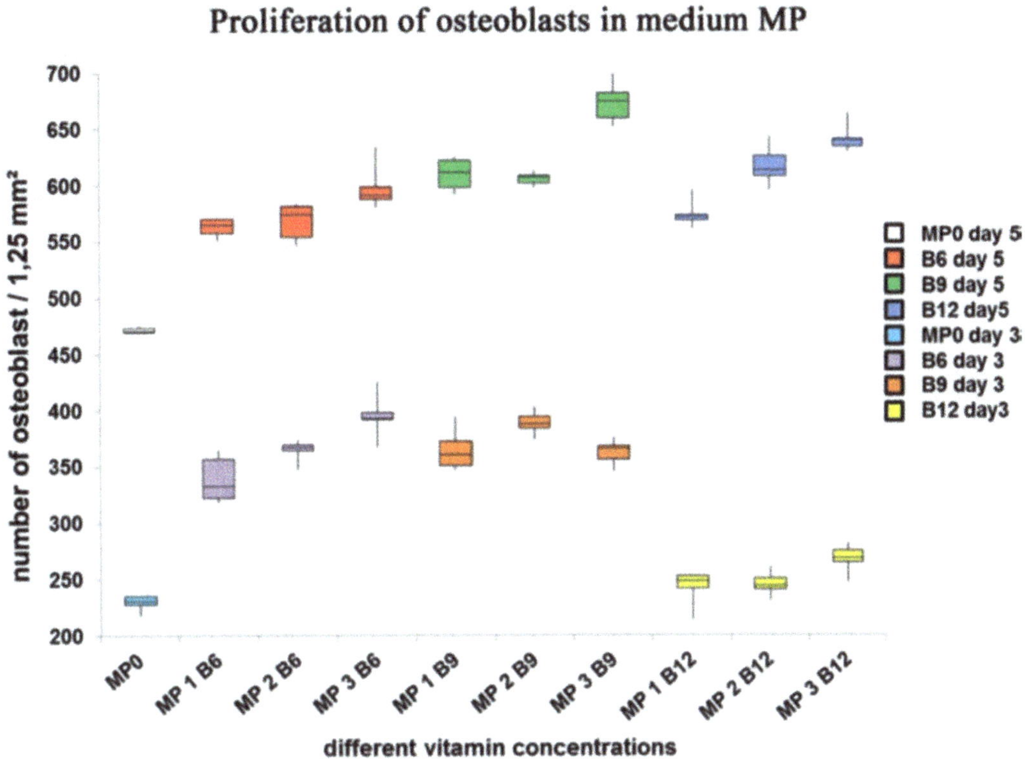

Fig. 13.1 Cell proliferation with B vitamin complex and single B vitamins in medium MP. Medium MP with B vitamin complex was used with different single vitamin B concentrations over 5 days. All groups started with nearly the same cell number at day 1 $p < 0.05$ (data not shown). An increase in cell number after 3 and 5 days was observed in all groups

(Axioplan 2, Carl Zeiss, Germany) and processed using AxioVision 3.1 software (Carl Zeiss, Germany).

Sixty thousand osteoblasts/cm^2 were seeded in 100 × 20 mm plastic petri dishes (TPP, Trasadingen, Schweiz). After cultivation for 14 days at 37 °C in an atmosphere of 5% CO_2 in the different media, osteoblastic cells were fixed with methanol and primary antibodies were used (diluted 1:100 with Blocking Solution): anti-collagen I (Biotrend, Cologne, Germany), anti-osteocalcin (TaKaRa Bio, MoBiTec, Goettingen, Germany), and anti-osteonectin (TaKaRa Bio, MoBiTec, Goettingen, Germany). Digital images were taken under standardized conditions by fluorescence microscopy (Axioplan 2 Carl Zeiss, Germany) and processed using the software AxioVision 3.1 (Carl Zeiss, Germany).

13.3 Results and Discussion

Proliferation of osteoblastic cells during the experiments was evaluated by cell number analysis during culture. Expression of marking proteins of osteogenic differentiation was assessed by immunohistochemistry. Proliferation and

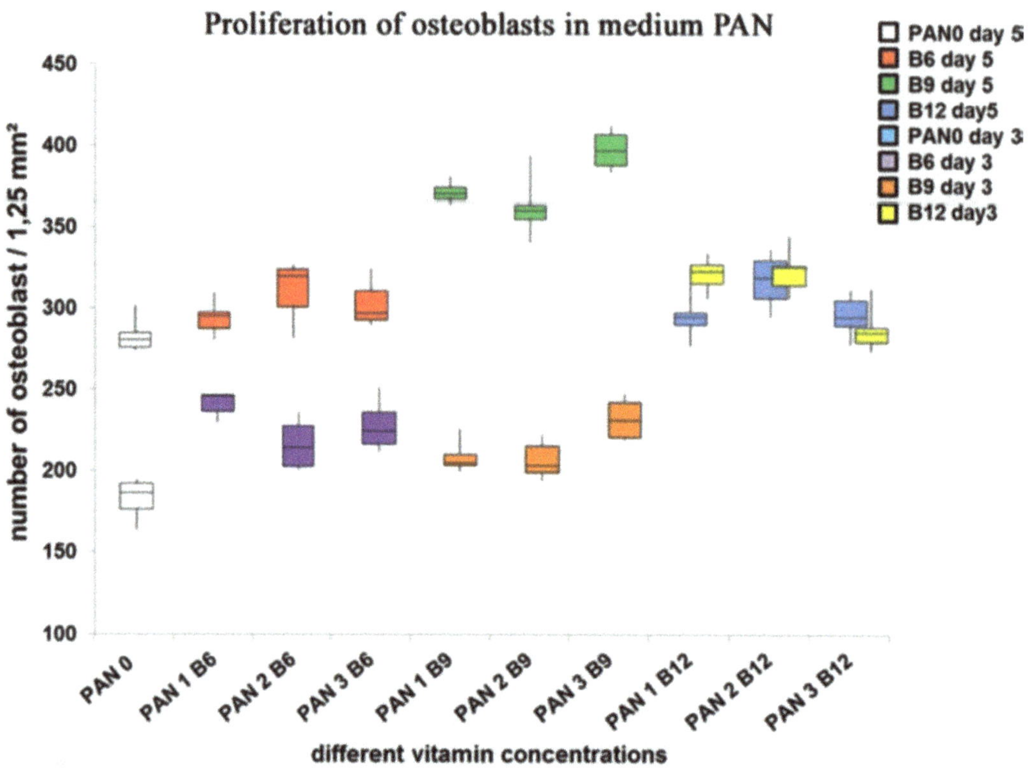

Fig. 13.2 Cell proliferations with single B vitamins in medium PAN. Medium PAN was used only with different single vitamin B concentrations over 3 and 5 days. All groups started with nearly the same cell number at day 1 $p < 0.05$ (data not shown). An increase in cell number after 3 and 5 days was observed in all groups

differentiation of osteoblasts enable the production of extracellular matrix (ECM) and is therefore the initial step in the formation of calcified tissue, especially bone.

This study mainly focuses on the elucidation of the metabolic pathways during biomineralization to get an idea of these processes in vivo and in vitro. Previous experiments with seven different B vitamins in different concentrations revealed a positive effect on cell proliferation with increasing concentrations caused by three B vitamins pyridoxal (B_6), folic acid (B_9), and cobalamine (B_{12}) (Dhonukshe-Rutten et al. 2003; Swart et al. 2016).

Characteristics of the B vitamins are:

- Essential nutrients that must be added to the body for normal cell formation, growth, and development
- Catalyzing and regulatory functions as cofactors and enzymes
- Being water-soluble, without danger of hypervitaminosis when overdosed

Under the conditions of the present study, the use of vitamin B_6, B_9, and B_{12} in different concentrations resulted in a significant increase of cell proliferation ($p < 0.05$). The negative control groups MP_0 and PAN_0 differed significantly from all other groups $MP_{1,2,3}$ and $PAN_{1,2,3}$ ($p < 0{,}05$) (Table 13.1, Figs. 13.1, 13.2, and 13.3).

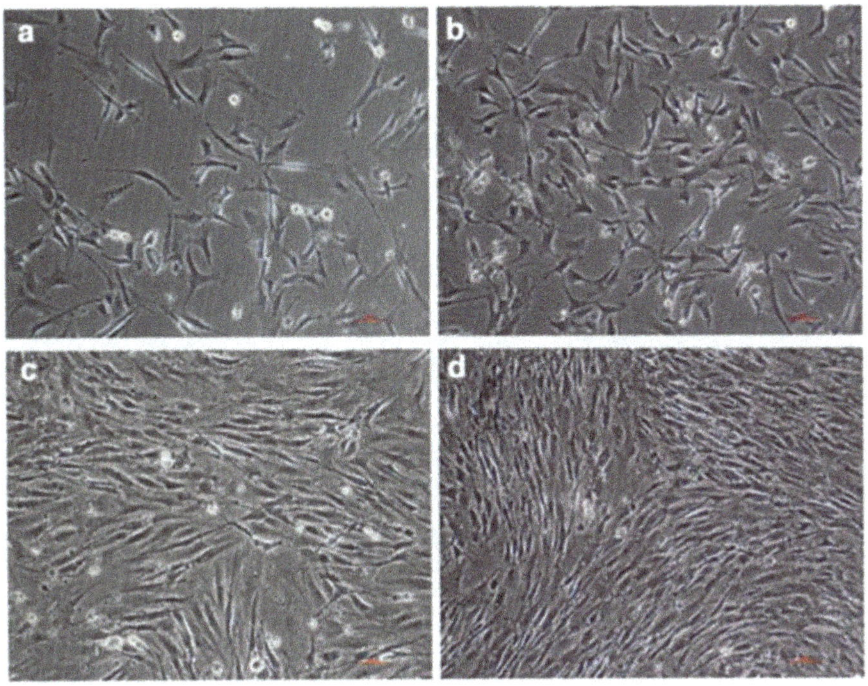

Fig. 13.3 Osteoblastic cells (**a**) after 3 days of incubation medium PAN_0; (**b**) after 3 days of incubation medium PAN_3 (with vitamin B_9); (**c**) after 5 days of incubation medium PAN_0, (**d**) after 5 days of incubation medium PAN_3 (with vitamin B_9)

Finally, supplementation of certain vitamins in an appropriate concentration significantly increased proliferation and improved growth of osteoblast-like cells. Probably, this increased cell growth leads to a superior wound healing and bone regeneration.

Using vitamin culture media to enhance proliferation and collagen formation (Herrmann et al. 2007) of osteoblast-like cells during culturing seems to be quite reasonable.

During different stages of differentiation, several proteins are synthesized by the osteoblasts (Roach 1994; Kim et al. 1996):

(a) Collagen type I, the main component of the ECM
(b) Non-collagenous proteins like alkaline phosphatase
(c) Osteonectin
(d) Later in the differentiation progress osteocalcin

While collagen type I as well as the protein marker osteonectin could be detected by immunohistochemistry at the end of the experiments (Fig. 13.4), none of the cell cultures showed any signs of osteocalcin expression. Neither the B vitamins nor the B vitamin complexes significantly stimulated the expression of the typical bone cell proteins.

Supplementation of other vitamins, e.g., ascorbic acid, supports the synthesis of collagen, and the ECM (extracellular matrix) (Urban et al. 2012) seemed to have a positive effect compared to vitamin-free cultures (Najeeb et al. 2016; Fratoni and Brandi 2015; Zhaoli Dai and Koh 2015). Bioactive vitamins placed on implant sur-

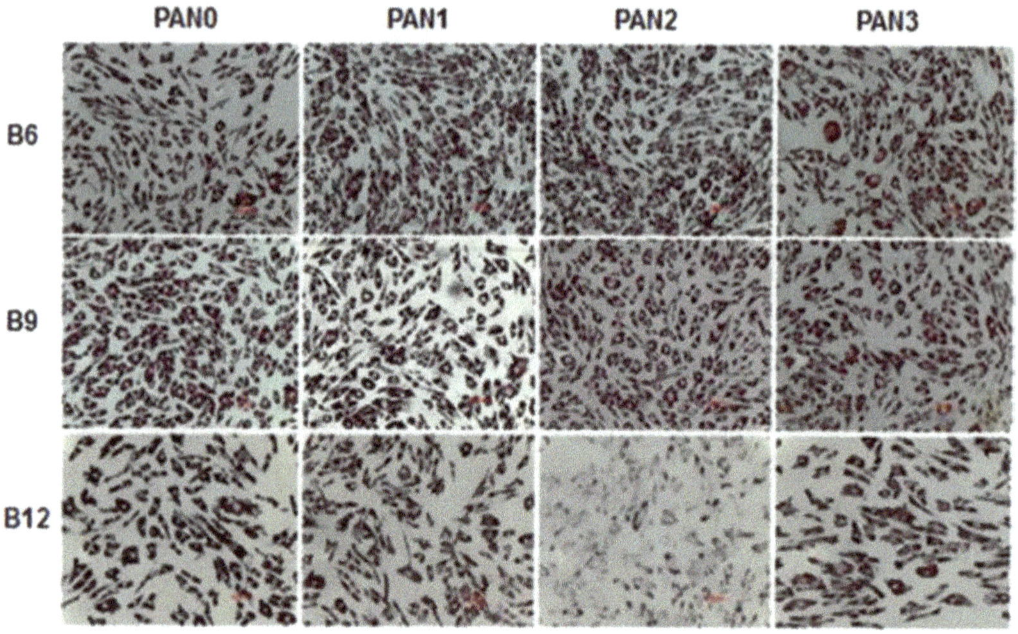

Fig. 13.4 Immunohistochemical analyses of collagen (primary antibody "anti-collagen I (Biotrend, Cologne, Germany)") in medium PAN with single vitamins B_6, B_9, and B_{12}

face may positively affect wound healing due to direct transmission into surrounding tissue. Mixing those vitamins into bone-substitute materials could be another beneficial aspect in bone regeneration by diffusion into the wound (Bartold et al. 2016). Further investigations should follow with the aim to increase supportive effects of vitamins on biological processes such as wound healing, bone regeneration, and revised healing of bone implants.

Acknowledgment Financial support of the Arbeitsgemeinschaft für Elektronenoptik e.V., Germany, is gratefully acknowledged.

References

Avenell A, Mak JCS, O'Connell D (2014) Vitamin D and vitamin D analogues for preventing fractures in post-menopausal women and older men. Cochrane Database Syst Rev (4) Art. No.: CD000227

Bartold PM, Gronthos S, Ivanovski S, Fisher A, Hutmacher DW (2016) Tissue engineered periodontal products. J Periodontal Res 51:1–15

Dhonukshe-Rutten RA, Lips P, de Jong N, Chin A, Paw MJM, Hiddink GJ, van Dusseldorp M, de Groot LC, van Staveren WA et al (2003) Vitamin B_{12} status is associated with bone mineral content and bone mineral density in frail elderly women but not in men. J Nutr 133(3):801–807

Elste V, Troesch B, Eggersdorfer M, Weber P (2017) Emerging evidence on neutrophil motility supporting its usefulness to define vitamin C intake requirements. Nutrients 9(5):503

Fratoni V, Brandi ML (2015) B vitamins, homocysteine and bone health. Nutrients 7:2176–2192

Herrmann M, Umanskaya N, Traber L, Schmidt-Gayk H, Menke W, Lanzer G, Lenhart M, Schmidt JP, Herrmann W (2007) The effect of B-vitamins on biochemical bone turnover Osteocalcin und Kollagen Typ I markers and bone mineral density in osteoporotic patients: a 1-year double blind placebo controlled trial. Clin Chem Lab Med 45(12):1785–1792

Herrmann W, Kirsch SH, Kruse V, Eckert R, Gräber S, Geisel J, Obeid R (2013) One year B and D vitamins supplementation improves metabolic bone markers. Clin Chem Lab Med 51(3):639–647

Javed F, Malmstrom H, Kellesarian SV, Al-Kheraif AA, Vohra F, Romanos GE (2016) Efficacy of vitamin D3 supplementation on osseointegration of implants. Implant Dent 25(2):281–287

Jones SJ, Boyde A (1977) The migration of osteoblasts. Cell Tissue Res 184:179–193

Kim GS, Kim CH, Park JY, Lee KU, Park CS (1996) Effects of vitamin B_{12} on cell proliferation and cellular alkaline phosphatase activity in human bone marrow stromal osteoprogenitor cells and UMRI06 osteoblastic cells. Metabolism 45:1443–1446

Masse PG, Jougleux JL, Tranchant CC, Dosy J, Caissie M, Coburn SP (2010) Enhancement of calcium/vitamin D supplement efficacy by administering concomitantly three nutrients essential to bone collagen matrix for the treatment of osteopenia in mid-dle-aged women: a one-year follow-up. J Clin Biochem Nutr 46(1):20–29

Najeeb S, Zafar MS, Khurshid Z, Zohaib S, Almas K (2016) The role of nutrition in perio-dontal health: an update. Nutrients 8:530

Owen TA, Aronow M, Shalhoub V, Barone LM, Wilming L, Tassinari MS, Kennedy MB, Pockwinse S, Lian JB, Stein GS (1990) Progressive development of the rat osteoblast phenotype in vitro: reciprocal relationships in expression of genes associated with osteoblast proliferation and differentiation during formation of the bone extracellular matrix. J Cell Physiol 143:420–430

Roach HI (1994) Why does bone matrix contain non-collagenous proteins? The possible roles of osteocalcin, osteonectin, osteopontin and bone sialoprotein in bone mineralisation and resorption. Cell Biol Int 18:617–628

Swart KM, Ham AC, van Wijngaarden JP, Enneman AW, van Dijk SC, Sohl E, Brouwer-Brolsma EM, van der Zwaluw NL, Zillikens MC, Dhonukshe-Rutten RA, van der Velde N, Brug J, Uitterlinden AG, de Groot LC, Lips P, van Schoor NM (2016) A randomized controlled trial to examine the effect of 2-year vitamin B_{12} and folic acid supplementation on physical performance, strength, and falling: additional findings from the B-PROOF study. Calcif Tissue Int 98(1):18–27

Urban K, Höhling HJ, Lüttenberg B, Szuwart T, Plate U (2012) An in vitro study of osteo-blast vitality influenced by the vitamins C and E. Head Face Med 8(25)

Vandenbroucke A, Luyten F, Flamaing J, Gielen E (2017) Pharmacological treatment of osteoporosis in the oldest old. Clin Interv Aging 12:1065–1077

Zhaoli Dai Z, Koh WP (2015) Review B-vitamins and bone health–a review of the current evidence. Nutrients 7:3322–3346

Chapter 14
Rice Plant Biomineralization: Electron Microscopic Study on Plant Opals and Exploration of Organic Matrices Involved in Biosilica Formation

Noriaki Ozaki, Takuya Ishida, Akiyoshi Osawa, Yumi Sasaki, Hiromi Sato, Michio Suzuki, Keiju Okano, and Yuko Yoshizawa

Abstract Biologically formed amorphous silica (biosilica) is widely found in diatoms, marine sponges, terrestrial plants, and bacteria, some of which have been well characterized. Although rice plants produce large amounts of biosilica (plant opal) in their leaf blades and rice husks, the molecular mechanism of biomineralization is still poorly understood. In the present study, we investigated the fundamental properties of plant opal in leaf blades of the rice plants (*Oryza sativa*) by scanning electron microscopy (SEM) equipped with energy-dispersive X-ray spectroscopy. The number of fan-shaped plant opal increases in the motor cells (bubble-shaped epidermal cells) during heading time. High-resolution SEM analysis revealed that the plant opals are composed of nanoparticles, as is the case with diatom silica and siliceous spicule of sponge. Organic matrices in biominerals have been considered to control mineralization. Biosilicas in diatom and marine sponge are formed under ambient conditions using organic matrices, unique proteins, and long-chain polyamines. In this study, we report the establishment of purification method of plant opals from rice leaf blades. Finally, we succeeded in extracting organic matrices from the purified plant opal.

Keywords Biomineralization · Biosilica · Organic matrix · Plant opal · Rice plant

---

N. Ozaki (✉) · T. Ishida · A. Osawa · Y. Sasaki · H. Sato · K. Okano · Y. Yoshizawa
Department of Biotechnology, Faculty of Bioresource Sciences, Akita Prefectural University, Akita, Japan
e-mail: ozanor@akita-pu.ac.jp; m14g005@akita-pu.ac.jp; keijuo@akita-pu.ac.jp; yyoshizawak@akita-pu.ac.jp

M. Suzuki
Department of Applied Biological Chemistry, Graduate School of Agricultural and Life Sciences, The University of Tokyo, Tokyo, Japan
e-mail: amichiwo@mail.ecc.u-tokyo.ac.jp

K. Endo et al. (eds.), *Biomineralization*,
https://doi.org/10.1007/978-981-13-1002-7_14

14.1 Introduction

Biomineralization is widespread phenomenon by which organisms produce minerals by using organic matrices under ambient conditions (Lowenstam and Weiner 1989). The resulting minerals, termed biominerals, have a specific morphology and demonstrate excellent physical properties. Biogenic amorphous silica (biosilica) is known as one of the representative biominerals. Biosilica is widely observed in skeleton of diatoms, spicules of marine sponges, spore coats of bacteria, and epicuticles of certain higher plants. As in the case of other biominerals, organic matrices in biosilicas are thought to be associated with silica formation. Until now, in diatoms, glass sponges, and certain facultative bacteria, several organic matrices involved in silica formation have previously been identified, such as unique proteins (silaffin, glassin, and CotB1) and long-chain polyamines (LCPAs) (Sumper and Kröger 2004; Shimizu et al. 2015; Matsunaga et al. 2007; Motomura et al. 2016). These matrices are highly charged and have been shown to promote silica formation from monosilicic acid solution near a neutral pH. On the other hand, there are few studies on silica formation of higher plants. The best-known example of silicon accumulating plants, rice plants (*Oryza sativa*), produces a large amount of biosilicas (plant opal) in their leaf blades and rice husks. Silicon uptake mechanism from soil is transporter mediated and energy dependent (Ma et al. 2006). Plant opal deposition has been shown to improve disease resistance, light interception, and mechanical properties (Ma and Takahashi 2002). Despite the importance of plant opal in rice plants, information on the molecular mechanisms involved in plant opal formation is very limited. To date, there are no published reports on organic matrices from plant opal of rice, as far as we know. In the present work, we have investigated the fundamental properties of plant opals by microscopic analyses and extracted an organic matrix from fan-shaped plant opals.

14.2 Materials and Methods

14.2.1 Plant Materials and Microscopy

The leaf blades of rice plants (*Oryza sativa* cv. Akita-sake-komachi) were collected from paddy field in Akita Prefectural University. Optical microscope (BX51, Olympus) and field emission SEM (SU-8010, Hitachi) were used to analyze the microstructure of leaf blades and morphology of plant opals. The chemical composition of silica was confirmed with an energy-dispersive X-ray spectroscope (EDX; EMAX x-act, HORIBA). Prior to counting the number of fan-shaped opal, the leaf blade was incinerated at 550 °C. The ashed sample was carefully placed on Superfrost micro slides (Matsunami) and observed with the optical microscope.

14.2.2 Extraction of Organic Matrices from Plant Opals

Plant opals were separated from mature leaves according to the method of Setoguchi et al. (1990) with slight modifications. After washing with distilled water, rice leaf blades were cut into small pieces and ground with a mixer mill. The homogenate was passed through a nylon mesh filter of 258 μm pore size (NB60, Atflon). The filtrate containing plant opals is put on a watch glass, and heavier fan-shaped plant opals were separated from lighter small leaf fragment by a series of decantation. Cell walls bound to fan-shaped plant opals were removed by sulfuric acid and cellulase (Onozuka R-10, Wako, Osaka) treatments. The resulting fan-shaped opals were suspended in 4 M hydrogen fluoride (HF) solution and left for 2 h at room temperature. After centrifugation for 10 min at 2000 *g*, the supernatant was subjected to dialysis (Float-A-Lyzer, Spectra-Por) against distilled water. The dialysate (HF-soluble fraction) was lyophilized and the resulting organic matrices were subjected to tricine-SDS-PAGE. Organic matrices were detected by Coomassie Brilliant blue (CBB; EzStain AQua, ATTO) and silver (SilverXpress, Thermo Fisher) staining. The HF-soluble fraction passed through the 30 kDa molecular weight cutoff filter (Amicon Ultra 15, Millipore) was used to raise antibody in rabbits through a commercial source. Another set of sample was subjected to SDS-PAGE and subsequent blotting to a PVDF membrane. The membrane was blocked with 5% skim milk diluted in TBS (Tris-buffered saline; 50 mM Tris, 0.85% NaCl, pH 7.2) with Tween 20 (0.05%) for 1 h and then incubated in the primary antibody solution (1:100) for 1 h at room temperature. After washing, it was incubated in 1:3000 diluted solution of AP-conjugated goat anti-rabbit IgG secondary antibody (Bio-Rad) for 1 h at room temperature. The target protein was visualized using a BCIP/NBT substrate system (Bio-Rad).

14.3 Results and Discussion

14.3.1 Morphology and Function of Plant Opals

Representative SEM micrographs of several types of plant opal from rice leaf blades are shown in Fig. 14.1. SEM-EDX analysis proved that all types of plant opals were composed of silicon, oxygen, and carbon (data not shown). The surface of leaf blades consists of silicified cells, called long cells making plate-shaped opals (Fig. 14.1a), prickle hair (Fig. 14.1b), and short cells making dumbbell-shaped opals (Fig. 14.1c). Our preliminary study revealed that plant opals on leaf surface are formed and silicified within 2 weeks after germination (data not shown). The possible function of these opals on the leaf surface is considered to protect against biotic and abiotic stress, such as pathogenic bacteria and dryness. Only the

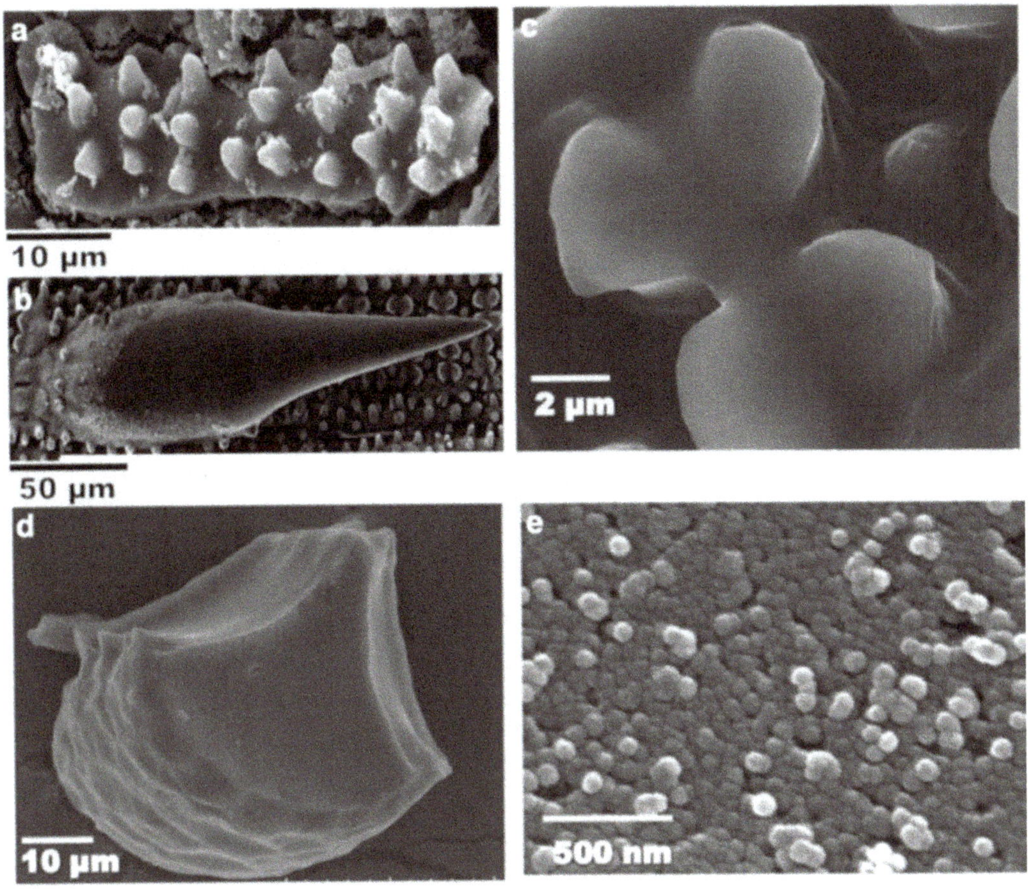

Fig. 14.1 Representative scanning electron microscope (SEM) micrographs of plant opals in rice leaf blades. (**a**) Plate-shaped opal. (**b**) Silicified prickle hair. (**c**) Dumbbell-shaped opals. (**d**) Purified fan-shaped opal. (**e**) Silica nanoparticles constituting fan-shaped opal

fan-shaped plant opal (Fig. 14.1d) is formed inside the leaf blade. Our research group confirmed that fan-shaped opal contains highest concentration of silica (Sato et al. 2017). Based on higher magnification image of fan-shaped opals, we found that the opal comprised fine particles with several tens of nanometer in diameter (Fig. 14.1e). Similar silica nanoparticles are also found in the spicules of marine sponges (Aizenberg et al. 2005)

In order to investigate the formation period of the fan-shaped opal, we collected rice leaves from July to October. To count the number of opals, each collected leaf blades were treated by calcination at 550 °C. The optical micrograph of surface of leaf blade after calcination is shown in Fig. 14.2a. Fan-shaped plant opals (arrowheads) were observed in the motor cells between the veins of the leaf (white dotted line) and were aligned like a backbone. As shown in Fig. 14.2b, the number of fan-shaped opals sharply increased around the heading time. The heading time (dotted line) in Akita prefecture was early August with strong sunlight. Although the function of the fan-shaped opal had not been clarified (Kaufman et al. 1979;

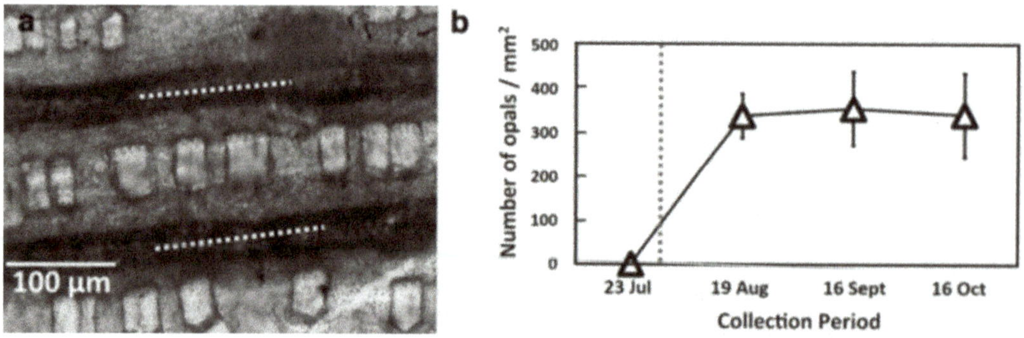

Fig. 14.2 Fan-shaped plant opal formation in the flag leaf of rice. (**a**) Optical micrograph of surface of ashed leaf blade. White dotted lines indicate vascular bundle. When looking at fan-shaped opals from another angle, it looks like rectangle structures (arrowheads). (**b**) Time course of formation of fan-shaped plant opals. Dotted line indicates the heading time (ear-forming period). The number of fan-shaped opal was measured by counting rectangle structures (arrowhead in **a**)

Agarie et al. 1996), we suggested the possibility that fan-shaped opals have a role in guiding light to chloroplast by optical simulation and actual optical experiment (Sato et al. 2016). Another possibility is that the fan-shaped opals formed inside the leaf play a role like a bone and improve the posture for light interception (Ma and Takahashi 2002). In either case, the fan-shaped opal may promote photosynthesis necessary for panicle formation.

14.3.2 *Organic Matrices from Separated Plant Opals*

Although organic matrices from biosilica are considered to play important roles in silica formation, there are few reports about organic compounds in plant opal (phytolith) of higher plants (Elbaum et al. 2009). It was difficult to extract organic matrices from opals, due to complex structure consisting of cuticle and silica layer. So, we developed a novel silica purification method and succeeded in extracting organic matrices from the separated plant opal. Cell walls bound to the silica were decomposed by successive treatments with sulfuric acid and cellulase. The HF-soluble fraction from opals was subjected to tricine-SDS-PAGE. At least two main bands (arrowheads) were detected using CBB staining (Fig. 14.3a). On the other hand, only one band was stained with silver staining (Fig. 14.3b, arrowhead). From these results, the band with an apparent molecular mass of 10 kDa is referred to as the HF-soluble protein. Only the 10 kDa protein strongly reacted with the antibody raised against the fraction containing HF-soluble protein (Fig. 14.3c, arrowhead), indicating that the antibody was highly specific to this protein. The amino acid sequence analysis by LC-MS/MS and immunohistochemical analysis of this protein are in progress. Detailed results will be reported elsewhere.

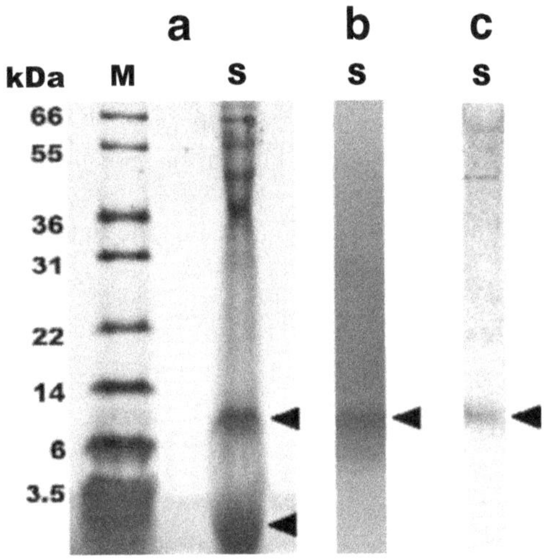

Fig. 14.3 Tricine-SDS-PAGE (12.5%) and Western blot analyses of the HF-soluble organic matrices extracted from fan-shaped plant opals. (**a**) Two major bands (arrowheads) were detected by CBB staining. (**b**) Only one band (arrowhead) was positive for silver staining. (**c**) Western blotting with an anti-HF-soluble proteins antiserum. Only one immunoreactive band was detected at about 10 kDa. *M* molecular mass standards. *S* HF-soluble fraction

References

Agarie S, Agata W, Uchida H, Kubota F, Kaufman PB (1996) Function of silica bodies in the epidermal system of rice (*Oryza sativa* L.): testing the window hypothesis. J Exp Bot 47:655–660

Aizenberg J, Weaver JC, Thanawala MS, Sundar VC, Morse DE, Fratzl P (2005) Skelton of *Euplectella* sp: structural hierarchy from nanoscale to the macroscale. Science 309:275–278

Elbaum R, Melamed-Bessudo C, Tuross N, Levy A, Winer S (2009) New methods to isolate organic materials from silicified phytolith reveal fragmented glycoproteins but no DNA. Quat Int 193:11–19

Kaufman PB, Takeoka Y, Carlson TJ, Bigelow WC, Jones JD, Morre PH, Ghosheh NS (1979) Studies on silica deposition in sugarcane, using scanning electron microscopy, energy dispersive X-ray analysis, neutron activation analysis, and light microscopy. Phytomorphology 29:185–193

Lowenstam HA, Weiner S (1989) On biomineralization. Oxford University Press, London

Ma JF, Takahashi E (2002) Functions of silicon in plant growth. In: Soil, fertilizer, and plant silicon research in Japan. Elsevier Science, Amsterdam

Ma JF, Tamai K, Yamaji N, Mitani N, Konishi S, Katsuhara M, Ishiguro M, Murata Y, Yano M (2006) A silicon transporter in rice. Nature 440:688–691

Matsunaga S, Sakai R, Jimbo M, Kamiya H (2007) Long-chain polyamines (LCPAs) from marine sponge: possible implication in spicule formation. Chem Biochem 8:1729–1735

Motomura K, Ikeda T, Matsuyama S, Mohamed A, Tanaka T, Ishida T, Hirota R, Kuroda A (2016) The C-terminal zwitterionic sequence of CotB1 is essential for biosilicification of the *Bacillus cereus* spore coat. J Bacteriol 198:276–282

Sato K, Yamauchi A, Ozaki N, Ishigure T, Oaki Y, Imai H (2016) Optical properties of biosilicas in rice plants. RSC Adv 6:109168–109173

Sato K, Ozaki N, Nakanishi K, Sugahara Y, Oaki Y, Salinas C, Herrera S, Kisailus D, Imai H (2017) Effects of nanostructured biosilica on rice plant mechanics. RSC Adv 7:13065–13071

Setoguchi H, Okazaki M, Suga S (1990) Calcification in higher plants with special reference to cystoliths. In: Origin, evolution, and modern aspects of biomineralization in plants and animals. Plenum Press, New York

Shimizu K, Amano T, Bari MR, Weaver JC, Arima J, Mori N (2015) Glassin, a histidine-rich protein from the siliceous skeletal system of the marine sponge Euplectella, directs silica polycondensation. PNAS 112:11449–11454

Sumper M, Kröger N (2004) Silica formation in diatoms: the function of long-chain polyamines and silaffins. J Mater Chem 14:2059–2065

Chapter 15
DMP1 Binds Specifically to Type I Collagen and Regulates Mineral Nucleation and Growth

Anne George, Elizabeth Guirado, and Yinghua Chen

Abstract Extracellular matrix of bone and dentin is highly complex and involves a dynamic process of deposition and removal. Cells are the main architect that build this designer matrix that is highly specialized to calcified tissues. Osteoblasts or odontoblasts secrete both collagen and noncollagenous proteins in a temporal and spatial manner. Type I collagen self-assembles and forms a fabric-like template onto which noncollagenous proteins and mineral bind in a well-regulated manner. Dentin matrix protein 1 (DMP1) is one such noncollagenous protein that contains several acidic groups that can bind calcium ions which in turn binds phosphate and initiates the calcification process. In this study, we demonstrate that DMP1 is localized at specific sites on the self-assembled collagen matrix of dentin. In vitro nucleation studies on demineralized and deproteinized dentin slice adsorbed with DMP1 show bundles of well-ordered needle-shaped nanohydroxyapatite deposited on the dentin matrix. The nucleated mineral structures had uniform length and width and their long axis was oriented parallel to the collagen fibril axis. Overall, the physiologically self-assembled collagen and DMP1 mediated ordered deposition of nanocrystalline HAP.

Keywords Dentin matrix protein 1 · Collagen · Hydroxyapatite · Mineralization · Extracellular matrix

15.1 Introduction

Biological composites such as bone, dentin, and cementum consist of a crystalline inorganic phase mainly carbonated hydroxyapatite embedded within a biopolymeric organic matrix (Veis 1993; Veis and Dorvee 2013). The cells that produce these mineralized matrices exert a regulatory and exquisite control over the minerals they deposit, creating materials of varied shapes, sizes, and high tensile strength.

A. George (✉) · E. Guirado · Y. Chen
Brodie Tooth Development Genetics & Regenerative Medicine Research Laboratory, Department of Oral Biology, University of Illinois at Chicago, Chicago, IL, USA
e-mail: anneg@uic.edu; eguira@uic.edu; yinghua@uic.edu

K. Endo et al. (eds.), *Biomineralization*,
https://doi.org/10.1007/978-981-13-1002-7_15

The stereospecific interaction of macromolecules with biominerals represents a unique phenomenon in nature (Addadi et al. 2001; Grzesiak et al. 2017).

Mineralized tissue formation results from the coordinated activity of highly differentiated cells. During the differentiation process, these cells secrete an extracellular matrix which performs various functions (Grzesiak et al. 2017; Hirata et al. 2005; Kang et al. 2015). A distinct feature of the ECM in calcified tissues is that it contains both crystal growth promoters and inhibitors (Goldberg and Smith 2004). Components in the ECM are involved in directing the deposition of specific calcium phosphate polymorphs during the formation of the calcified matrix.

The deposition of extracellular matrix and subsequent mineralization are a temporal and spatial event. They are assembled from a collagenous fibrillar network containing small amounts of tissue-specific regulatory proteins and other widely circulatory proteins. Phosphoproteins are one of the major component groups among the noncollagenous proteins found in all calcified tissues (Ravindran and George 2014). They have been postulated to play an important role in the initiation of calcification and possibly in the regulation of crystal growth. These regulatory proteins are responsible for controlled crystal growth within the collagenous matrix.

Dentin matrix protein (DMP1) is an example of a regulatory protein localized in the ECM of bone and dentin (George et al. 1993, 1994, 1995; He and George 2004). Understanding the players and the mechanism by which the extracellular matrix calcifies is important to understand the function of mineralized biological tissues. In the current study, we demonstrate that DMP1 is localized to specific sites on the dense physiologically arranged collagen fibrils of demineralized dentin matrix. Using a demineralized and deproteinized dentin slice, we demonstrate that adsorbed recombinant DMP1 can promote the deposition of organized nanocrystalline hydroxyapatite ribbons. Modeling of DMP1 shows that the protein could have a flexible carboxyl terminal domain, which might help in binding collagen and Ca^{2+} in the ECM.

15.2 Methods

15.2.1 Expression of Recombinant DMP1 Protein

Full-length rat recombinant DMP1 was produced as previously published (Bedran-Russo et al. 2013; Srinivasan et al. 1999). BSA (bovine serum albumin) was used as a negative control.

15.2.2 Preparation of Demineralized Dentin Wafers for Immunogold Labeling

Third molars without caries were selected and kept frozen following approval of the Institutional Review Board at the University of Illinois at Chicago (protocol 2009-0198). Coronal dentin cross-sections 1.5 mm thick were cut from each tooth and further sectioned to produce 250-μm-thick slices using a hydrated diamond blade saw (IsoMet 1000, Buehler, Lake Bluff, IL, USA). These slices represent the samples hereinafter referred to as dentin wafers.

Wafers measuring 1.5 × 3 × 0.250 mm thick were placed together in 14% EDTA at 4 °C for 10 days. Demineralization was verified by X-ray microradiography (MX-20 Faxitron, LLC, Lincolnshire, IL). These dentin wafers were dehydrated in a series of ethanol from 30% to 100%, trimmed, and embedded in epoxy resin, and ultrathin sections 70 nm were placed on 300 mesh formvar-coated nickel grids.

Grid-mounted tissue sections were processed for colloidal gold immunohistochemistry by incubating the sections with rabbit primary antibody against DMP1 (1:250) as published before. After which the sections were incubated with anti-rabbit IgG colloidal gold particles (10 nm gold particles) and washed. For controls, the sections were incubated with 20 nm gold-conjugated anti-rabbit IgG. All the sections were imaged either unstained or stained with uranyl acetate and imaged using JEOL JEM 1220 Electron Microscope and digital images obtained using Erlangshen ESW 1000w 785 camera.

15.2.3 *Preparation of Demineralized and Deproteinized Dentin Wafers for Nucleation Experiments*

Demineralized dentin wafers were subjected to treatment with 1 M NaCl for 1 h at room temperature to disrupt loosely bound noncollagenous proteins. Samples were then incubated in 0.25% trypsin-EDTA twice for 4 h at 37 °C to remove strongly bound, endogenous noncollagenous proteins. These wafers were cryosectioned to 5 μm, stained with Stains-All® (Sigma-Aldrich), and imaged to confirm the completeness of removal of noncollagenous proteins (Padovano et al. 2015).

In vitro nucleation was performed as reported earlier for 14 days (He et al. 2003). At the end of the time point, samples were washed and dehydrated by passing through a series of graded ethanol solutions, 30%, 50%, 90%, and 100% for 10 min each. The samples were finally dehydrated by immersing them in a solution of hexamethyldisilazane embedded in epoxy resin, and ultrathin sections of 70 nm were placed on copper TEM grid and examined in a JEOL JEM 1220 TEM (JEOL Ltd., Tokyo, JAPAN) Gatan accelerating voltage of 60 kV. Images were recorded using a CCD camera (Gatan Inc., Pleasanton, CA).

15.2.4 *Modeling of DMP1*

The I-TASSER (Iterative Threading ASSEmbly Refinement) server was used for DMP1 3D structure prediction (Roy et al. 2010; Yang et al. 2015; Yang and Zhang 2015a, b; Zhang 2009). The polypeptide strand was built by using human DMP1 sequence data from NCBI protein database (NP_004398.1). The program uses ab initio *modeling* as well as the LOMETS multiple threading program to retrieve proteins with similar folds from the PDB library. Replica-exchange Monte Carlo simulations generated a pool of protein structures from which low free-energy states were selected. Iterative template fragment assembly simulations identified the top five near-native models. C scores between −5 and 2 are assigned to these models, with more positive scores indicating greater confidence.

15.3 Results

15.3.1 DMP1 Binds to Densely Packed Collagen Fibrils of the Dentin Matrix

Immunogold labeling experiment showed that gold particles were distributed specifically over the dense collagen fibril of the demineralized dentin matrix (Fig. 15.1a). Demineralization of dentin led to the dissolution of the mineral only and did not alter the antigenic properties of DMP1 in the matrix. Staining the dentin slice with uranyl acetate and lead citrate showed that DMP1 was localized on the collagen matrix. Image presented in Fig. 15.1b shows that the labeling was mostly localized at the edge of the 67 nm periodic band of type I collagen. This region would correspond to the gap region of the self-assembled collagen matrix.

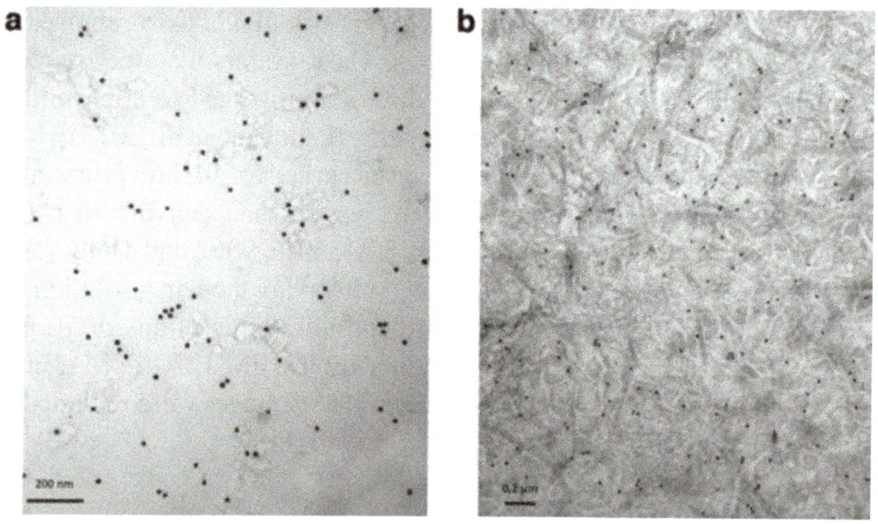

Fig. 15.1 Localization of DMP1 on the dentin wafer. (**a**) Unstained transmission electron micrograph of the demineralized dentin slice on which immunogold labeling with anti-DMP1 was performed prior to TEM. Scale bar represents 200 nm. (**b**) Same experiment wherein the dentin slice was stained with uranyl acetate and lead citrate. Scale bar represents 0.2 μm

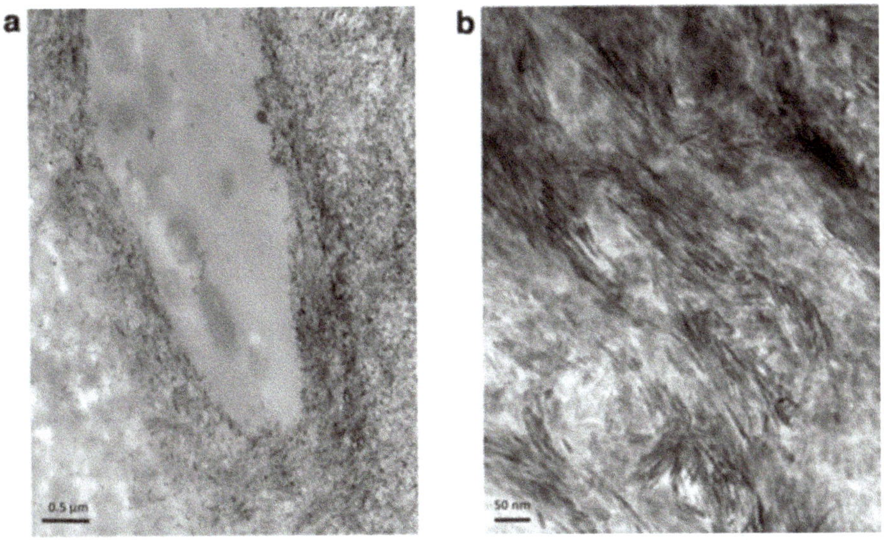

Fig. 15.2 Structural morphology of DMP1 mediated mineral deposition: (**a**) transmission electron microscopy (TEM) image of DMP1 mediated HA nanocrystal on demineralized and deproteinized dentin slice. Scale bar represents 0.5 µm. (**b**) Higher magnification image showing bands of closely aligned mineral fibers aligned parallel to the collagen fibrils. Scale bar represents 50 nm

15.3.2 Structural Characterization of the Mineral Deposited on the Collagen Matrix of Dentin

In vitro nucleation studies showed that demineralized and deproteinized dentin slices adsorbed with DMP1 initiated calcium phosphate deposition. At the end of 14 days, TEM analysis showed the presence of nanostructured mineral structures which were aligned to the dentin collagen fibrils (Fig. 15.2). At low magnification (Fig. 15.2a), it was apparent that the dentin slice was coated with electron-dense calcium phosphate mineral, particularly concentrated around the dentinal tubule. The high magnification image (Fig. 15.2b) shows that the dark electron-dense deposits are bundles of mineral lamellae which are about 3–5 nm apart. The needle-like mineral lamellae were all oriented with their long axis nearly parallel to the collagen fibrils. Selected area electron diffraction analysis (SAED) of the acicular deposits (Fig. 15.3a) showed the presence of nanocrystalline hydroxyapatite as they displayed the 002 reflection pattern (Fig. 15.3b).

15.3.3 Computation and Ab Initio Models of DMP1

Computer modeling was used to gain insight into the molecular shape of DMP1. Two predicted models are shown in Fig. 15.4a, b. Of these, (b) represents the highest scoring model C-score of (−1.59), while, model a had a C-score of (−2.54).

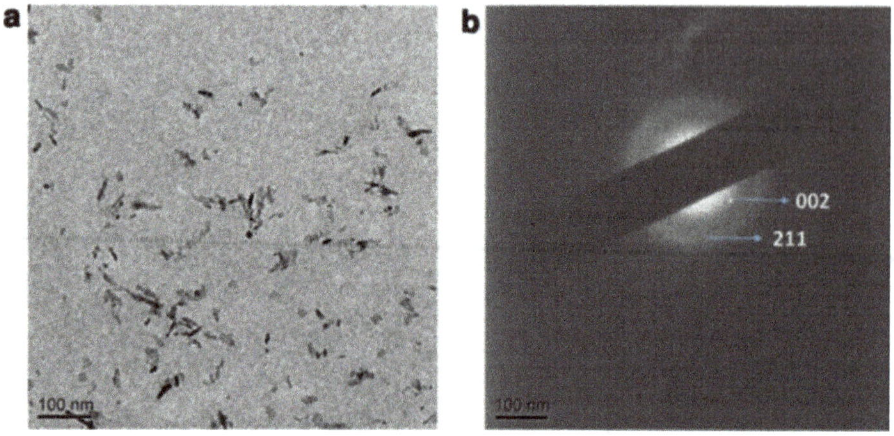

Fig. 15.3 Characterization of the Ca-P deposits: (**a**) TEM image shows nanocrystalline Ca-P deposits with acicular morphology. (**b**) Selected area electron diffraction pattern indexed to nanocrystalline HAP. Note that the 002 reflections are in the process of forming arcs indicating preferred orientation of the c-axis of the HAP parallel to that of the collagen fibrils

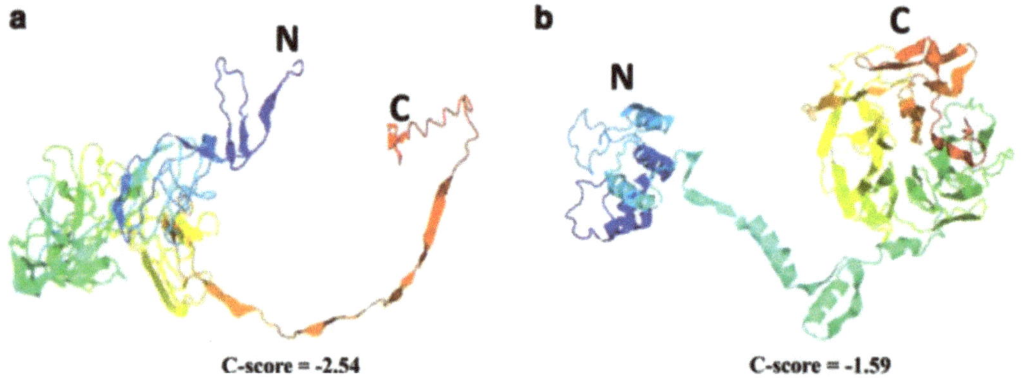

Fig. 15.4 Energy-minimized models of full-length DMP1: the I-TASSER (Iterative Threading ASSEmbly Refinement) server was used for DMP1 3D structure prediction (NP_004398.1). The program uses ab initio modeling as well as the LOMETS multiple threading program to retrieve proteins with similar folds from the PDB library

Model a shows a "globular" N-terminus with an "extended arm" at the C-terminus. However, Model b with a lower free-energy shows that the C-terminus had the propensity to fold into beta sheets, while the N-terminus remained globular.

15.4 Discussion

The constituents of the extracellular matrix of bone and dentin are responsible for modulating nucleation of apatite nanoparticles and their growth into micrometer-sized crystals. The organic matrix mainly consists of type I collagen which forms the template that directs ordered deposition of mineral crystals. The rest of the components of the organic matrix consist of noncollagenous proteins, lipids, and proteoglycans. Each of these classes of macromolecules play decisive roles in the controlled growth of HAP on the collagen matrix.

In this study, we used the demineralized and deproteinized dentin slice as a template to demonstrate the role of extracellular dentin matrix protein 1, a member of the noncollagenous class of proteins in calcified tissues. The processed dentin slice contains fibrillar cross-linked collagen arranged in a three-dimensional supramolecular architecture.

We first showed the spatial localization of DMP1 on the demineralized collagen matrix. Demineralization was able to expose the epitope site for the antibody to bind to DMP1. Gold particles were specifically localized on the collagen fibril. As DMP1 is a calcium-binding protein, there is a good possibility that some might be removed from the dentin matrix during the process of demineralization. Specific localization of DMP1 on the collagen template suggests that initiation of mineral deposition would be site specific.

In vitro nucleation experiments conducted on the dentin wafer adsorbed with DMP1 show abundant Ca-P deposits around the dentinal tubule. Higher magnification of the deposits shows that nucleation is not a random event, but the process is initiated in spatially distinct nucleation sites. Closer inspection shows that the nanocrystals are deposited as bundles of mineral structures in a highly organized manner with their c-axis oriented nearly parallel to the collagen fibrils. The nanocrystalline deposits had nearly similar length and widths suggesting that the self-assembled collagen fibrils could dictate the morphology and growth of the mineral deposits. The mineral structures were characterized as nanocrystalline HAP. McNally et al. also reported the presence of similar rigid hydroxyapatite struts encased in the collagen matrix of the human femoral bone (McNally et al. 2012). In a new model for the ultrastructure of bone based on TEM analysis, Schwarcz reports the presence of stacks of mineral lamellae packed around the fibrils and that the lamellae are spaced less than 1 nm apart (Schwarcz 2015). Similar ultrastructure of the mineral phase was observed in this study.

With the use of molecular modeling, we have demonstrated that DMP1 contains a flexible loop between the C- and N-termini where the proteolytic cleavage site resides. The stringent model (Fig. 15.4b) showed that C-DMP1 had the propensity to form beta sheets. This could be envisaged as DMP1 in the presence of calcium adopts a beta sheet structure (He et al. 2003). We have shown that the C-terminal portion of DMP1 is highly acidic due to abundant glutamic acid residues along with serines which could be phosphorylated, thereby increasing the negative charge (He et al. 2005). We have also demonstrated that intermolecular assembly of the peptides at the C-terminus in the presence of calcium ions was important to form a stereospecific template for hydroxyapatite nucleation. It is possible that the nanocrystalline hydroxyapatite fibrillar deposits observed in this study could be dependent on the beta sheet conformation of C-DMP1 and the confined gap regions present in the three-dimensional supramolecular architecture of self-assembled type I collagen.

Overall, this study demonstrates that biomineralization is a complex cell-mediated process and the DMP1 has an intimate relationship with the collagen matrix. Such an interaction dictates the site-specific nucleation of Ca-P nanocrystalline hydroxyapatite. Subsequently, other proteins in the ECM might be responsible for crystal fusion and controlled growth of the initially nucleated crystals.

Acknowledgments This work was supported by National Institutes of Health Grant DE 11657 and the Brodie Endowment Fund (AG). "This work made use of instruments in the Electron Microscopy Service (Research Resources Center, UIC."

References

Addadi L, Weiner S, Geva M (2001) On how proteins interact with crystals and their effect on crystal formation. Z Kardiol 90(3):92–98

Bedran-Russo AK, Ravindran S, George (2013) A imaging analysis of early DMP1 mediated dentine remineralization. Arch Oral Biol 58:254–260

George A, Sabsay B, Simonian PA, Veis A (1993) Characterization of a novel dentin matrix acidic phosphoprotein. Implications for induction of biomineralization. J Biol Chem 268:12624–12630

George A, Gui J, Jenkins NA, Gilbert DJ, Copeland NG, Veis A (1994) In situ localization and chromosomal mapping of the AG1 (Dmp1) gene. J Histochem Cytochem 42:1527–1531

George A, Silberstein R, Veis A (1995) In situ hybridization shows Dmp1 (AG1) to be a developmentally regulated dentin-specific protein produced by mature odontoblasts. Connect Tissue Res 33:67–72

Goldberg M, Smith AJ (2004) Cells and extracellular matrices of dentin and pulp: a biological basis for repair and tissue engineering. Crit Rev Oral Biol Med 15:13–27

Grzesiak J, Smieszek A, Marycz K (2017) Ultrastructural changes during osteogenic differentiation in mesenchymal stromal cells cultured in alginate hydrogel. Cell Biosci 7:2

He G, George A (2004) Dentin matrix protein 1 immobilized on type I collagen fibrils facilitates apatite deposition in vitro. J Biol Chem 279:11649–11656

He G, Dahl T, Veis A, George A (2003) Dentin matrix protein 1 initiates hydroxyapatite formation in vitro. Connect Tissue Res 44(1):240–245

He G, Gajjeraman S, Schultz D, Cookson D, Qin C, Butler WT, Hao J, George A (2005) Spatially and temporally controlled biomineralization is facilitated by interaction between self-assembled dentin matrix protein 1 and calcium phosphate nuclei in solution. Biochemistry 44:16140–11614

Hirata I, Nomura Y, Tabata H, Miake Y, Yanagisawa T, Okazaki M (2005) SEM observation of collagen fibrils secreted from the body surface of osteoblasts on a CO3apatite-collagen sponge. Dent Mater J 24:460–464

Kang H, Shih YR, Varghese S (2015) Biomineralized matrices dominate soluble cues to direct osteogenic differentiation of human mesenchymal stem cells through adenosine signaling. Biomacromolecules 16:1050–1061

McNally EA, Schwarcz HP, Botton GA, Arsenault AL (2012) A model for the ultrastructure of bone based on electron microscopy of ion-milled sections. PLoS One 7:e29258

Padovano JD, Ravindran S, Snee PT, Ramachandran A, Bedran-Russo AK, George A (2015) DMP1-derived peptides promote remineralization of human dentin. J Dent Res 94:608–614

Ravindran S, George A (2014) Multifunctional ECM proteins in bone and teeth. Exp Cell Res 325:148–154

Roy A, Kucukural A, Zhang Y (2010) I-TASSER: a unified platform for automated protein structure and function prediction. Nat Protoc 5:725–738

Schwarcz HP (2015) The ultrastructure of bone as revealed in electron microscopy of ion-milled sections. Semin Cell Dev Biol 46:44–50
Srinivasan R, Chen B, Gorski JP, George A (1999) Recombinant expression and characterization of dentin matrix protein 1. Connect Tissue Res 40:251–258
Veis A (1993) Mineral-matrix interactions in bone and dentin. J Bone Miner Res 8(2):S493–S497
Veis A, Dorvee JR (2013) Biomineralization mechanisms: a new paradigm for crystal nucleation in organic matrices. Calcif Tissue Int 93:307–315
Yang J, Zhang Y (2015a) I-TASSER server: new development for protein structure and function predictions. Nucleic Acids Res 43:W174–W181
Yang J, Zhang Y (2015b) Protein structure and function prediction using I-TASSER. Curr Protoc Bioinformatics 52 5(8):1–15
Yang J, Yan R, Roy A, Xu D, Poisson J, Zhang Y (2015) The I-TASSER suite: protein structure and function prediction. Nat Methods 12:7–8
Zhang Y (2009) I-TASSER: fully automated protein structure prediction in CASP8. Proteins 77(9):100–113

Chapter 16
Exploration of Genes Associated with Sponge Silicon Biomineralization in the Whole Genome Sequence of the Hexactinellid *Euplectella curvistellata*

Katsuhiko Shimizu, Hiroki Kobayashi, Michika Nishi, Masatoshi Tsukahara, Tomohiro Bito, and Jiro Arima

Abstract Silicatein is the first protein isolated from the silicon biominerals and characterized as constituent of the axial filament in the silica spicules of the demosponge *Tethya aurantia*, by significant sequence similarity with cathepsin L, an animal lysosomal protease, and as a catalyst of silica polycondensation at neutral pH and room temperature. This protein was then identified in a wide range of the class Demospongiae and in some species of the class Hexactinellida. Our attempt to isolate silicatein from the silica skeleton of *Euplectella* was unsuccessful, but instead we discovered glassin, a protein directing acceleration of silica polycondensation and sharing no significant relationship with any proteins including silicatein. The present study aims to verify the existence of silicatein by exploring the whole genome DNA sequence database of *E. curvistellata* with the sequence similarity search. Although we identified the sequences of glassin, cathepsin L and chitin synthetase, an enzyme synthesizing chitin, which has already been found in the silicon biominer-

K. Shimizu (✉)
Platform for Community-Based Research and Education, Tottori University, Tottori, Japan
e-mail: kshimizu@tottori-u.ac.jp

H. Kobayashi
The United Graduate School of Agricultural Sciences, Tottori University, Tottori, Japan

M. Nishi
Faculty of Agriculture, Tottori University, Tottori, Japan
e-mail: B14A3142U@edu.tottori-u.ac.jp

M. Tsukahara
BioJet Ltd, Uruma, Okinawa, Japan
e-mail: tsuka@biojet.jp

T. Bito · J. Arima
Faculty of Agriculture, Tottori University, Tottori, Japan
e-mail: bito@muses.tottori-u.ac.jp; arima@muses.tottori-u.ac.jp

K. Endo et al. (eds.), *Biomineralization*,
https://doi.org/10.1007/978-981-13-1002-7_16

als in *E. aspergillum*, silicatein failed to be identified. Our result indicates that silicatein is not essential for poriferan silicon biomineralization in the presence of glassin.

Keywords biosilicification · Silica · Silicatein · Glassin · Chitin

16.1 Introduction

Silicon biominerals are produced by the living organisms through physiological activities in contrast to silicon-based manmade products, often manufactured through processes with high energy consumption and harsh impacts on the environment. Understanding of the mechanisms on silicon biomineralization is expected to offer the prospect of developing environmentally benign routes to synthesize silicon-based materials. Silicon biominerals generally contain a small amount of organic substances, which may help production of silicon biominerals at physiological conditions.

Phylum Porifera (sponges) consists of four classes, Hexactinellida (glass sponges), Demospongiae (demosponges), Calcarea (calcareous sponges), and Homoscleromorpha, among which Hexactinellida, Demospongiae, and Homoscleromorpha produce silica biominerals while calcium carbonate biominerals occur in Calcarea.

The demosponge *Tethya aurantia* produces a large quantity of silicon biomineral in a form of silica as needlelike structures or spicules, allowing us to isolate and analyze the organic molecules occluded in the biomineral. Silicatein, the first protein isolated from silicon biomineral and characterized, constitutes the axial filament in the spicules; shares significant sequence similarity with cathepsin L, an animal lysosomal protease; and catalyzes silica polycondensation at neutral pH and room temperature (Shimizu et al. 1998; Cha et al. 1999). This protein and its gene were then identified in a wide range of the class Demospongiae (Krasko et al. 2000; Pozzolini et al. 2004; Funayama et al. 2005; Müller et al. 2007). In addition, PCR products encoding a partial silicatein sequences were amplified in the class Hexactinellida including *Crateromorpha meyeri* (Müller et al. 2008a), *Monorhaphis chuni* (Müller et al. 2008b), and *Euplectella aspergillum* (unpublished data. The sequence was deposited to GenBank database by Müller et al. in 2011. The accession number FR748156). Our attempt to isolate silicatein from the silica skeleton of the *E. aspergillum* and *E. curvistellata* was unsuccessful, but instead we discovered glassin as a protein directing acceleration of silica polycondensation (Shimizu et al. 2015). Sequences encoding silicatein have not identified from the transcriptome analysis of *Aphrocallistes vastus* by Riesgo et al. (2015). Veremeichik et al. (2011) tried to isolate silicatein genes from *Pheronema raphanus*, *Aulosaccus schulzei*, and *Bathydorus levis*, resulting in only identification of *Aulosaccus* sp. silicatein-like sequence with cysteine at the catalytic residue instead of serine as seen in silicateins of other species. Collectively, the existence of silicateins has been unsettled in Hexactinellida.

The present study aims to verify the existence of genetic information on silicatein by exploring the whole genome DNA sequence database of *E. curvistellata* with the sequence similarity search and discusses on relationship of silicatein and glassin in silicon biomineralization of Porifera.

16.2 Materials and Methods

Live specimens of *E. curvistellata* were collected at a depth of 236 m at 32°30 N, 129°10 E in the East China Sea on March 4, 2012, as described previously (Shimizu et al. 2015) and then stored in ethanol at −20 °C. Genomic DNA was extracted from the specimen stored in ethanol with DNeasy Blood & Tissue Kit (QIAGEN, Hilden, Germany). The genomic DNA library was prepared from mechanically fragmented genomic DNA with TruSeq DNA prep kit (Illumina, San Diego, CA, USA). Then, the library was sequenced with MiSeq (Illumina) three times. The raw reads were trimmed and assembled using Genomics Workbench (CLC Bio Inc., Aarhus, Denmark). Sequence similarities were analyzed with NCBI BLAST program.

16.3 Results and Discussion

16.3.1 Construction of Whole Genome DNA Library of E. curvistellata

The library of *E. curvistellata* whole genome DNA was constructed with the next-generation DNA sequencer. Total three runs of sequencing gave rise to 27,939,250 reads, being assembled to 442,583 contigs with the average length of 427 and the median length of 420 (Table 16.1). The longest contig covers 145,960 while the shortest is 18 nucleotides. Total number of the nucleotides reached to 190,209,345. This number can be roughly considered as a genome size of the species, with fairly matching to that of *Amphimedon queenslandica*, being 167 Mbp (Srivastava et al. 2010).

To evaluate the quality of the library, we run the blast program with *Aphrocallistes vastus* Cox3 gene (GenBank accession no. EU000309.1) (Rosengarten et al. 2008) as a query. As a result, we obtained the single contig_1075 containing not only Cox3 gene but also the whole mitochondrion DNA sequence, 19,700 bp. This result indicates that the library is qualitatively sound and can be useful for gene searching.

Table 16.1 Summary of whole genome sequencing and assembly

Reads	Number of contigs	Maximum contig (base)	Minimum contig (base)	N50 (base)	Average length (base)	Total length (base)
27,939,250	442,583	145,960	18	420	427	190,209,345

16.3.2 Search for Silicatein Gene

The axial filament was obtained in the intact form by dissolving the silica spicules of *T. aurantia* (Shimizu et al. 1998). Although the axial filament was observed in the cross section of *Euplectella* silica spicules under the scanning electron microscope (Weaver et al. 2007), the axial filaments or any filamentous materials were not obtained in our attempt. The extract contained proteins, but these proteins had no silicatein sequences as long as we examined. On the other hand, a partial silicatein cDNA from *E. aspergillum* was archived in DNA sequence database (FR748156) (Table 16.2). In addition, silicateins or silicatein-like sequences have been reported from the hexactinellid sponges *Aulosaccus* sp. (Veremeichik et al. 2011), *C. meyeri* (Müller et al. 2008a), and *M. chuni* (Müller et al. 2008b).

To verify the silicatein sequence in *E. curvistellata* genome, the local blast program was executed with these hexactinellid silicatein sequences as well as *T. aurantia* silicateins as queries and *E. curvistellata* genomic DNA library as a database. For the partial silicatein cDNA from *E. aspergillum*, no contig with E values less than 10 was hit. Similarly, no hit was obtained when *T. aurantia* silicateins α (AF032117) and β (AF098670), *Aulosaccus* sp. silicatein-like (ACU86976), *C. meyeri* silicatein (CAP49202), and *M. chuni* silicatein (CAZ04880) were used as queries.

The amino acid sequence KNSWG was widely conserved in silicateins and cathepsin L; 296–300 of *T. aurantia* silicatein α (Shimizu et al. 1998, AF032117), 296–300 of *Suberites domuncula* silicatein (Krasko et al. 2000, AJ272013), 292–

Table 16.2 Identification of the genes related to hexactinellid biosilica

Protein	Previous description	*E. curvistellata* genome search
Silicatein	*C. meyeri* (Müller et al. 2008a; CAP49202) *M. chuni* (Müller et al. 2008b; CAZ04880) *E. aspergillum* (Müller et al. 2011; FR748156) No silicatein gene in *A. vastus* (Riesgo et al. 2015)	No hit with queries as follows: *E. aspergillum* (Müller et al. 2011; FR748156) *T. aurantia* silicateins α and β (Shimizu et al. 1998; AF032117, and AF098670, respectively) *Aulosaccus* sp. silicatein-like (Veremeichik et al. 2011; ACU86976) *C. meyeri* (Müller et al. 2008a; CAP49202) *M. chuni* (Müller et al. 2008b; CAZ04880)
Cathepsin L	The gene identified in *A. vastus* transcriptome data (Riesgo et al. 2015)	1343 bp (324 AAs) composed of four exons in contig_50860 (306 bp) and contig_7,117 (8869 bp)
Glassin	A protein occluded in spicules of *Euplectella* (Shimizu et al. 2015)	1638 bp (546 AAs) in contig_14,569 (2400 bp) and contig_22,997 (1331 bp)
Chitin	Fluorescent dye staining, X-ray diffraction, chemical analysis (Ehrlich and Worch 2007)	Chitin synthase gene 4335 bp ORF (1445 AAs) in contig_18,557 (12,682bp)

296 of *S. domuncula* cathepsin L (Müller et al. 2003, AJ784224), and 299–303 human cathepsin L (Gal and Gottesman 1988, X12451). In the case of this sequence used as a query, contig_7,117 (8869 bp) was hit. The contig contains the stop codon, but not the first Met. The 5′ region, contig_50860, was obtained by running blast program with the contig_7,117 as a query. Total length of the coding region is 1343 bp composed of 4 exons coding 324 amino acid residues and 3 introns. The predicted protein sequence is more similar to those of sponge and human cathepsin L than silicateins. In addition, cysteine at the position corresponding to the catalytic residue and the surrounding sequences in cathepsin L are conserved in the contig, indicating that the gene encodes cathepsin L but not silicatein. The boundaries of all the four exons in the cathepsin L of *E. curvistellata* are identical to those of exon 2/ exon 3, exon 3/exon 4, and exon 4/exon 5 in human cathepsin L gene consists of eight exons and seven introns (Chauhan et al. 1993), suggesting that the exon-intron structure of cathepsin L in *E. curvistellata* is conserved in the human gene.

The result of our blast search for silicatein in *E. curvistellata* genome is consistent with the fact that the silicatein or silicatein-like proteins were not obtained in dissolution of silica spicules. Previous transcriptome analysis concluded that any silicatein gene was identified in the hexactinellid *A. vastus* (Riesgo et al. 2015). It is unlikely that silicatein exists in all species of the class Hexactinellida. However, further research should be performed using the hexactinellid species which have been reported to have the evidence for the existence of silicateins before the conclusion is drawn.

16.3.3 Search of Genes Associated with Silicon Biomineralization

Genes for glassin were assigned by conducting the similarity research with glassin cDNA as a query. The two contigs 14,569 and 22,997 cover 5′ and 3′ regions of glassin gene, respectively, while overlapping each other. Some mismatches were observed in the overlapped and 3′ regions, indicating the assembly in complicated sequences including the repetitive sequences is incomplete. Therefore, further refinement on the library may be required.

Ehrlich and Worch (2007) reported chitin in *E. aspergillum* as an organic component of their silicious skeletal systems. A gene encoding chitin synthase was searched using *A. queenslandica* chitin synthase2 and 3-like protein sequences (XP_011402997 and XP_003389565, respectively) as queries, and contig_18,557 (12,682 bp) containing 4335 bp open reading flame encoding 1445 amino acid residues was obtained. Our result suggests that *Euplectella* is capable of chitin synthesis and thus is consistent with previous observation on occurrence of chitin in *Euplectella*.

16.4 Conclusion

The present study aims to verify the existence of genetic information on silicatein by exploring the whole genome DNA sequence database of *E. curvistellata* with the sequence similarity search. We identified the sequences of glassin, cathepsin L and chitin synthetase, an enzyme synthesizing chitin, which has already been found in the silicon biominerals in *E. aspergillum* (Ehrlich and Worch 2007). However, silicatein failed to be identified in the genome data consistent with the previous extraction experiment (Shimizu et al. 2015). Although PCR products encoding partial silicatein sequences have been amplified in some hexactinellid sponges (Müller et al. 2008a, b), silicatein was not identified in the transcriptome analysis of *A. vastus* (Riesgo et al. 2015). Collectively, the existence of silicatein is not evident in Hexactinellid. At least, silicatein is not essential and glassin is responsible for silicon biomineralization in *E. curvistellata*. Therefore, the evidences imply that there are at least two ways for silicon biomineralization in Porifera in terms of usage of the protein for silica polymerization, silicatein or glassin, and that the selection of either protein depends on the species but not on the taxonomic classes.

Acknowledgment This work is supported by JSPS Kakenhi grant number 15 K06581.

References

Cha JN, Shimizu K, Zhou Y, Christiansen SC, Chmelka BF, Stucky GD, Morse DE (1999) Silicatein filaments and subunits from a marine sponge direct the polymerization of silica and silicones in vitro. PNAS 96:361–365

Chauhan SS, Popescu NC, Ray D, Fleischmann R, Gottesman MM, Troen BR (1993) Cloning, genomic organization, and chromosomal localization of human cathepsin L. J Biol Chem 268:1039–1045

Ehrlich H, Worch H (2007) Sponges as natural composites: from biomimetic potential to development of new biomaterials. In: Hajdu E (ed) Porifera research: biodiversity, innovation & sustainability, vol 28. Museu Nacional, Rio de Janeiro, pp 217–223

Funayama N, Nakatsukasa M, Kuraku S, Takechi K, Dohi M, Iwabe N, Miyata T, Agata K (2005) Isolation of Ef silicatein and Ef lectin as molecular markers of sclerocytes and cells involved in innate immunity in the freshwater sponge Ephydatia fluviatilis. Zool Sci 22:1113–1122

Gal S, Gottesman MM (1988) Isolation and sequence of a cDNA for human pro-(cathepsin L). Biochem J 253:303–306

Krasko A, Lorenz B, Batel R, Schröder HC, Müller IM, Müller WEG (2000) Expression of silicatein and collagen genes in the marine sponge Suberites domuncula is controlled by silicate and myotrophin. Eur J Biochem 267:4878–4887

Müller WEG, Krasko A, Le Pennec G, Schröder HC (2003) Biochemistry and cell biology of silica formation in sponges. Microsc Res Tech 62:368–377

Müller WEG, Schloßmacher U, Eckert C, Krasko A, Boreiko A, Ushijima H, Wolf SE, Tremel W, Müller IM, Schröder HC (2007) Analysis of the axial filament in spicules of the demosponge Geodia cydonium: different silicatein composition in microscleres (asters) and megascleres (oxeas and triaenes). Eur J Cell Biol 86:473–487

Müller WEG, Wang X, Kropf K, Boreiko A, Schloßmacher U, Brandt D, Schröder HC, Wiens M (2008a) Silicatein expression in the hexactinellid Crateromorpha meyeri: the lead marker gene restricted to siliceous sponges. Cell Tissue Res 333:339–351

Müller WEG, Boreiko A, Schloßmacher U, Wang X, Eckert C, Kropf K, Li J, Schröder HC (2008b) Identification of a silicatein (-related) protease in the giant spicules of the deep-sea hexactinellid Monorhaphis chuni. J Exp Biol 211:300–309

Pozzolini M, Sturla L, Cerrano C, Bavestrello G, Camardella L, Parodi AM, Raheli F, Benatti U, Müller WEG, Giovine M (2004) Molecular cloning of silicatein gene from marine sponge Petrosia ficiformis (Porifera, Demospongiae) and development of primmorphs as a model for biosilicification studies. Mar Biotechnol 6:594–603

Riesgo A, Maldonado M, López-Legentil S, Giribet G (2015) A proposal for the evolution of Cathepsin and Silicatein in sponges. J Mol Evol 80:278–291

Rosengarten RD, Sperling EA, Moreno MA, Leys SP, Dellaporta SL (2008) The mitochondrial genome of the hexactinellid sponge Aphrocallistes vastus: evidence for programmed translational frameshifting. J BMC Genomics 9(33)

Shimizu K, Cha J, Stucky GD, Morse DE (1998) Silicatein alpha: Cathepsin L-like protein in sponge biosilica. Proc Natl Acad Sci U S A 95:6234–6238

Shimizu K, Amano T, Bari Md R, Weaver JC, Arima J, Mori N (2015) Glassin, a histidine-rich protein from the silicious skeletal system of the marine sponge Euplectella directs silica polycondensation. Proc Nat Acad Sci USA 112:11449–11454

Srivastava M, Simakov O, Chapman J, Fahey B, Gauthier MEA, Mitros T, Richards GS, Conaco C, Dacre M, Hellsten U et al (2010) The Amphimedon queenslandica genome and the evolution of animal complexity. Nature 466:720–726

Veremeichik GN, Shkryl YN, Bulgakov VP, Shedko SV, Kozhemyako VB, Kovalchuk SN, Krasokhin VB, Zhuravlev YN, Kulchin YN (2011) Occurrence of a silicatein gene in glass sponges (Hexactinellida: Porifera). Mar Biotechnol 13:810–819

Weaver JC, Aizenberg J, Fantner GE, Kisailus D, Woesz A, Allen P, Fields K, Porter MJ, Zok FW, Hansma PK, Fratzl P, Morse DE (2007) Hierarchical assembly of the siliceous skeletal lattice of the hexactinellid sponge Euplectella aspergillum. J Struct Biol 158:93–106

Part III
Genome-Based Analysis of Biomineralization

Chapter 17
The Origin and Early Evolution of SCPP Genes and Tissue Mineralization in Vertebrates

Kazuhiko Kawasaki

Abstract Various secretory calcium-binding phosphoprotein (SCPP) genes are involved in the formation of the bone, dentin, enamel, and enameloid in bony vertebrates. By contrast, no SCPP gene is found in cartilaginous vertebrates. In order to explain this difference, I investigated the origin and early evolution of SCPP genes. First, I examined the phylogeny of *SPARC*-family genes that include evolutionary precursors of SCPP genes. Then, I analyzed the genomic arrangement of the SCPP genes and three *SPARC*-family genes, *SPARCL1*, *SPARCL1L1*, and *SPARCR1*. The results are consistent with our previous hypothesis that an SCPP gene-like structure arose in the 5′ half of *SPARCL1L1* in a common ancestor of jawed vertebrates, at about the same time as the origin of mineralized skeleton. It is possible that cartilaginous vertebrates secondarily lost early SCPP genes, while bony vertebrates gained various new SCPP genes. Some of these new SCPP genes appear to have specifically involved in scale formation; however, these scale genes were lost in tetrapods.

Keywords SCPP genes · SPARC gene family · Mineralized skeleton · Bony vertebrates · Cartilaginous vertebrates · Jawed vertebrates · Scale formation · Gene duplication · Genome duplication · Vertebrate evolution

17.1 Introduction

Among cardinal traits evolved in vertebrates is mineralized skeleton, which arose in a common ancestor of jawed vertebrates after the divergence of the lineage leading to modern jawless vertebrates (Fig. 17.1) (Donoghue and Sansom 2002). The bone, dentin, enamel, and enameloid are principal mineralized skeletal tissues (Donoghue and Sansom 2002). Among these tissues, the bone was secondarily lost in cartilaginous vertebrates (Eames et al. 2007), and enamel is thought to have originated in bony vertebrates (Schultze 2016).

K. Kawasaki (✉)
Department of Anthropology, Pennsylvania State University, University Park, PA, USA
e-mail: kuk2@psu.edu

K. Endo et al. (eds.), *Biomineralization*,
https://doi.org/10.1007/978-981-13-1002-7_17

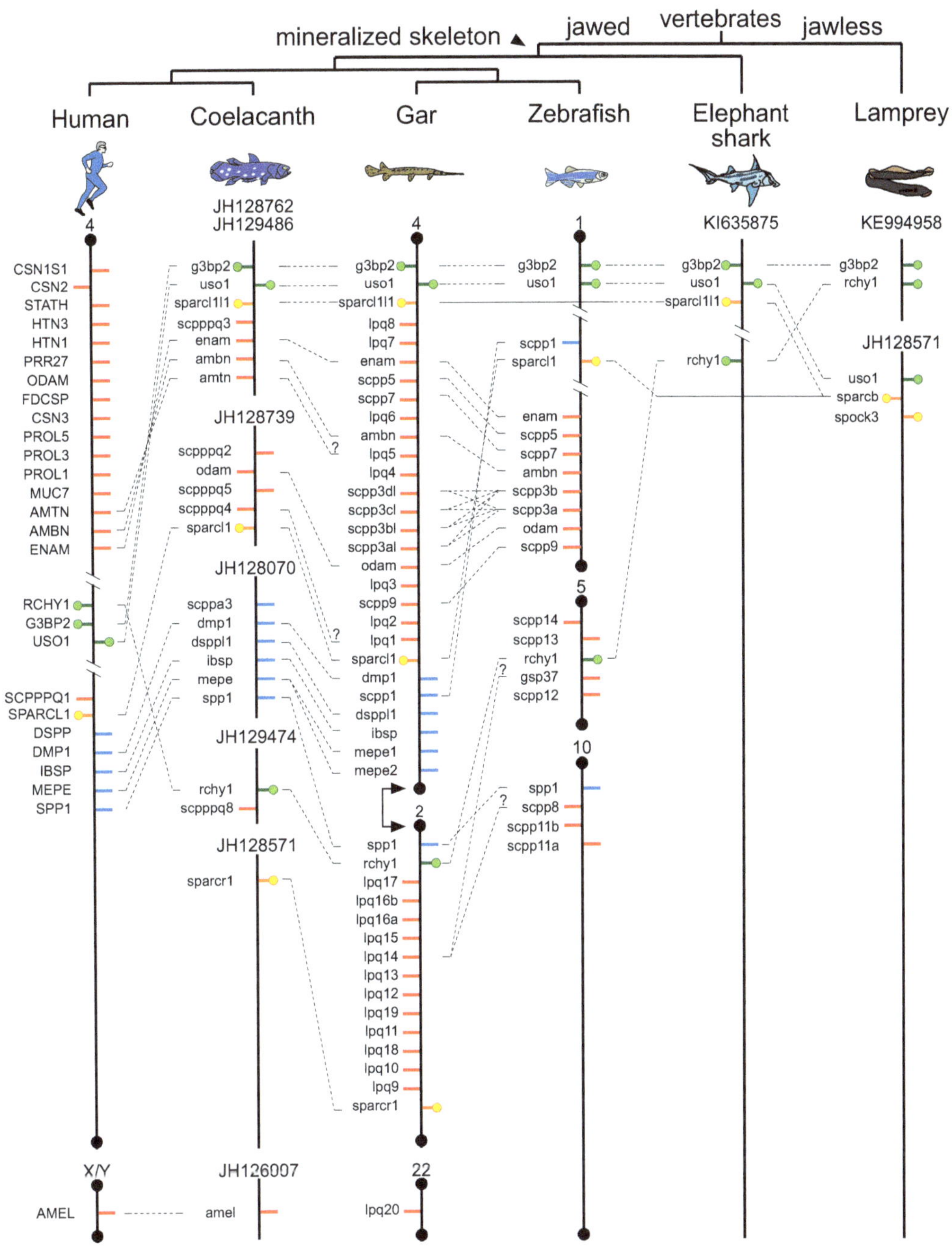

Fig. 17.1 The arrangement of SCPP genes, *SPARC* family genes, *USO1*, *G3BP2*, and *RCHY1* in the human, coelacanth, gar, zebrafish, elephant shark, and lamprey genomes. The phylogeny of these vertebrates and the origin of mineralized skeleton are shown on the top. Vertical bars represent chromosomes or contigs (names on the top). Regions separated by >200 kilobases are shown by double slashes. Horizontal bars represent P/Q-rich SCPP genes (red), acidic SCPP genes (blue), *SPARC*-family genes (yellow, circled), and other genes (green, circled). Genes with different transcriptional directions are shown on different sides (right, plus strand; left, minus strand). Orthologs are connected with a dashed line (a question mark represents unconfirmed orthologs). See Kawasaki et al. (2017) for more details, including lamprey *spock3*

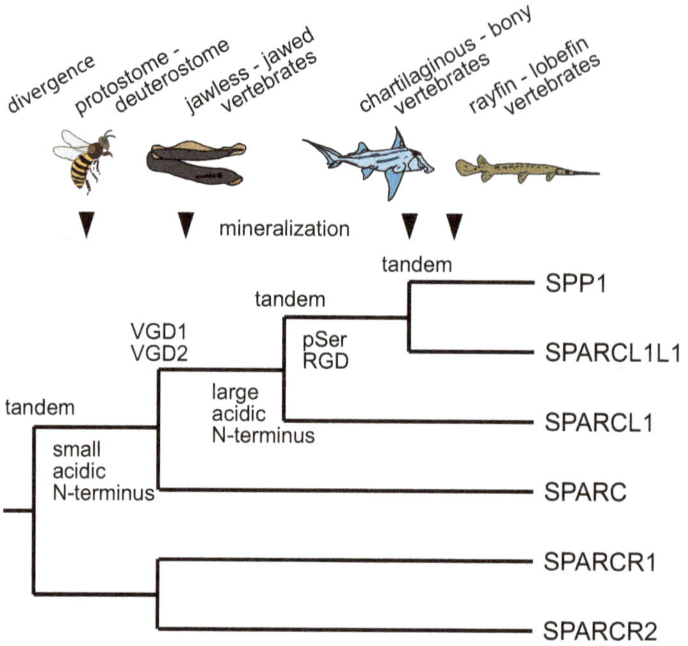

Fig. 17.2 Duplication history of *SPARC*-family genes and *SPP1*. Correlations of gene duplications (tandem or VGD1/VGD2), the divergence of animal clades (arrowhead), and the origin of skeletal mineralization are shown on the top (not in scale). Newly evolved characteristics are shown under the stem

In bony vertebrates, formation of mineralized tissues involves various secretory calcium-binding phosphoprotein (SCPP) genes, which arose by gene duplication and form gene clusters (Fig. 17.1) (Kawasaki and Weiss 2003). Two types of SCPP genes are known; one encodes acidic SCPPs and the other Pro and Glu (P/Q)-rich SCPPs. Most acidic SCPP genes are employed in the formation of the bone and/or dentin, whereas many P/Q-rich SCPP genes are expressed during the enamel and/or enameloid formation (Kawasaki 2011). In contrast to bony vertebrates, no SCPP gene is found in the genomes of cartilaginous vertebrates (Venkatesh et al. 2014). In order to explain this difference, I investigated the origin and early evolution of SCPP genes.

SCPP genes evolve rapidly, but all SCPP genes retain a characteristic exon-intron structure, which allows us to identify SCPP genes without relying on sequence similarities (Kawasaki and Weiss 2003). This characteristic exon-intron structure is also found in the 5′ half of the *SPARC*-like 1 (*SPARCL1*) and *SPARCL1*-like 1 (*SPARCL1L1*), both located adjacent to SCPP genes in the genomes of coelacanth and gar (Fig. 17.1) (Kawasaki et al. 2004, 2017). Moreover, the 5′ half of elephant shark *sparcl1l1* is highly similar to *SPP1* and other acidic SCPP genes, encoding an extremely acidic sequence, a cluster of Ser-Xaa-Glu (Xaa represents any amino acids, and the Ser residue is thought to be phosphorylated) near the N-terminus, and one or more Arg-Gly-Asp (RGD) integrin-binding sequences (Fig. 17.2). Based on these findings, we proposed that SCPP genes arose from the 5′ half of *SPARCL1L1* (Kawasaki et al. 2017).

The 3′ half of *SPARCL1* and *SPARCL1L1* encodes evolutionarily conserved amino acid sequences, known as the follistatin-like (FS) domain and the extracellular calcium-binding EF-hand (EC) motif (Bradshaw 2012). Genes encoding the

FS domain and the EC motif constitute the *SPARC* gene family, which includes *SPARC*, *SPARCL1*, *SPARCL1L1*, and two *SPARC*-related genes, *SPARCR1* and *SPARCR2* (Kawasaki et al. 2017). Previous studies suggested the duplication history of these genes (Fig. 17.2) (Bertrand et al. 2013; Torres-Núñez et al. 2015; Kawasaki et al. 2017). A tandem duplication split the *SPARC* and *SPARCR* lineages before the divergence of protostomes and deuterostomes. In the *SPARC* lineage, *SPARC* and the common ancestor of *SPARCL1* and *SPARCL1L1* arose in two vertebrate genome duplications (VGD1/VGD2) (Ohno 1970), thought to have occurred in the common ancestor of jawless vertebrates and jawed vertebrates (Kuraku et al. 2009). In the *SPARCR* lineage, *SPARCR1* and *SPARCR2* originated also in VGD1/VGD2. *SPARCL1* and *SPARCL1L1* arose subsequently by tandem duplication in the common ancestor of cartilaginous vertebrates and bony vertebrates (Fig. 17.2).

Duplicated *SPARC* family genes appear to have differentiated asymmetrically; while one duplicate maintained ancient characteristics, the other duplicate obtained new characteristics. The new characteristics, encoded by the differentiated genes, include a small N-terminal acidic domain arisen early in the *SPARC* lineage, a large N-terminal acidic domain in the common ancestor of *SPARCL1* and *SPARCL1L1*, and a cluster of phospho-Ser (pSer) residues in the N-terminus and an RGD integrin-binding sequence in *SPARCL1L1* (Fig. 17.2) (Kawasaki et al. 2017). We hypothesized that the most derived characteristics arose in *SPARCL1L1* evolved into *SPP*1 and other acidic SCPP genes (Fig. 17.2). This hypothesis infers that an *SPP1*-like structure originated in the common ancestor of jawed vertebrates, at about the same time as the origin of skeletal mineralization (Fig. 17.2) (Kawasaki et al. 2017). In the present study, I reexamined this hypothesis and analyzed the genomic arrangement of SCPP genes and their adjacent genes.

17.2 Materials and Methods

In the present study, four genes were added to our previous analysis (Kawasaki et al. 2017). These genes are *sparcl1* in the whale shark and Asian arowana (GenBank XM_020510428.1 and XM_018735764.1, respectively) and *sparc* in the Pacific hagfish and gray bichir (reconstructed from GenBank SRX2541845 and SRX796491, respectively). Amino acid sequences of the FS domain and the EC motif, deduced from the nucleotide sequences, were used to construct a maximum likelihood (ML) tree and a Bayesian inference (BI) tree, as described previously (Kawasaki et al. 2017). I considered 95% or higher bootstrap values in the ML tree and 95% or higher posterior probabilities in the BI tree as statistically significant.

17.3 Results and Discussion

17.3.1 Phylogenetic Analysis

Among the newly analyzed genes, the whale shark gene, annotated as "*sparcl1*," was clustered with elephant shark *sparcl1l1* (100% in the BI tree; Fig. 17.3). Elephant shark *sparcl1l1* is characterized by a large exon, which encodes a highly acidic sequence and is flanked by a phase-0 intron at the 5′ border and a phase-1 intron at the 3′ border (Kawasaki et al. 2017). A similar large exon was also identified in this whale shark gene (649–1243 nucleotides of XM_020510428.1), but not known from any other *SPARC* family genes. Based on these findings, I consider this whale shark gene as the *SPARCL1L1* ortholog. Unfortunately, exons 1, 2, 3, and the 5′ end of exon 4 of whale shark *sparcl1l*1 were not identified, and details of these exons remain to be elucidated.

Similar to our previous analysis (Kawasaki et al. 2017), *SPARC* genes in all jawed vertebrates formed a single cluster (95% and 100% in the ML and BI trees, respectively), whereas the phylogeny between *SPARCL1L1* in cartilaginous vertebrates, *SPARCL1L1* in bony vertebrates, and *SPARCL1* in bony vertebrates was not resolved by significant statistical supports (Fig. 17.3). This result suggests a close phylogenetic relationship of *SPARCL1* and *SPARCL1L1*.

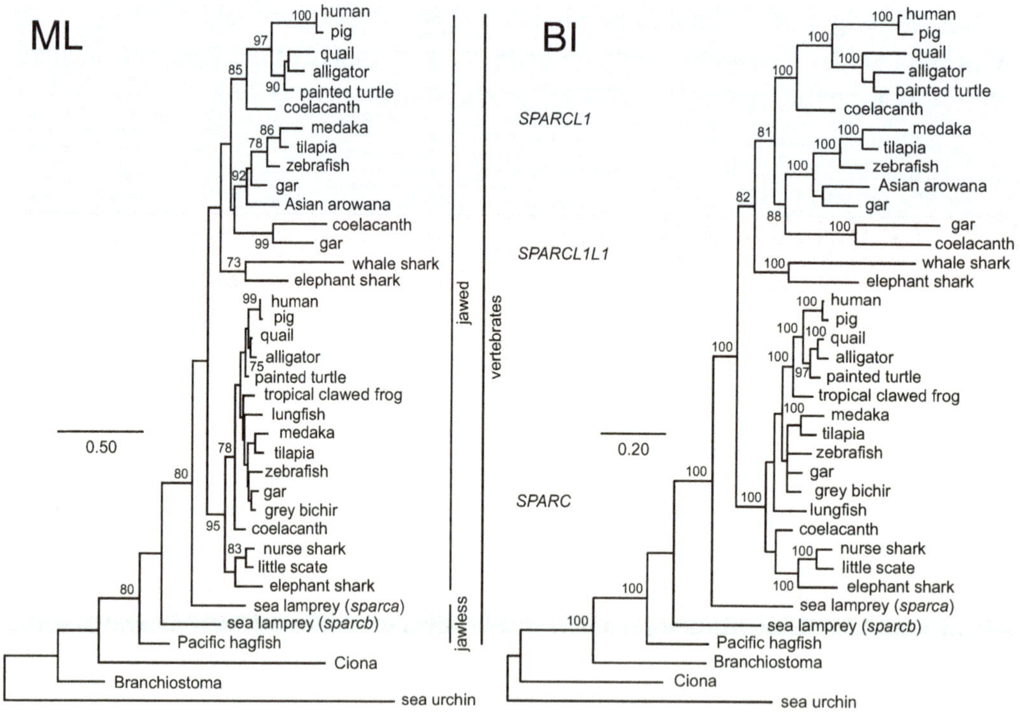

Fig. 17.3 Phylogenetic trees constructed by the ML and BI methods. Different colors show *SPARC*, *SPARCL1*, *SPARCL1L1*, and *sparcb*. Non-vertebrate *SPARC* genes are the common ancestor of *SPARC*, *SPARCL1*, and *SPARCL1L1*. Bootstrap values of >70% in the ML tree, and posterior probabilities of >80% in the BI tree are shown at the node. Vertical bars indicate genes in jawed and jawless vertebrates. Horizontal bars represent scales

In the present study, I used three jawless vertebrate genes, *sparca* and *sparcb* in lampreys and a hagfish gene. I tentatively call this hagfish gene *sparc*, because this gene encodes a small N-terminal acidic domain (71 residues), similar to *SPARC* in jawed vertebrates (Kawasaki et al. 2004). In the BI tree, *SPARC*, *SPARCL1*, and *SPARCL1L1* in all jawed vertebrates formed a cluster (100%), and this cluster was most closely related to *sparca* (100%; Fig. 17.3), which is thought to be orthologous to *SPARC* (Kawasaki et al. 2017). However, the ML tree did not well support this relationship and did not resolve the phylogeny of these genes, *sparcb*, and hagfish *sparc* (80% or less; Fig. 17.3).

17.3.2 Arrangements of SCPP Genes and SPARC Family Genes in Vertebrate Genomes

In the genome of the elephant shark, gar, and coelacanth, *g3bp2*, *uso1*, and *sparcl1l1* are clustered, and their order and directions are conserved (Fig. 17.1). The arrangement of these genes suggests that the last common ancestor of jawed vertebrates had a similar cluster. In the lamprey genome, *sparcb* is located adjacent to *uso1*, which reinforces our previous hypothesis that *sparcb* is co-orthologous to *SPARCL1* and *SPARCL1L1* (Fig. 17.1) (Kawasaki et al. 2017). Unlike *SPARCL1* or *SPARCL1L1*, *sparcb* encodes a small N-terminal acidic domain, similar to *SPARC* (Kawasaki et al. 2017). This is presumably because the large N-terminal acidic domain evolved in the common ancestor of *SPARCL1* and *SPARCL1L1* in the jawed vertebrate lineage after the divergence of the lineage leading to modern jawless vertebrates (Fig. 17.2).

The phylogeny of *sparcb* as a co-ortholog of *SPARCL1* and *SPARCL1L1* is not consistent with the topology of the phylogenetic trees; *sparcb*, *SPARC* (including *sparca*), *SPARCL1*, and *SPARCL1L1* are intermingled (Fig. 17.3). The size of the encoded N-terminal acidic domain is small in *SPARC* and *sparcb* but large in *SPARCL1* and *SPARCL1L1*, suggesting an asymmetrical functional divergence of the common ancestor of *SPARCL1* and *SPARCL1L1*. The functional divergence probably led to differential sequence changes, which may partly explain the low resolution of these genes in the phylogenetic analysis.

In the gar genome, *sparcl1l1*, 18 P/Q-rich SCPP genes, *sparcl1*, and six acidic SCPP genes are clustered on chromosome 4, while *spp1*, *rchy1*, 12 P/Q-rich SCPP genes, and *sparcr1* form a cluster on chromosome 2 (Fig. 17.1). Adjacent locations of *MEPE* and *SPP1* in the human and coelacanth genomes suggest that these two large SCPP gene clusters in the gar genome were originally connected to each other (double arrow in Fig. 17.1). The original cluster was presumably composed of *sparcl1l1*, P/Q-rich SCPP genes, *sparcl1*, acidic SCPP genes, *rchy1*, P/Q-rich SCPP genes, and *sparcr1* in this order. The arrangement of the orthologs of these genes in the coelacanth genome suggests that the last common ancestor of bony vertebrates had a similar gene cluster, containing at least five acidic and three P/Q-rich SCPP genes (Fig. 17.1).

It was shown that two zebrafish SCPP gene clusters, located on chromosomes 5 and 10, originated by the teleost genome duplication (Braasch et al. 2016). The locations of *spp1* and *rchy1* in the gar and zebrafish genomes suggest that these two zebrafish SCPP gene clusters are co-orthologons of the SCPP gene cluster on gar chromosome 2 (Fig. 17.1). Twelve P/Q-rich SCPP genes are found on gar chromosome 2 and seven P/Q-rich SCPP genes on zebrafish chromosomes 5 and 10 (Fig. 17.1). By contrast, only *scpppq8* (XR_322354.2) was identified in the syntenic region in the coelacanth genome and none in the tetrapod genomes (Fig. 17.1). Among these P/Q-rich SCPP genes, the only gene investigated to date is *gsp37*, which encodes a matrix protein of the surface layer of scales (Miyabe et al. 2012). Moreover, expression of ten P/Q-rich SCPP genes on gar chromosome 2 was detected in the skin that overlies scales but not in the teeth or bone (Kawasaki et al. 2017). Interestingly, both coelacanth *scpppq8* and zebrafish *gsp37* encode similar sequence elements, including a cluster of pSer residues, a Cys residue (rare in SCPP genes), and an RGD integrin-binding sequence. These findings suggest that one or more P/Q-rich SCPP genes involved primarily in scale formation arose in the common ancestor of bony vertebrates and that these scale SCPP genes were secondarily lost in tetrapods.

In summary, the present analysis is consistent with our previous hypothesis (Kawasaki et al. 2017): an *SPP1*-like structure originated in the 5′ half of *SPARCL1L1* in a common ancestor of jawed vertebrates, roughly contemporaneous with the origin of skeletal mineralization. It is possible that early SCPP genes were secondarily lost in cartilaginous vertebrates, while common ancestors of bony vertebrates gained various acidic and P/Q-rich SCPP genes. Some of these P/Q-rich SCPP genes may have specifically involved in scale formation, but these scale genes were lost in tetrapods.

Acknowledgments I am grateful to Prof. Joan Richtsmeier at Penn State for encouragement and Prof. Hiromichi Nagasawa at the University of Tokyo for inviting me to BiominXIV. This work was made possible by the financial support from the Department of Anthropology at Penn State and from the National Institute of Health (P01HD078233).

References

Bertrand S, Fuentealba J, Aze A, Hudson C, Yasuo H, Torrejon M et al (2013) A dynamic history of gene duplications and losses characterizes the evolution of the SPARC family in eumetazoans. Proc Biol Sci 280:20122963

Braasch I, Gehrke AR, Smith JJ, Kawasaki K, Manousaki T, Pasquier J et al (2016) The spotted gar genome illuminates vertebrate evolution and facilitates human-teleost comparisons. Nat Genet 48:427–437

Bradshaw AD (2012) Diverse biological functions of the SPARC family of proteins. Int J Biochem Cell Biol 44:480–488

Donoghue PCJ, Sansom IJ (2002) Origin and early evolution of vertebrate skeletonization. Microsc Res Tech 59:352–372

Eames BF, Allen N, Young J, Kaplan A, Helms JA, Schneider RA (2007) Skeletogenesis in the swell shark *Cephaloscyllium ventriosum*. J Anat 210:542–554

Kawasaki K (2011) The SCPP gene family and the complexity of hard tissues in vertebrates. Cells Tissues Organs 194:108–112

Kawasaki K, Weiss KM (2003) Mineralized tissue and vertebrate evolution: the secretory calcium-binding phosphoprotein gene cluster. Proc Natl Acad Sci U S A 100:4060–4065

Kawasaki K, Suzuki T, Weiss KM (2004) Genetic basis for the evolution of vertebrate mineralized tissue. Proc Natl Acad Sci U S A 101:11356–11361

Kawasaki K, Mikami M, Nakatomi M, Braasch I, Batzel P, Postlethwait JH et al (2017) SCPP genes and their relatives in gar: rapid expansion of mineralization genes in osteichthyans. J Exp Zool B Mol Dev Evol 328:645–665

Kuraku S, Meyer A, Kuratani S (2009) Timing of genome duplications relative to the origin of the vertebrates: did cyclostomes diverge before or after? Mol Biol Evol 26:47–59

Miyabe K, Tokunaga H, Endo H, Inoue H, Suzuki M, Tsutsui N et al (2012) GSP-37, a novel goldfish scale matrix protein: identification, localization and functional analysis. Faraday Discuss 159:463–481

Ohno S (1970) Evolution by gene duplication. Springer, New York

Schultze HP (2016) Scales, enamel, cosmine, ganoine, and early osteichthyans. C R Palevol 15:83–102

Torres-Núñez E, Suarez-Bregua P, Cal L, Cal R, Cerdá-Reverter JM, Rotllant J (2015) Molecular cloning and characterization of the matricellular protein Sparc/osteonectin in flatfish, *Scophthalmus maximus*, and its developmental stage-dependent transcriptional regulation during metamorphosis. Gene 568:129–139

Venkatesh B, Lee AP, Ravi V, Maurya AK, Lian MM, Swann JB et al (2014) Elephant shark genome provides unique insights into gnathostome evolution. Nature 505:174–179

Part IV
Evolution in Biomineralization

Chapter 18
Immunolocalization of Enamel Matrix Protein-Like Proteins in the Tooth Enameloid of Actinopterygian Bony Fish

Ichiro Sasagawa, Shunya Oka, Masato Mikami, Hiroyuki Yokosuka, and Mikio Ishiyama

Abstract Tooth enameloid in bony fish is a well-mineralized tissue resembling enamel in mammals. It was assumed that the dental epithelial cells are deeply involved in the formation of enameloid. However, unlike enamel matrix which fully consists of several ectodermal enamel matrix proteins (EMPs), whether enameloid matrix contains ectodermal EMPs has been debated for a long time. In the present study, transmission electron microscopy-based immunohistochemical examinations, using the protein A-gold method with antibodies and antiserum against mammalian amelogenin, were performed in order to search for EMP-like proteins in the cap enameloid of basic actinopterygians, *Polypterus* and gar. Positive immunoreactivity was detected in the cap enameloid matrix just before the appearance of many crystallites along collagen fibrils, indicating that the cap enameloid contains EMP-like proteins. Immunolabelling was usually found along the collagen fibrils but was not seen on the electron-dense fibrous structures. Therefore, it is conceivable that the ectodermal EMP-like proteins in cap enameloid are involved in crystallite formation along collagen fibrils.

I. Sasagawa (✉)
Advanced Research Center, The Nippon Dental University, Niigata, Japan
e-mail: ichsasgw@ngt.ndu.ac.jp

S. Oka
Department of Biology, The Nippon Dental University, Niigata, Japan
e-mail: okashun@ngt.ndu.ac.jp

M. Mikami
Department of Microbiology, The Nippon Dental University, Niigata, Japan
e-mail: mikami@ngt.ndu.ac.jp

H. Yokosuka · M. Ishiyama
Department of Histology, School of Life Dentistry at Niigata, The Nippon Dental University, Niigata, Japan
e-mail: yokosuka@ngt.ndu.ac.jp; ishiyama@ngt.ndu.ac.jp

K. Endo et al. (eds.), *Biomineralization*,
https://doi.org/10.1007/978-981-13-1002-7_18

Keywords Bony fish · Enameloid · Enamel matrix protein · Immunohistochemistry · Tooth · Transmission electron microscopy

18.1 Introduction

Cap enameloid is a well-mineralized tissue that occupies the tooth tip of actinopterygians (ray-finned bony fish) and corresponds to mammalian tooth enamel. Enameloid is an attractive tissue for elucidating biomineralization in fish and evolution of dental hard tissues in early vertebrates because its process of formation is different from that of mammalian enamel. Unlike amelogenesis in mammals, enameloid is formed by both odontoblasts and dental epithelial cells. Most of the organic matrix, including abundant collagen fibrils, is provided by odontoblasts during the matrix formation stage of enameloid, and many odontoblast processes are present in the matrix. Therefore, enameloid is homologous to the outermost layer of dentin. Dental epithelial cells are mainly engaged in the degeneration and removal of organic matrix and in the formation of large crystals during the maturation stage of enameloid formation (Sasagawa and Ishiyama 2005a, b).

The pattern of mineralization in enameloid is accordingly different from that in enamel. The mineralization process in cap enameloid is summarized as follows. During the matrix formation stage, many matrix vesicles (MVs) and electron-dense fibrous structures (EDFSs) that are probably derived from MVs (Sasagawa and Ishiyama 2003) are observed in the collagen-rich enameloid matrix. MVs are often the first sites at which crystallites appear. Then, many slender crystallites are deposited along the collagen fibrils in the enameloid, in a manner similar to the dentin and bone, during the mineralization stage. During the next maturation stage, the dental epithelial cells remove the degenerated organic matrix, including collagen fibrils, from enameloid and supply inorganic ions to boost crystal growth, like the maturation stage of amelogenesis in mammals. In matured enameloid, bundles are formed from thick elongated crystals that become twisted with each other, which are thought to keep the structure of degenerated collagen fibrils. However, the presence of ectodermal EMPs in enameloid is an unsolved question, in spite of expected active participation of the inner dental epithelial (IDE) cells.

Polypterus and gar possess both collar enamel in their teeth and ganoine in the scales, other than cap enameloid (Fig. 18.1a). EMP-like proteins were detected in collar enamel and the ganoine layer by means of immunohistochemistry (Sasagawa et al. 2012, 2014, 2016). It was assumed that the collar enamel and the ganoine are an ectodermal element, and EMP-like proteins play an important role in biomineralization in these tissues. Therefore, those species might be a suitable model for examining the localization of EMP-like proteins in cap enameloid. However, available data are limited concerning the ectodermal EMP-like protein in cap enameloid of *Polypterus* and gar. Concerning gar, transmission electron microscopy (TEM)-based immunohistochemistry recently detected EMP-like proteins in enameloid matrix (Sasagawa et al. in prep). In the present preliminary study, we report the fine structure of the initial mineralization and immunolocalization of EMP-like proteins in the enameloid matrix of *Polypterus*, in addition to gar.

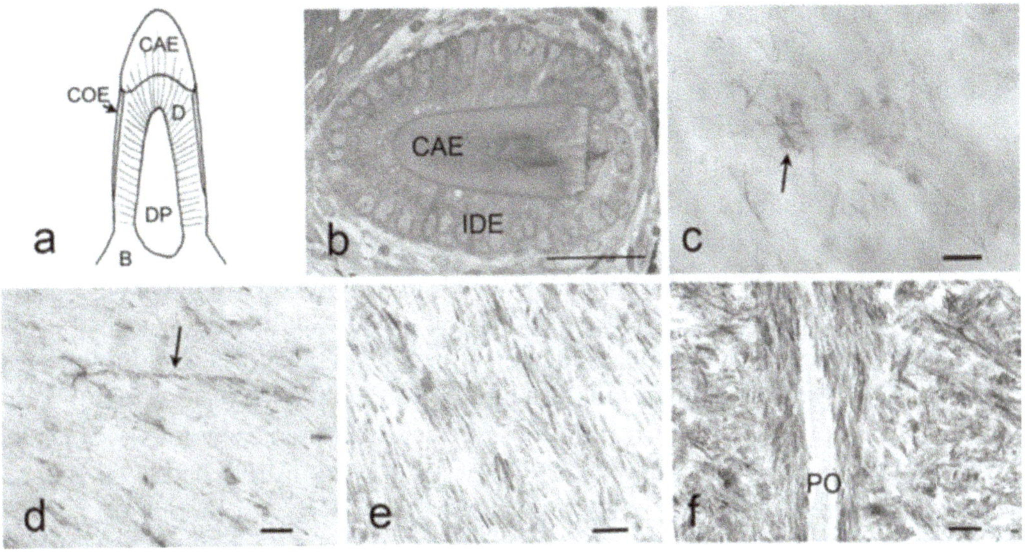

Fig. 18.1 (**a**) Schematic sketch of the structure of erupted teeth in *Polypterus* (Modified after Sasagawa et al. 2013). (**b–f**) Light (**b**) and transmission electron (**c–f**) micrographs showing enameloid formation during the early stage of mineralization (**b**, **c**) and the late stage of mineralization (**d–f**), in *Polypterus*. (**b**) Histological section of a tooth germ stained with TB. Mineralization has not started yet. (**c**) EDFSs that may originate from MV (arrow). (**d**) Initial fine crystallites found on EDFSs (arrow) and collagen fibrils. (**e**) Crystallites oriented along the collagen fibrils. (**f**) Slender crystallites form bundles and seem to align in the direction of collagen fibrils. *B* bone, *CAE* cap enameloid, *COE* collar enamel, *D* dentin, *DP* dental pulp, *IDE* inner dental epithelium, *PO* a process of odontoblast. Bar = 50 µm (**b**), 200 nm (**c**, **f**), 100 nm (**d**, **e**)

18.2 Materials and Methods

The actinopterygian fish *Polypterus*, *Polypterus senegalus* (three specimens, total length 9.5–19 cm), and gars, *Lepisosteus oculatus* (three specimens, total length 16–55 cm), were used in the present study. Local university animal care committees approved the euthanasia and all other animal procedures.

We subjected the tooth germs during the stages of enameloid formation to TEM observations and TEM-based immunohistochemical examinations using antibodies against mammalian amelogenins (AMEL). An affinity-purified, polyclonal anti-27 kDa bovine AMEL antibody (BAA) (Shimokawa et al. 1984) and anti-25 kDa porcine AMEL antiserum (PAA) (Uchida et al. 1989, 1991) were used in the present study. In previous studies, positive immunoreactivity with the anti-BAA and anti-PAA has been detected in the collar enamel of teeth and ganoine of ganoid scales in gar and the collar enamel of teeth in *Polypterus*, respectively (Sasagawa et al. 2012, 2014, 2016). For the immunohistochemical analyses, jaws containing tooth germs were placed in 4% paraformaldehyde-0.2% glutaraldehyde fixative (0.05 M 4-(2-hydroxyethyl)-1- piperazineethanesulfonic acid (HEPES) buffer, pH 7.4) for 3 h at 4 °C. The specimens were then dehydrated with N, N-dimethylformamide and embedded in LR-White resin (LR-W, London Resin, Reading, UK) at −20 °C. The protein A-gold (PAG) method was employed for immunohistochemical analyses.

For TEM immunohistochemistry, ultrathin sections of the tooth germs obtained from LR-W resin blocks were mounted on nickel grids. The specimens were floated on a drop of 1% NGS for 15 min and then incubated overnight on a drop of the relevant antibody or antiserum diluted 1:200–1:400 with BSA-PBS. The sections were then washed and transferred onto a drop of PAG conjugate (5 nm gold, EMPAG5, BBI) diluted 1:10 with BSA-PBS for 30 min after being treated with 1% NGS for 10 min. These sections were stained with platinum blue (TI blue, Nissin EM, Tokyo, Japan) and lead citrate (TI-Pb) and often stained with phosphotungstic acid (PTA) in addition to TI-Pb (TI-Pb-PTA) and then examined in a TEM (JEM-1010, JEOL). Negative controls were performed by incubating sections in PBS lacking antibody or antiserum, or in normal rabbit serum (NRS) instead of antibody or antiserum. For TEM studies, ultrathin sections were mainly stained with lead citrate alone and examined using a TEM. Semi-thin sections that had been stained with 0.1% toluidine blue (TB) were also prepared for light microscopy. Details of the methods were described in previous reports (Sasagawa et al. 2012, 2014, 2016).

18.3 Results

Formation of cap enameloid is divided into three stages, namely, matrix formation, mineralization and maturation, according to morphological studies. In the present study, we mainly examined the stage of mineralization (Fig. 18.1b).

18.3.1 Initial Mineralization of Enameloid in Polypterus

In the TEM observation, abundant collagen fibrils were visible in the enameloid matrix during the early stage of enameloid mineralization. Many EDFSs and a few MVs were also observed in the enameloid matrix. There were no crystallites in the EDFSs, MVs and collagen fibrils, during the early stage (Fig. 18.1c). During the late stage of mineralization, fine, slender crystallites were found in both the EDFSs and collagen fibrils (Fig. 18.1d). In area where mineralization process is more advanced, many marked slender crystallites accumulated along the collagen fibrils (Fig. 18.1e) and formed bundles that aligned in the direction of the collagen fibrils (Fig. 18.1f). Afterwards, the crystallites increased in size, associated with the degeneration and removal of collagen fibrils.

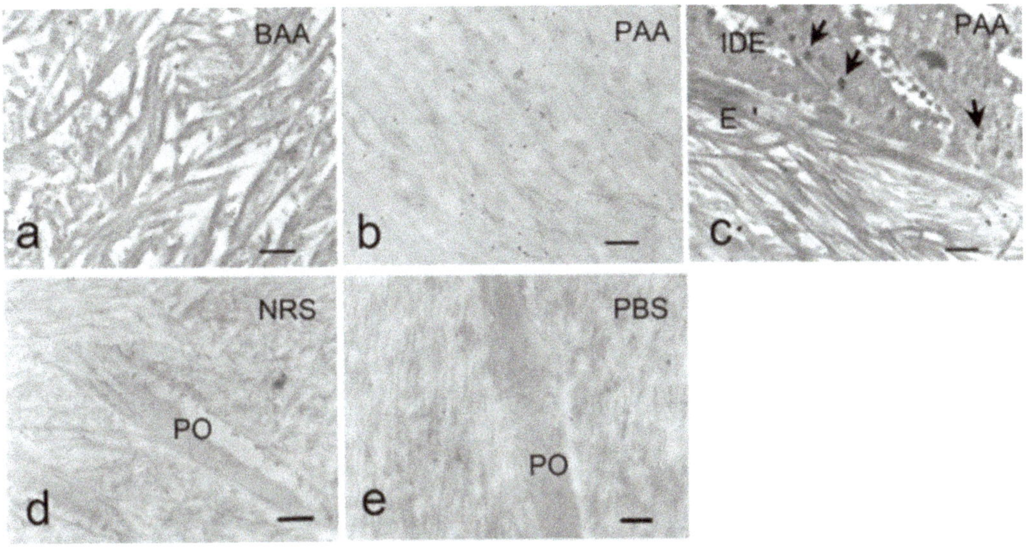

Fig. 18.2 Transmission electron micrographs of immunohistochemistry in gar, PAG method using an anti-bovine AMEL antibody (BAA) and an anti-porcine AMEL antiserum (PAA). (**a**) Many PAG particles are found on the collagen fibrils, BAA, stained with Ti-Pb-PTA. (**b**) Few PAG particles are seen on the electron-dense fibrous substances, PAA, Ti-Pb. (**c**) PAG particles are found in the granules (arrows) in the IDE cells, PAA, Ti-Pb-PTA. (**d**, **e**) Control sections incubated in NRS instead of antibodies (**d**) or in PBS lacking antibodies (**e**), Ti-Pb. *E* enameloid, *PO* a process of odontoblast. Bar = 500 nm (**a**–**e**)

18.3.2 Immunohistochemical Localization of EMP-Like Proteins in Enameloid Matrix

18.3.2.1 Gar

During the early stage of mineralization, a number of PAG particles were observed in the enameloid matrix, in which crystallites did not appear yet. Most of the PAG particles were observed on the collagen fibrils (Figs. 18.2a, c). The EDFSs showed no immunoreactivity (Fig. 18.2b). Only a few PAG particles were seen in predentin. In the IDE cells, electron-dense granules in the distal cytoplasm often contained PAG particles (Fig. 18.2c). Only a few PAG particles were seen in the negative control sections (Fig. 18.2d, e). During the late stage of mineralization, when many fine crystallites were visible along collagen fibrils, only a few PAG particles were found in the enameloid. During the former stage of matrix formation and the subsequent stage of maturation, little immunolabelling by the antibodies was found in the tooth germs (data not shown).

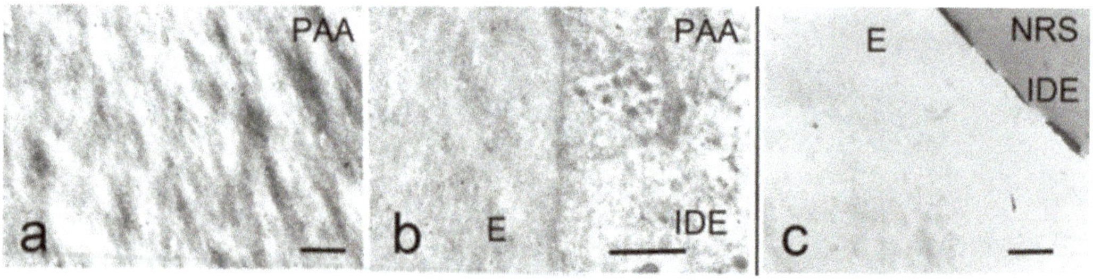

Fig. 18.3 Transmission electron micrographs of immunohistochemistry in *Polypterus*, PAG method using an anti-porcine AMEL antiserum (PAA), stained with Ti-Pb-PTA. (**a**) PAG particles are found on the collagen fibrils in the enameloid. (**b**) PAG particles are also visible in the granules of the IDE cells (IDE). (**c**) Control sections incubated in NRS instead of antibodies, in the early stage of enameloid maturation, Ti-Pb. Bar = 500 nm (**a**–**c**)

18.3.2.2 *Polypterus*

In the enameloid matrix during the early stage of mineralization, many PAG particles were found along the collagen fibrils (Fig. 18.3a). The EDFSs exhibited no immunoreactivity. Immunoreactivity was also detected in the granules of IDE cells (Fig. 18.3b). During the late stage of mineralization, in which many slender crystallites accumulated along the collagen fibrils, immunolabelling was scarcely found in the enameloid (data not shown). Only weak labelling was visible in the negative control sections by NRS (Fig. 18.3c, Sasagawa et al. 2012)

18.4 Discussion

Positive immunolabelling by the antibodies against mammalian AMEL was detected in the enameloid matrix during the early stage of enameloid mineralization. The results indicated that EMP-like proteins are present in the matrix of enameloid in *Polypterus* and gar. Immunoreactivity was also found in the granules of IDE cells, indicating that EMP-like proteins were secreted from IDE cells. During the stage of enameloid matrix formation, immunolabelling was hardly found in enameloid matrix. EMP-like proteins might exist in the matrix just before the appearance of crystallites along collagen fibrils in the enameloid mineralization stage. Immunoreactivity was scarcely detected in the mineralizing enameloid matrix, in which fine crystallites were deposited along collagen fibrils, during the late stage of mineralization, suggesting that the EMP-like proteins had degenerated or had been removed. EMP-like proteins are probably present for a short period during the stage of mineralization (Fig. 18.4).

PAG particles were mainly observed on collagen fibrils in the enameloid. It is possible that the EMP-like proteins are involved in mineralization along the collagen fibrils in enameloid, because the initial crystallites appeared in collagen fibrils in the subsequent substage. On the other hand, EDFSs exhibited no immunolabelling. It is likely that EDFSs are not the structure that contains EMP-like proteins. In

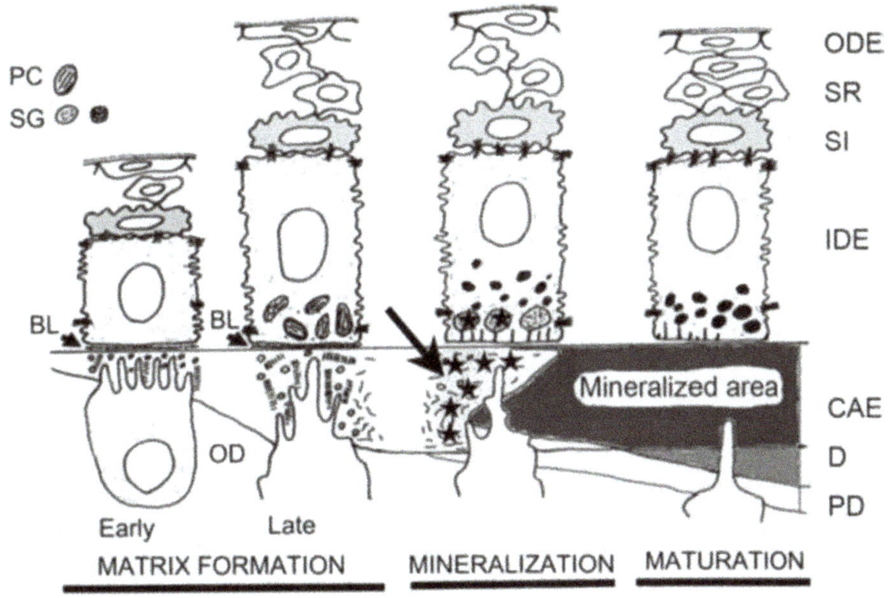

Fig. 18.4 Schematic drawings showing IDE cells during three stages of enameloid formation in gar (Modified from Sasagawa and Ishiyama 2005a). The long arrow and solid stars indicate positions of positive immunoreactivity for anti-mammalian AMEL antibodies. *BL* basal lamina, *CAE* cap enameloid, *D* dentin, *IDE* inner dental epithelial cells, *OD* odontoblasts, *ODE* outer dental epithelial cells, *PC* procollagen granule, *PD* predentin, *SG* secretory granule, *SI* stratum intermedium, *SR* stellate reticulum

a previous morphological study using TEM (Sasagawa and Ishiyama 2003), it was assumed that the EDFSs were the site of initial mineralization in cap enameloid. However, in the present TEM study, fine crystallites seemed to appear at both the EDFSs and collagen fibrils simultaneously. Because this phenomenon was observed in the enameloid matrix of gar (Sasagawa et al. in prep), this initial mineralization process in the enameloid seems to be very similar in *Polypterus* and gar. Even if the EDFSs are one of the sites of initial mineralization, the EDFSs might not be related to crystallite formation along the collagen fibrils in enameloid.

In mammals, AMEL occupies approximately 90% of EMPs. It is assumed that AMEL plays an important part in producing the structure of the enamel layer and to encourage crystal growth during amelogenesis. In *Polypterus* and gar, EMP-like proteins have been detected in the collar enamel and ganoine by several immunohistochemical studies using anti-mammalian AMEL antibodies (Ishiyama et al. 1999; Sasagawa et al. 2012, 2014, 2016; Zylberberg et al. 1997). According to recent genetic analyses, however, gars do not have an AMEL gene, but ameloblastin, enamelin, and many other secretory calcium-binding phosphoprotein (SCPP) genes are present and are expressed in both teeth and scales (Qu et al. 2015; Braasch et al. 2016). It is likely that the EMP-like proteins in actinopterygian fish have epitopes similar to mammalian AMEL, and the anti-mammalian AMEL antibodies may have cross-reacted with these proteins. It is probable that the EMP-like proteins detected in enameloid matrix are SCPPs (Kawasaki et al. 2017).

Acknowledgements The authors wish to thank Dr. T. Uchida of Hiroshima University and Dr. H. Shimokawa of Tokyo Medical and Dental University for donations of the antibodies against porcine AMEL (TU) and the antibody against bovine AMEL (HS). This study was supported in part by Grants-in-Aid for Scientific Research No. 16591844 and 21592329 from the Ministry of Education, Science, Sports, and Culture, Japan, and by a Research Promotion Grant (NDUF-13-10, NDUF-14-12, NDU Grants N-15015) from The Nippon Dental University.

Conflict of Interest The author declares no conflicts of interest associated with this manuscript.

References

Braasch I, Gehrke AR, Smith JJ, Kawasaki K, Manousaki T, Pasquier J, Amores A, Desvignes T, Batzel P, Catchen J, Berlin AM, Campbell MS, Barrell D, Martin KJ, Mulley JF, Ravi V, Lee AP, Nakamura T, Chalopin D, Fan S, Wcisel D, Canestro C, Sydes J, Beaudry FEG, Sun Y, Hertel J, Beam MJ, Fasold M, Ishiyama M, Johnson J, Kehr S, Lara M, Letaw JH, Litman GW, Litman RT, Mikami M, Ota T, Saha NR, Williams L, Stadler PF, Wang H, Taylor JS, Fontenot Q, Ferrara A, Searle SMJ, Aken B, Yandel M, Schneider I, Yoder JA, Volff J-N, Meyer A, Amemiya CT, Venkatesh B, Holland PWH, Guiguen Y, Bobe J, Shubin NH, Palma FD, Alfoldi J, Lindblad-Toh K, Postlethwait JH (2016) The spotted gar genome illuminates vertebrate evolution and facilitates human-teleost comparisons. Nat Genet 48:427–437

Ishiyama M, Inage T, Shimokawa H (1999) An immunocytochemical study of amelogenin proteins in the developing tooth enamel of the gar-pike, *Lepisosteus oculatus* (Holostei, Actinopterygii). Arch Histol Cytol 62:191–197

Kawasaki K, Mikami M, Nakatomi M, Braasch I, Batzel P, Postlethwait JH, Sato A, Sasagawa I, Ishiyama M (2017) SCPP genes and their ancestors in gar: rapid expansion of mineralization genes in osteichthyans. J Exp Zool (Mol Dev Evol) 328B:645–665

Qu Q, Haitina T, Zue M, Ahlberg PE (2015) New genomic and fossil data illuminate the origin of enamel. Nature 526:108–111

Sasagawa I, Ishiyama M (2003) Fine structural observations of the initial mineralization during enameloid formation in gar-pikes, *Lepisosteus oculatus*, and polypterus, *Polypterus senegalus*, bony fish. In: Kobayashi I, Ozawa H (eds) Biomineralization(BIOM2001); formation, diversity, evolution and application. Proceedings of the 8th international symposium on biomineralizations. Tokai University Press, Kanagawa, pp 381–385

Sasagawa I, Ishiyama M (2005a) Fine structural and cytochemical mapping of enamel organ during the enameloid formation stages in gars, *Lepisosteus oculatus*, Actinopterygii. Archs Oral Biol 50:373–391

Sasagawa I, Ishiyama M (2005b) Fine structural and cytochemical observations on the dental epithelial cells during cap enameloid formation stages in *Polypterus senegalus*, a bony fish (Actinopterygii). Connect Tissue Res 46:33–52

Sasagawa I, Yokosuka H, Ishiyama M, Mikami M, Shimokawa H, Uchida T (2012) Fine structural and immunohistochemical detection of collar enamel in the teeth of *Polypterus senegalus,* an actinopterygian fish. Cell Tissue Res 347:369–381

Sasagawa I, Ishiyama M, Yokosuka H, Mikami M (2013) Teeth and ganoid scales in *Polypterus* and *Lepisosteus,* the basic actinopterygian fish: an approach to understand the origin of the tooth enamel. J Oral Biosci 55:76–84

Sasagawa I, Ishiyama M, Yokosuka H, Mikami M, Shimokawa H, Uchida T (2014) Immunohistochemical and western blot analyses of collar enamel in the jaw teeth of gars, *Lepisosteus oculates,* an actinopterygian fish. Connect Tissue Res 55:225–233

Sasagawa I, Oka S, Mikami M, Yokosuka H, Ishiyama M, Imai A, Shimokawa H, Uchida T (2016) Immunohistochemical and western blot analyses of ganoine in the ganoid scales of *Lepisosteus oculatus*, an actinopterygian fish. J Exp Zool (Mol Dev Evol) 326B:193–209

Sasagawa I, Ishiyama M, Yokosuka H, Mikami M, Oka S, Shimokawa H, Uchida T (in prep) Immunolocalization of enamel matrix protein-like proteins in the tooth enameloid of spotted gar, *Lepisosteus oculatus,* an actinopterygian bony fish

Shimokawa H, Wassmer P, Sobel ME, Termine JD (1984) Characterization of cell-free translation products of mRNA from bovine ameloblasts by monoclonal and polyclonal antibodies. In: Fearnhead RW, Suga S (eds) Tooth enamel IV. Elsevier, Amsterdam, pp 161–166

Uchida T, Tanabe T, Fukae M (1989) Immunocytochemical localization of amelogenins in the deciduous tooth germs of the human fetus. Arch Histol Cytol 52:543–552

Uchida T, Tanabe T, Fukae M, Shimizu M, Yamada M, Miake K, Kobayashi S (1991) Immunochemical and immunohistochemical studies, using antisera against porcine 25 kDa amelogenin, 89 kDa enamelin and the 13-17 kDa nonamelogenins, on immature enamel of the pig and rat. Histochemistry 96:129–138

Zylberberg L, Sire J-Y, Nanci A (1997) Immunodetection of amelogenin-like proteins in the ganoine of experimentally regenerating scales of *Calamoichys calabaricus,* a primitive actinopterygian fish. Anat Rec 249:86–95

Chapter 19
Geographical and Seasonal Variations of the Shell Microstructures in the Bivalve *Scapharca broughtonii*

Kozue Nishida and Takenori Sasaki

Abstract Cyclical ontogenetic changes of shell microstructures have been observed in the subfamily Anadarinae (Mollusca: Bivalvia, Arcidae) including fossil taxa. The changes in the bloody clam *Scapharca broughtonii* are controlled by temperature, which fluctuates seasonally, and can be used to determine the age of the individuals and to reconstruct paleoenvironments. In this study, samples of *S. broughtonii* from eight localities covering broad geographical regions at various latitudes in Japan, Korea, and Russia were examined to assess the utility of time series variations in microstructures for paleoenvironmental and paleoecological studies. All specimens showed cyclical changes in the relative thickness of the composite prismatic and crossed lamellar structures in the outer layer with ontogenetic progression, and thus, this feature can be used as a proxy for water temperature of their habitats. Specimens from southern latitudes showed higher annual shell growth rates than northern specimens, suggesting that low temperatures arrest shell growth in *S. broughtonii* and play a key role in determining the longevity and body size in *S. broughtonii*. In long-lived individuals from the four northernmost localities, the relative thickness of the composite prismatic structure tended to decrease as the individuals aged, which may be a consequence of declining physiological activity, such as organic matrix secretion.

Keywords Shell microstructure · Geographic variation · Water temperature · Growth rate · Age determination · Bivalve · *Scapharca broughtonii* · Temperate species

---

K. Nishida (✉)
Ibaraki College, National Institute of Technology, Ibaraki, Japan

Japan Society for the Promotion of Science (JSPS), Tokyo, Japan
e-mail: nishida@gm.ibaraki-ct.ac.jp

T. Sasaki
The University Museum, The University of Tokyo, Bunkyo-ku, Tokyo, Japan
e-mail: sasaki@um.u-tokyo.ac.jp

K. Endo et al. (eds.), *Biomineralization*,
https://doi.org/10.1007/978-981-13-1002-7_19

19.1 Introduction

Shell microstructures of molluscs are highly diversified (Carter 1990), and the shell microstructures formed by a single individual can differ, depending on phylogenetic (Taylor et al. 1969; Shimamoto 1986; Sato and Sasaki 2015), crystallographic (Ubukata 2001; Checa et al. 2009, 2013), and environmental (Carter 1980; Kennish 1980; Lutz and Clark 1984) factors. Recently, Nishida et al. (2012) reported seasonal changes in the relative thickness of the two microstructures (composite prismatic and crossed lamellar structures) in the outer layer of the bloody clam *Scapharca broughtonii*. The composite prismatic and crossed lamellar structures of the outer layer are formed on the exterior and interior sides, respectively (Fig. 19.1), with the composite prismatic structure being thicker at lower water temperatures (Nishida et al. 2012). Nishida et al. (2015) observed shell microstructures in cultured specimens of *S. broughtonii* reared at five different temperatures, demonstrating experimentally the thermal dependency of the mode of shell microstructural formation in this species. Cyclical changes in microstructures with ontogeny have been observed in the subfamily Anadarinae (Mollusca: Bivalvia, Arcidae), including fossil taxa (Kobayashi and Kamiya 1968; Kobayashi 1976a, 1976b; Nishida et al. 2012), and can be useful for age determination and temperature reconstruction. Knowledge on geographical variations in shell microstructural formation in *S. broughtonii* remains limited (Nishida et al. 2012). Thus, samples of *S. broughtonii* were collected for this study from eight localities at various latitudes in Japan, Russia, and Korea to assess the utility of the cyclic thickness fluctuation in shell microstructures in paleoenvironmental and paleoecological studies.

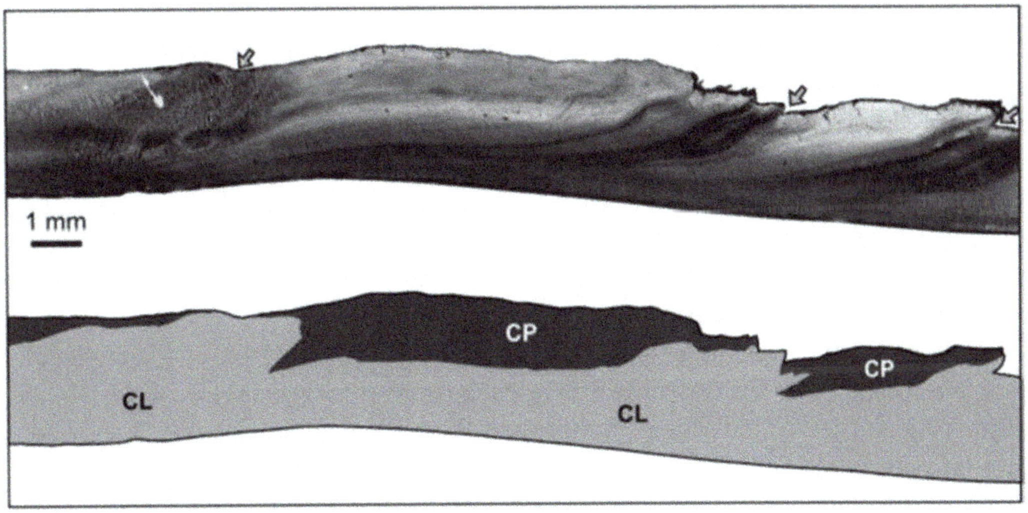

Fig. 19.1 An optical micrograph of the acetate peel of radial section of the outer layer near the outer shell margin in the specimen SB-IN3-01 collected at locality 4. With the growth toward to the right, fluctuations are observed in the relative thickness of the composite prismatic and crossed lamellar structures of the outer layer. Gray arrows indicate growth breaks. Abbreviations: CL, crossed lamellar layer; CP, composite prismatic layer

19.2 Materials and Methods

We examined *S. broughtonii* shells collected from six sites in Japan (Localities 1, 2, 4, 5, 7, 8), one site in Russia (Locality 3), and one site in Korea (Locality 6) (Table 19.1, Fig. 19.2). Of the 12 specimens collected from Localities 2–6 and 8, 9 were collected by dredge operations, and the remaining 3 specimens were likely collected also by dredging. The specimens at Locality 1 were cultured in a net, and the specimens at Locality 7 were cultured in a cage. Shell microstructures of those 14 specimens were prepared by the acetate peel method (Kennish et al. 1980), and then the thickness of the composite prismatic and crossed lamellar structures and the total thickness of the outer layer were measured at approximately 1-mm intervals following Nishida et al. (2012) with ImageJ/NIH image analysis software (version 1.45; http://imagej.nih.gov/ij/). Data of three specimens from Localities 1, 2, and 7 (SB-MT3, SB-YR-101-1, and SB-KM10b-2, respectively) reported in Nishida et al. (2012) were used for comparison with the data obtained in this study. According to Nishida et al. (2012), the age of each individual could be estimated by the number of the growth break (summer break) intervals and the positive peaks observed in the relative thickness of the crossed lamellar structure.

19.3 Results

The relative thickness of the composite prismatic and crossed lamellar structures in the outer layer of each specimen changed cyclically with ontogeny (Figs. 19.2 and 19.3). The ratio of the composite prismatic structure thickness to the total outer layer thickness was 0% at the minimum and had a maximum value as high as 58–80% (Figs. 19.2 and 19.3). For all specimens, the intervals between the cycle of relative thickness fluctuation of the two structures shortened with ontogeny, and the range of fluctuation in the relative thickness of the composite prismatic structure decreased in specimens older than 4 years (Figs. 19.2 and 19.3). In the specimens from Vladivostok (SB-RU11–01, SB-RU11-02; Fig. 19.2), the relative thickness of the composite prismatic structure fluctuated seasonally during earlier growth stages, while the fluctuations became smaller at later growth stages until the cyclic changes in the relative thickness became almost indiscernible.

To examine the variations in annual growth of individuals from the same localities, we compared at least two specimens each for four localities (Localities 1–3, 7; Figs. 19.3 and 19.4). Individuals cultured in the same cage at Locality 7 showed a similar pattern of microstructural changes (Fig. 19.3c, d). In contrast, growth patterns of the individuals cultured at Locality 1 showed considerable variations (Fig. 19.3a, b).

Growth curves for the specimens from the eight localities are shown in Fig. 19.2. The annual shell growth rate was higher in the specimens from southern localities than in those from northern localities, corresponding to the general increase in water

Table 19.1 Specimens of *S. broughtonii* examined in this study. All specimens are registered at the Department of Historical Geology and Paleontology, University Museum, The University of Tokyo (UMUT). Asterisks indicate specimens reported by Nishida et al. (2012); specimens 1, 2a, 2b, 3a, and 3b in Nishida et al. (2012) are identified as specimens SB-MT3, SB-YU101–1, SB-YR102–4, SB-KM10b-2, and SB-KM10b-3, respectively, in this study

Locality number	Sampling site	Sampling method	Depth	Collection date	Number of specimens	Specimen number	Collection number
Locality 1	Mutsu Bay, Aomori Prefecture	Cultured in net	5–10 m	20 September 2010	$N = 2$	SB-MT3*	UMUT RM31012
						SB-MT4	UMUT RM32670
Locality 2	(2–1) at 38°05’ N, 140°58′ E, Miyagi Prefecture, in the Pacific Ocean	Dredge	22–23 m	28 December 2010	$N = 3$	SB-YR101–1*	UMUT RM31013
						SB-YR101–4	UMUT RM32671
						SB-YR101–11	UMUT RM32672
	(2–2) at 38°09’ N, 140°59′ E, Miyagi Prefecture, in the Pacific Ocean	Dredge	22–23 m	28 December 2010	$N = 3$	SB-YR102–2	UMUT RM32673
						SB-YR102–4*	UMUT RM31014
						SB-YR102–9	UMUT RM32674
Locality 3	Off Vladivostok, Sea of Japan	Dredge?	–	July 2011	$N = 2$	SB-RU11–01	UMUT RM32675
						SB-RU11–02	UMUT RM32676
Locality 4	Nanao Bay, Ishikawa Prefecture, Sea of Japan	Dredge	30 m	01 November 2011	$N = 1$	SB-IN3–01	UMUT RM32677
Locality 5	Kohama Bay, Fukui Prefecture, Sea of Japan	Dredge	4–5 m	24–27 February 2011	$N = 2$	SB-FK1	UMUT RM32678
						SB-FK2	UMUT RM32679
Locality 6	Jinhae-gu, Sea of Japan, Korea	Dredge?	–	29 June 2011	$N = 1$	SB-KOT-3	UMUT RM32680

(continued)

Table 19.1 (continued)

Locality number	Sampling site	Sampling method	Depth	Collection date	Number of specimens	Specimen number	Collection number
Locality 7	At 33°58’ N, 131°50′ E off Kudamatsu city, Yamaguchi Prefecture, in the Seto Island Sea	Cultured in cage	10 m	22 December 2010	$N = 2$	SB-KM10b-2*	UMUT RM31015
						SB-KM10b-3*	UMUT RM31016
Locality 8	Tachibana Bay, Nagasaki Prefecture	Dredge	22–23 m	11 January 2011	$N = 1$	SB-NT1	UMUT RM32681

temperature (Figs. 19.1, 19.4 and 19.5). Nishida et al. (2012) reported that shell growth of the field-collected specimens of *S. broughtonii* was probably arrested at temperatures below 12 °C. The length of time in a year when the water temperature was above 12 °C was longer in the south than in the north (Fig. 19.2b).

19.4 Discussion

All specimens showed cyclical ontogenetic changes in the relative thickness of the two structures (composite prismatic and crossed lamellar structures) in the outer shell layer. Thus, this character of shell microstructure in this species can be applied as a proxy of water temperature in different geographic regions. The annual shell growth rate was higher in southern specimens than in northern specimens (Fig. 19.5), probably due to the shorter duration of temperatures below 12 °C, a temperature range in which shell growth is reported to be arrested (Nishida et al. 2012). The specimens from Locality 8 (water temperature range 16–26 °C) probably grew all year round. On the other hand, the specimens from Locality 4 (0–25 °C) may form shells only for a period of approximately 4 months. Thus, low temperatures below 12 °C are suggested to play a key role in the longevity and shell size in *S. broughtonii*.

Nishida et al. (2015) suggested that the faster growth at lower temperatures is achieved by dominantly building the composite prismatic structure, probably as an adaptive strategy to precipitate shells under cold water environments. However, as the composite prismatic structure is physically weaker than the crossed lamellar structure (Taylor and Layman 1972; Currey 1976), it is disadvantageous for maintaining the shell mechanical strength. Thus, a trade-off between growth and physical characteristics (e.g., strength) should be considered in investigations of thermal

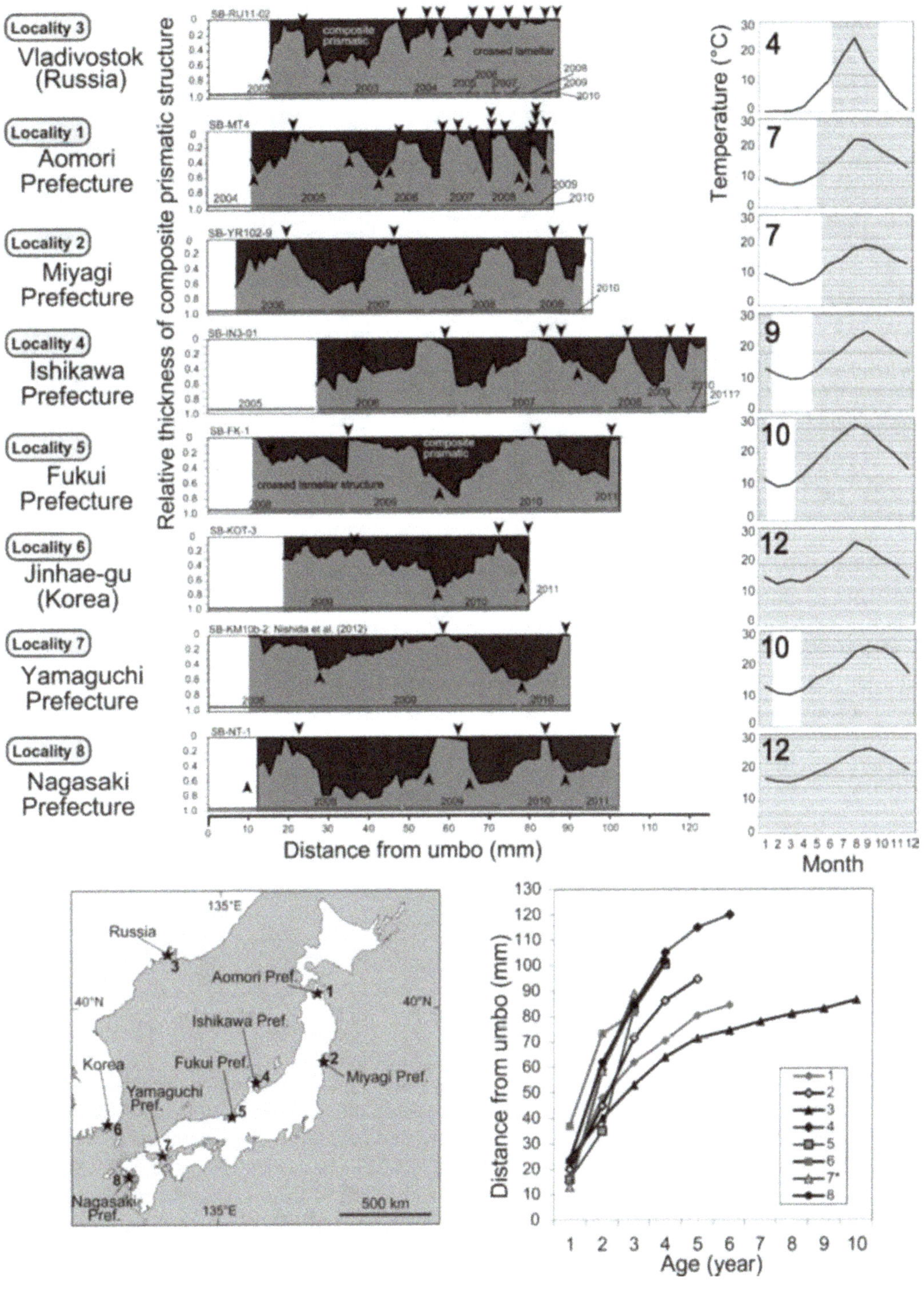

Fig. 19.2 The growth curves and changes in the relative thickness of the two structures in the outer layer at eight localities arranged from north to south along the coasts of Japan, Russia, and Korea. Arrow heads indicate growth breaks; black, gray, and white areas indicate composite prismatic structure, crossed lamellar structure, and missing sections of the outer layer, respectively, and the growth years are indicated by horizontal bars. The water temperature data are from the Japan Oceanographic Data Center (JODC, http://www.data.jma.go.jp/obd/stats/etrn/index.php). Water temperature at each of the eight localities is shown with gray shading on months with water temperature above 12 °C and the number indicating the number of months with water temperature above 12 °C. The growth curve of Locality 7 is for the reference specimen cited from Nishida et al. (2012)

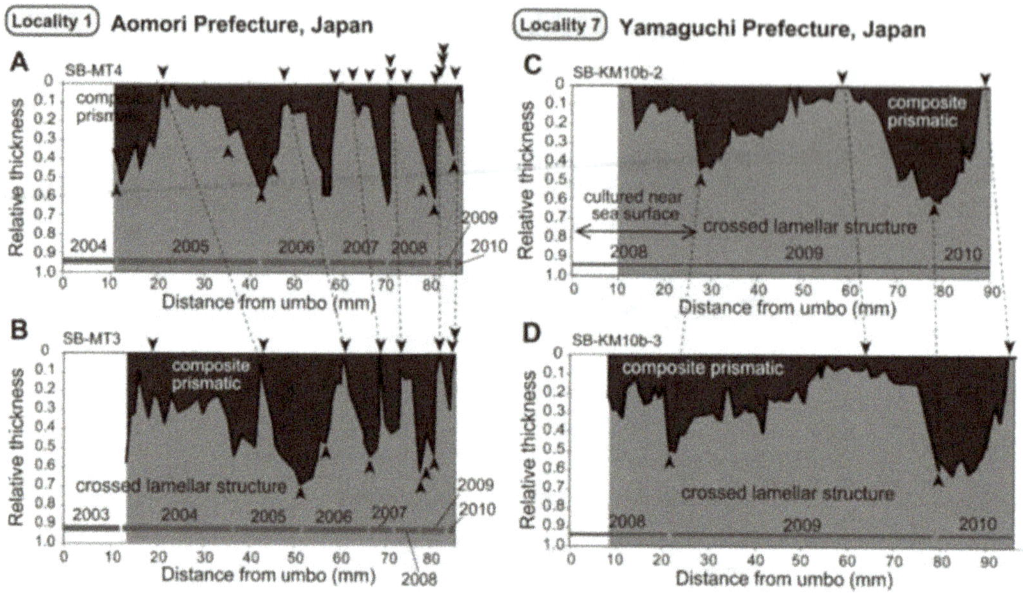

Fig. 19.3 Differences in shell microstructural records between two cultured individuals reared in the same localities. (**a**) Specimen SB-MT4 at Locality 1. (**b**) Specimen SB-MT3 at Locality 1, reported by Nishida et al. (2012). (**c**) Specimen SB-KM10b-2 at Locality 7, reported by Nishida et al. (2012). (**d**) Specimen SB-KM10b-3 at Locality 7. Arrows indicate growth breaks in the outer shell surface; black, gray, and white areas indicate composite prismatic structure, crossed lamellar structure, and missing sections of the outer layer, respectively

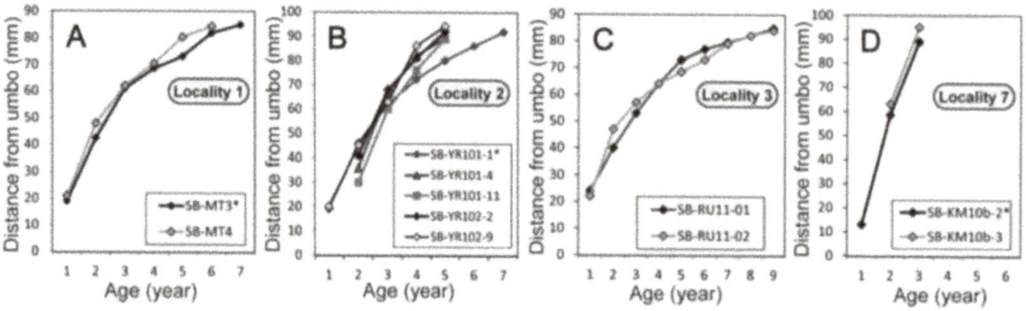

Fig. 19.4 Growth curves of the specimens from Localities 1, 2, 3, and 7 drawn based on the intervals of the summer growth breaks and the positive peaks in the thicknesses of the crossed lamellar structure. Asterisks indicate specimens reported by Nishida et al. (2012); specimens 1, 2a, and 3a in Nishida et al. (2012) are identified as specimens SB-MT3, SB-YU101–1, and SB-KM10b-2, respectively, in this study. (**a**) Specimens SB-MT3 and SB-MT4 from Locality 1. (**b**) Specimens SB-YR101–1, SB-YR101–4, SB-YR101–11, SB-YR102–2, and SB-YR102–9 from Locality 2. (**c**) Specimens SB-RU11–01 and SB-RU11–02 from Locality 3. (**d**) Specimens SB-KM10b-2 and SB-KM10b-3 from Locality 7

adaptation of microstructures in molluscs. The growth strategy of *S. broughtonii* inferred by shell growth patterns and microstructures (e.g., to reach a larger body size and/or maturity faster) might be important in the growth stage before maturity. In long-lived specimens from Localities 1–4, the relative thickness of the composite prismatic structure tended to decrease as the individuals aged (Figs. 19.2 and 19.3).

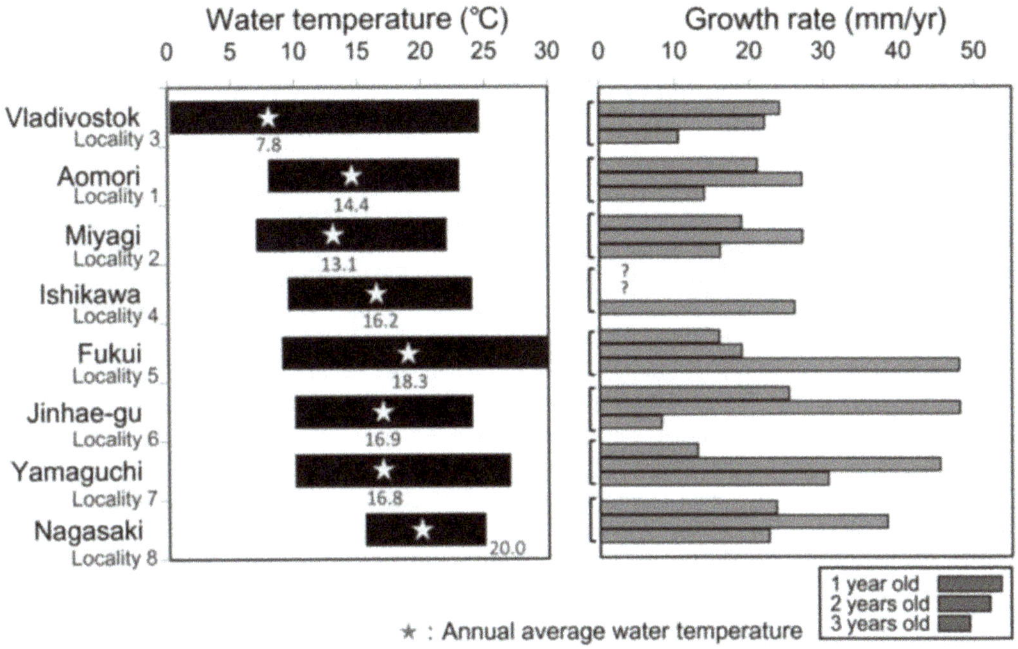

Fig. 19.5 Observed water temperature and estimated annual shell growth rates at eight localities arranged from north to south. The temperature data are from the Japan Oceanographic Data Center (JODC, http://www.data.jma.go.jp/obd/stats/etrn/index.php). The average annual seawater temperature at the eight localities approximately ranges from 7.8 to 20.0 °C. Annual shell growth rate was estimated from growth curves in Fig. 19.2. Annual growth rates of 1- and 2-year-old specimens at Locality 4 were not estimated because no summer growth break was observed in the shell surface of the 1-year-old specimen

Although the primary factor controlling the relative thickness of the two structures in the outer layer would be the seasonal changes in water temperature, physiological factors related to aging may also control microstructural formation in *S. broughtonii*. Palmer (1983) suggested that the cost of shell production is cheaper in organic-rich shells than in organic-poor shells. Composite prismatic structure in bivalve shells is richer in organics than is the crossed lamellar structure (Taylor and Layman 1972; Nishida et al. 2015) and, thus, after sexual maturity, a decrease in the volume of composite prismatic structure in shells may be accompanied by a decline in physiological activity, such as organic matrix secretion. Age-related changes in shell microstructures may show a trade-off between growth and physiological factors attributable to aging. At later growth stages of the individuals from Locality 3, the relative thickness of the composite prismatic structure became thinner with aging until cyclic changes in the relative thickness were almost indiscernible. Because this region is in the northern limit for this species, energetic cost might be needed not only for shell microstructural formation but also other physiological demands.

Differences observed in cultivation experiments may also have some effect. Patterns of the relative thickness of the two shell structures were more variable in the specimens from Locality 1, where they were cultured in a net hanging in the water column above the seafloor than in those from Locality 7, where they were cultured in a cage resting on the bottom sediment. Yurimoto et al. (2007) reported a lower monthly shell growth rate in the individuals of *Scapharca kagoshimensis* cultivated in hanging nets than in those cultivated in cages on the seafloor and attributed this difference to buffeting of the suspended individuals by waves. Thus, the specimens from Locality 7 likely experienced less growth stress than those from Locality 1.

Acknowledgments We thank Kazuyoshi Endo, Toshihiro Kogure, Takanobu Tsuihiji, Hodaka Kawahata, Atsushi Suzuki, Toyoho Ishimura, and paleobiology seminar members of University of Tokyo for their suggestions on research methods and their comments; Yuji Kuyama, Makoto Fukui (Kudamatsu Institute of Mariculture, Yamaguchi Prefecture, Japan), and the other members of this institute; Shizuka Murakami (Kudamatsu City, Yamaguchi Prefecture, Japan), Hiroyuki Izumo (Miyagi Federation of Fisheries Cooperative Associations, Yuriage branch), and the other members of this association; Shoji Ohhasi (Nagasaki Prefecture Fisheries Technology Institute, Nagasaki Prefecture, Japan), Kei Senbokuya (Ishikawa Prefecture Fisheries Technology Institute, Ishikawa Prefecture, Japan), and the other members of these institutes for the donated specimens; and the members of FORTE Co. Ltd. for English editing. This study was supported by Mikimoto Fund for Marine Ecology and KAKENHI 24654167, 17K14413, 17J11417 funded by JSPS.

References

Carter JG (1980) Environmental and biological controls of bivalve shell mineralogy and microstructure, in skeletal growth of aquatic organisms: biological records of environmental change (topics in geobiology). In: Rhoads DC, Lutz RA (eds) Skeletal growth of aquatic organisms: biological records of environmental change. Plenum Publishing Corp, New York, pp 69–113

Carter JG (1990) Glossary of skeletal biomineralization. In: Carter JG (ed) Skeletal biomineralization: patterns, processes and evolutionary trends, 1. Van Nostrand Reinhold, New York, pp 609–661

Checa AG, Sánchez-Navas A, Rodríguez-Navarro A (2009) Crystal growth in the foliated aragonite of monoplacophorans (Mollusca). Cryst Growth Des 9:4574–4580

Checa AG, Bonarski JT, Willinger MG, Faryna M, Berent K, Kania B, González-Segura A, Pina CM, Pospiech J, Morawiec A (2013) Crystallographic orientation inhomogeneity and crystal splitting in biogenic calcite. J R Soc Interface 10:20130425

Currey JD (1976) Further studies on the mechanical properties of mollusc shell material. J Zool 180:445–453

Kennish MJ (1980) Shell microgrowth analysis: *Mercenaria mercenaria* as a type example for research in population dynamics. In: Rhoads DC, Lutz RA (eds) Skeletal growth of aquatic organisms: biological records of environmental change. Plenum Publishing Corp, New York, pp 255–294

Kennish MJ, Lutz RA, Rhoads DG (1980) Preparation of acetate peels and fractured sections for observation of growth patterns within the bivalve shell. In: Rhoads DC, Lutz RA (eds) Skeletal growth of aquatic organisms: biological records of environmental change. Plenum Publishing Corp, New York, pp 597–601

Kobayashi I (1976a) Internal structure of the outer shell layer of *Anadara olluscani* (Schrenck). Venus 35:63–72 (in Japanese)

Kobayashi I (1976b) The change of internal shell structure of *Anadara ninohensis* (Okuta) during the shell growth. J Geol Soc Jpn 82:441–447

Kobayashi I, Kamiya H (1968) Microscopic observations on the shell structure of bivalves-part III genus *Anadara*. J Geol Soc Jpn 74:351–362 (in Japanese with English abstract)

Lutz RA, Clark GR (1984) Seasonal and geographic variation in the shell microstructure of a salt marsh bivalve (*Geukensia demissa* (Dillwyn)). J Mar Res 42:943–956

Nishida K, Ishimura T, Suzuki A, Sasaki T (2012) Seasonal changes in the shell microstructure of the bloody clam, *Scapharca broughtonii* (Mollusca: Bivalvia: Arcidae). Palaeogeogr Palaeoclimatol Palaeoecol 363–364:99–108

Nishida K, Suzuki A, Isono R, Hayashi M, Watanabe Y, Yamamoto Y, Irie T, Nojiri Y, Mori C, Sato M, Sato K, Sasaki T (2015) Thermal dependency of shell growth, microstructure, and stable isotopes in laboratory-reared *Scapharca broughtonii* (Mollusca: Bivalvia). Geochem Geophys Geosyst 16:2395–2408

Palmer AR (1983) Relative cost of producing skeletal organic matrix versus calcification: evidence from marine gastropods. Mar Biol 75:287–292

Sato K, Sasaki T (2015) Shell microstructure of Protobranchia (Mollusca: Bivalvia): diversity, new microstructures and systematic implications. Malacologia 59:45–103

Shimamoto M (1986) Shell microstructure of the Veneridae (Bivalvia) and its phylogenetic implications. Sci Rep Tohoku Univ Ser 2(56):1–39

Taylor JD, Layman M (1972) The mechanical properties of bivalve (Mollusca) shell structures. Palaeontology 15:73–87

Taylor JD, Kennedy WJ, Hall A (1969) The shell structure and mineralogy of the Bivalvia, introduction, Nuculacea-Trigonacea. Bull Br Mus Nat Hist Zool 22:1–125

Ubukata T (2001) Nucleation and growth of crystals and formation of cellular pattern of prismatic shell microstructure in bivalve molluscs. Forma 16:141–154

Yurimoto T, Nasu H, Tabase N, Maeno Y (2007) Growth, survival and feeding of ark shell *Scapharca kagoshimensis* with hung and settled culture in Ariake Bay, Japan. Aquaculture Sci 55:535–540 (in Japanese with English abstract)

Part V
Biomineralization in Medical and Dental Sciences

Chapter 20
Enhancement of Bone Tissue Repair by Octacalcium Phosphate Crystallizing into Hydroxyapatite In Situ

Osamu Suzuki and Takahisa Anada

Abstract We have reported that octacalcium phosphate (OCP) enhances bone repair in critical-sized rat calvaria defects, while OCP is gradually crystallized to apatite structure. Our studies showed that:

1. OCP enhances differentiation of osteoblastic cells in two- and three-dimensional conditions.
2. OCP enhances osteoclast formation from bone marrow cells (macrophages) in the co-culture with osteoblasts by raising osteoclast-inducing factor (RANKL).
3. OCP enhances macrophages migration.
4. These cellular responses are brought about associated with the hydrolysis of OCP toward a nonstoichiometric Ca-deficient hydroxyapatite (HA), which is accompanied by physicochemical changes such as inorganic ion exchanges and serum proteins adsorption.

Combining OCP with natural polymers, such as collagen and gelatin, improves not only their moldabilities but also increases the osteoconductivity and the biodegradability in vivo. The hydrolysis of OCP may be involved in displaying bone regenerative capacity of OCP.

Keywords Octacalcium phosphate (OCP) · Hydroxyapatite·Hydrolysis · Osteoblasts · Osteoclasts · Bone substitute materials

20.1 Introduction

It has been advocated that octacalcium phosphate (OCP, $Ca_8H_2(PO_4)_6 \cdot 5H_2O$) could be a precursor phase to biological apatite crystals in the bone (Brown 1966) although there is still a controversy about whether OCP is actually present

O. Suzuki (✉) · T. Anada
Division of Craniofacial Function Engineering, Graduate School of Dentistry, Tohoku University, Sendai, Japan
e-mail: suzuki-o@m.tohoku.ac.jp; anada@m.tohoku.ac.jp

K. Endo et al. (eds.), *Biomineralization*,
https://doi.org/10.1007/978-981-13-1002-7_20

in bone mineralization (Rey et al. 2014). It has been reported that in a highly supersaturated calcium and phosphate solution with respect to hydroxyapatite (HA, $Ca_{10}(PO_4)_6(OH)_2$), amorphous calcium phosphate (ACP, $Ca_3(PO_4)_2 \cdot nH_2O$) is formed first, and then it transforms to an OCP-like phase before crystallizing to the thermodynamically most stable HA phase (Meyer et al. 1978) at physiological pH. ACP has been confirmed in growing chicken embryonic long bone (Kerschnitzki et al. 2016). The structure of the OCP-like phase has been suggested to resemble HA having a similar characteristics in X-ray diffraction (XRD) (Meyer et al. 1978). In fact, it has been shown that an apatite structure, having a solubility similar to OCP, can be synthesized in the presence of fluoride ions (Shiwaku et al. 2012). It has also been shown that ACP is aggregated as a cluster forms and then transforms to HA via a Ca-deficient OCP-like structure (Habraken et al. 2013) and that growing calcium phosphates involve the common cluster structure throughout the HA formation (Onuma et al. 2017). We hypothesized that the introduction of synthetic OCP into bone defects should lead to the enhancement of the initial deposition of bone matrix followed by additional bone formation (Suzuki et al. 1991). An experiment of onlay graft of OCP in the granule form onto mouse calvaria, in comparison with HA materials, was conducted to test the hypothesis and showed that OCP enhances the appearance of bone tissue around these granules more than those by HA materials (Suzuki et al. 1991). This review article summarizes how the OCP materials work in bone repair if placed in bone defects and in the vicinity of bone-tissue-related cells in vitro.

20.2 Bone-Bonding Property of OCP Implanted in Bone Defects

It has been proposed that direct bone bonding of ceramic materials is brought about through an apatite layer formation on the materials, thereby allowing chemical bonding between newly formed bone apatite crystals and the apatite formed on the materials (Kokubo 1991). Such direct bonding has been reported to occur in ceramic materials, such as glass ceramics (Hench et al. 1973; Kokubo 1991), HA (Aoki 1973), and β-tricalcium phosphate (β-TCP, $Ca_3(PO_4)_2$) (Kotani et al. 1991). The property is ascribed to the osteoconduction, which is defined as the bone formation taking place in orthotopic site (LeGeros 2002). We have found that when the tissue response was observed using undecalcified sections of the granules of OCP implantation onto mouse calvaria by transmission electron microscopy, newly formed bone crystals directly bonded to the surface of crystals in the OCP granules (Suzuki et al. 2008). From this observation, it was apparent that the OCP has an osteoconductive property (Oyane et al. 2012).

20.3 Hydrolysis from OCP to Ca-Deficient HA in Physiological Conditions

It is known that OCP is more soluble than β-TCP and HA and less soluble than dicalcium phosphate dihydrate (DCPD, $CaHPO_4 \cdot 2H_2O$) under neutral pH (Brown et al. 1981; Chow 2009). It is of interest to learn about whether OCP is actually converted to HA in vivo conditions. It has been expected that OCP is converted (hydrolyzed) to HA if placed in the in vivo environment (Suzuki et al. 1991). There is a general consensus that OCP is stacked by apatite layer alternatively with hydrated layers and that the hydrolysis is once initiated; it advances spontaneously and irreversibly (LeGeros et al. 1989; Suzuki et al. 1995a, b; Tomazic et al. 1989). The structural changes of OCP have been investigated because the laboratory synthesized OCP is a well-grown crystal (Kobayashi et al. 2014; Sakai et al. 2016; Suzuki et al. 1991, 2006a, b). Other investigations showed that OCP remained untransformed in simulated body fluid (SBF) even prolonged incubation (Ito et al. 2014) under supersaturated conditions with respect to HA theoretically estimated (Lu et al. 2005). The implantation of OCP in the bone and subcutaneous tissues promoted the structural changes in XRD (Suzuki et al. 1991, 1993, 2006b) and in Fourier transform infrared (FTIR) absorption from that of OCP to apatite structure with increasing Ca/P molar ratio (Sakai et al. 2016) and carbonate ion containment (Suzuki et al. 2009) although characteristics of OCP in XRD still remained (Sakai et al. 2016; Suzuki et al. 1991, 1993, 2006b). One of features in the structural changes of OCP by its implantation and incubation in physiological conditions is that the chemical composition of Ca/P molar ratio has never reached to that of a stoichiometric value (1.67) but tends to go to producing a Ca-deficiency, resulting in the formation of a Ca-deficient HA (Sakai et al. 2016; Suzuki et al. 1995b). OCP hydrolysis can be enhanced with experimentally given higher supersaturated conditions in vitro by promoting calcium ion consumption into the crystals and phosphate ion release from the crystals (Kobayashi et al. 2014; Sakai et al. 2016; Suzuki et al. 2006a), suggesting that in vivo environment could be providing such an ionic conditions. It has been reported that human serum is saturated with respect to OCP (Fidelman et al. 1987), which is not contradict to the proposition that HA can be grown on OCP template (Miake et al. 1993).

20.4 Osteoblastic Cell Response

It was observed that, when the granules of OCP were implanted onto mouse calvaria, the crystals of OCP were accumulated by circulating non-collagenous serum proteins, including α_2HS-glycoproteins and apolipoprotein E (Kaneko et al. 2011; Suzuki et al. 1993), the ultrastructure of which bears a close resemblance to the tissue structure so-called bone nodules, which is considered as the initial bone deposition locus in intramembranous bone development (Barradas et al. 2011; Suzuki et al. 1991). Osteoblasts then started to form a collagenous bone matrix around the bone nodule-like OCP-protein complex (Suzuki et al. 1991, 2008), indicating that OCP acts on a nucleus of bone formation. From these observations, it was hypothesized that OCP may activate osteoblastic cell activity on its surfaces. In order to test the hypothesis, mouse bone marrow stromal ST-2 cells were inoculated on OCP particles coated on plastic cell culture plate in comparison with HA materials (Anada et al. 2008; Suzuki et al. 2006b). mRNAs of osteoblast differentiation markers, such as alkaline phosphatase (ALP), type I collagen, and osterix, increased with increasing the dose of OCP (Anada et al. 2008).

20.5 Osteoclastic Cell Response

When OCP is placed in bone defects, OCP shows biodegradable characteristics that tend to be replaced with new bone (Honda et al. 2009; Imaizumi et al. 2006; Kikawa et al. 2009; Miyatake et al. 2009; Murakami et al. 2010; Suzuki 2013). It was ascertained that OCP hydrolysis is accompanied by a subtle reduction from a neutral pH to some extent acidic pH with the hydrolysis (Masuda et al. 2017), which may affect the cellular responses of immune cells (Hirayama et al. 2016). A histological examination showed that OCP enhanced macrophage migration (Hirayama et al. 2016) and multinucleated giant cells appearance around the surfaces (Honda et al. 2009; Imaizumi et al. 2006; Kikawa et al. 2009; Miyatake et al. 2009; Murakami et al. 2010; Suzuki 2013), where osteoblasts are forming new bone, more than HA (Suzuki 2013). The multinucleated giant cells were shown to be tartrate-resistant acid phosphatase (TRAP) positive osteoclast-like cells (Imaizumi et al. 2006), suggesting that OCP biodegrades through phagocytic resorption not by simple chemical dissolution. It is known that osteoclasts can be formed by the fusion of macrophages (Asagiri et al. 2007; Kong et al. 1999; Yasuda et al. 1999) so that the macrophage migration to OCP surfaces may be involved in the formation of osteoclast-like cells (Hirayama et al. 2016). An in vitro study in fact revealed that the multinucleated giant cells, expressing osteoclast marker genes such as TRAP and cathepsin K, can be formed on the surface of OCP but not on the surface of HA in the co-culture with osteoblasts (Takami et al. 2009). The osteoblasts cultured on OCP expressed receptor activator of NF-kappaB ligand (RANKL), an osteoclast differentiation factor (Takami et al. 2009). Calcium ion concentration in culture medium decreased in the presence of OCP, which corresponds to the change induced by OCP during its hydrolysis (Suzuki et al. 2006a), while the experimentally reduced calcium ion concentration induced RANKL mRNA expression of osteoblasts (Takami et al. 2009). These results suggest that the physicochemical environment induced by OCP brings about the biodegradable characteristics of this material through osteoclast differentiation from macrophages increasing through RANKL expressions by osteoblasts in the implanted OCP. The mechanism of physicochemical changes, including the protein adsorption, induced during the hydrolysis from

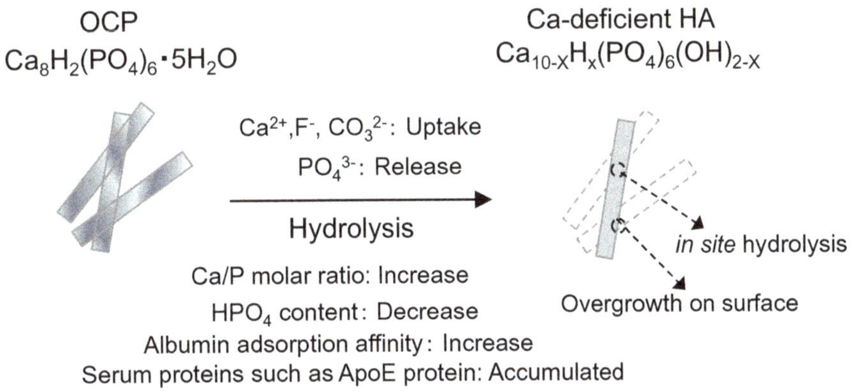

Fig. 20.1 Observed various physicochemical reactions caused during the hydrolysis of synthetic OCP placed in vivo(Suzuki et al. 1991, 2006b, 2008) and in vitro (Suzuki et al. 2006a, b) environments. OCP can be progressively hydrolyzed to Ca-deficient HA under a physiological environment via topotaxial conversion (in situ hydrolysis) and dissolution-reprecipitation (overgrowth of apatite on an OCP crystal surface) (Brown et al. 1981; Miyake et al. 1993; Suzuki et al. 1995b). Ca-deficient HA can be formed, and chemical composition change and surface reaction are promoted during the hydrolysis (Suzuki et al. 1995b, 2006b; Kaneko et al. 2011)

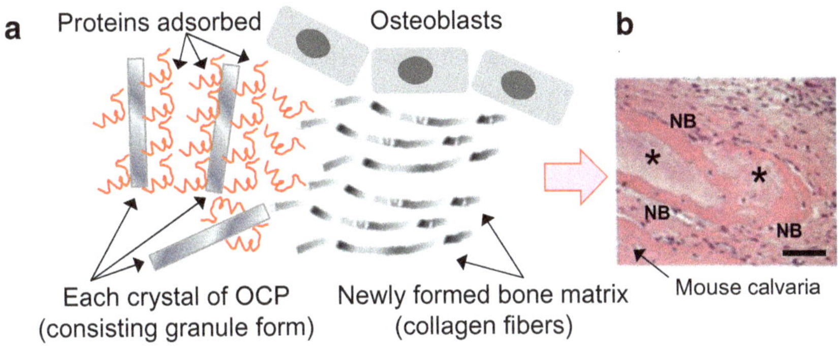

Fig. 20.2 Conceptual scheme of the beginning of bone formation from the synthetic OCP crystals implanted in bone tissue that is based on the ultrastructural observation (**a**) (Suzuki et al. 1991, 1993, 2008) and newly boned bone around OCP granules implanted onto mouse calvaria for 21 days (**b**). Right figure (**b**), decalcified histological section stained by hematoxylin and eosin. Asterisks (*): *OCP* granules, *NB* new bone; bar = 50 μm. (Reproduced from Fig. 2c in Acta Biomater 5:1756–1766, 2009 (Kikawa et al. 2009) with permissions from Elsevier Ltd)

OCP to Ca-deficient HA, is summarized in Fig. 20.1. The osteoblast differentiation stimulated by OCP, as a nucleus of the initial bone deposition, is summarized in Fig. 20.2.

20.6 Bone Substitute Materials

OCP cannot be sintered with keeping its crystalline phase, unlike HA and β-TCP, due to the inclusion of large amount of water molecules (Brown et al. 1962). The granules or the precipitates of OCP were combined with various natural polymers, such as collagen, gelatin, alginate, and hyaluronic acid, in order to acquire the moldability and improve the handling property (Fuji et al. 2009; Handa et al. 2012; Kamakura et al. 2006; Shiraishi et al. 2010; Suzuki et al. 2014). OCP/collagen was made of OCP granules mixed with re-constituted collagen matrix (Kamakura et al. 2006). OCP/gelatins were made of OCP granules mixed with re-constituted gelatin matrix (Saito et al. 2016) and OCP directly precipitated with gelatin molecules (Handa et al. 2012). OCP/collagen composite enhanced the bone formation more than OCP alone when compared in a rat critical-sized calvaria defect (Kamakura et al. 2006). Bone regeneration was augmented in a dose-dependent manner of OCP in the collagen matrix (Kawai et al. 2009), which corresponded to the tendency of increasing osteoblastic cell differentiation in vitro (Anada et al. 2008). After preclinical trial (Kawai et al. 2014), the OCP/collagen composite is under a company-initiative clinical trial in the field of oral surgery in Japan. The OCP-co-precipitated gelatin composite showed a highly biodegradable property in critical-sized rat calvaria defect (Handa et al. 2012) and also in rabbit tibia defect which is an orthopedic bone defect model (Chiba et al. 2016). The inclusion of OCP crystals in gelatin was shown to produce an oriented bone regarding newly formed collagen matrix (Ishiko-Uzuka et al. 2017). OCP/alginates were made of OCP granules mixed with a calcium-cross-linked re-constituted alginate matrix (Shiraishi et al. 2010) and OCP directly precipitated with alginate molecules (Fuji et al. 2009). The combining OCP with alginate allowed the composite to proliferate osteoblastic cells although the alginate is a material that does not have a cellular binding motif (Fuji et al. 2009). OCP/hyaluronic acids (HyAs) were made of OCP granules mixed with HyA medical products, having different molecular weights (Suzuki et al. 2014). OCP/HyAs acquired injectability and OCP combined with a lower molecular weight HyA and with a higher molecular weight HyA enhanced bone augmentation more than OCP alone when placed on the subperiosteal region of mouse calvaria through an osteoclastic resorption of OCP (Suzuki et al. 2014). Thus, the osteoconductive property and the handling property of OCP could be controlled by those natural polymers that are combined with OCP.

20.7 Conclusion

It seems likely that the enhancement of bone formation by OCP implantation is derived from its stimulatory capacity on osteoblastic cell activity during its crystallizing into Ca-deficient HA. OCP-based materials could be used as bone substitute materials in various bone defects.

Acknowledgments This study was supported in part by grants-in-aid (17076001, 23106010 17K19740 and 18H02981) from the Ministry of Education, Science, Sports, and Culture of Japan, the Uehara Memorial Foundation, the Suzuken Memorial Foundation, and the Iketani Science and Technology Foundation. The author thanks Emeritus Professor and former President of Japan Fine Ceramics Co. Ltd., S. Ito; Professors R. Kamijo, M. Nakamura, and M. Takami, Showa University;

Professor T. Katagiri, Saitama Medical School; Professors E. Itoi, S. Kamakura, T. Takahashi, and Emeritus; Professors M. Sakurai, M. Kagayama, and S. Echigo, Tohoku University; Drs. T. Kawai, and Y. Shiwaku, Tohoku University; and Dr. Y. Honda, Osaka Dental University.

References

Anada T et al (2008) Dose-dependent osteogenic effect of octacalcium phosphate on mouse bone marrow stromal cells. Tissue Eng Part A 14:965–978

Aoki H (1973) Synthetic apatite as an effective implant material *Kokubyo Gakkai zasshi*. J Stomatol Soc Jpn 40:277

Asagiri M et al (2007) The molecular understanding of osteoclast differentiation. Bone 40:251–264

Barradas AM et al (2011) Osteoinductive biomaterials: current knowledge of properties, experimental models and biological mechanisms. Eur Cell Mater 21:407–429 discussion 429

Brown W (1966) Crystal growth of bone mineral. Clin Orthop Relat Res 44:205–220

Brown WE et al (1962) Crystallographic and chemical relations between octacalcium phosphate and hydroxyapatite. Nature 196:1050–1055

Brown WE et al (1981) Crystal chemistry of octacalcium phosphate. Prog Cryst Growth Charact 4:59–87

Chiba S et al (2016) Effect of resorption rate and osteoconductivity of biodegradable calcium phosphate materials on the acquisition of natural bone strength in the repaired bone. J Biomed Mater Res A 104:2833–2842

Chow LC (2009) Next generation calcium phosphate-based biomaterials. Dent Mater J 28:1–10

Eidelman N et al (1987) Calcium phosphate saturation levels in ultrafiltered serum. Calcif Tissue Int 40:71–78

Fuji T et al (2009) Octacalcium phosphate-precipitated alginate scaffold for bone regeneration. Tissue Eng Part A 15:3525–3535

Habraken WJ et al (2013) Ion-association complexes unite classical and non-classical theories for the biomimetic nucleation of calcium phosphate. Nat Commun 4:1507

Handa T et al (2012) The effect of an octacalcium phosphate co-precipitated gelatin composite on the repair of critical-sized rat calvarial defects. Acta Biomater 8:1190–1200

Hench LL et al (1973) Direct chemical bond of bioactive glass-ceramic materials to bone and muscle. J Biomed Mater Res 7:25–42

Hirayama B et al (2016) Immune cell response and subsequent bone formation induced by implantation of octacalcium phosphate in a rat tibia defect. RSC Adv 6:57475–57484

Honda Y et al (2009) The effect of microstructure of octacalcium phosphate on the bone regenerative property. Tissue Eng Part A 15:1965–1973

Imaizumi H et al (2006) Comparative study on osteoconductivity by synthetic octacalcium phosphate and sintered hydroxyapatite in rabbit bone marrow. Calcif Tissue Int 78:45–54

Ishiko-Uzuka R et al (2017) Oriented bone regenerative capacity of octacalcium phosphate/gelatin composites obtained through two-step crystal preparation method. J Biomed Mater Res B Appl Biomater 105:1029–1039

Ito N et al (2014) Importance of nucleation in transformation of octacalcium phosphate to hydroxyapatite. Mater Sci Eng C Mater Biol Appl 40:121–126

Kamakura S et al (2006) Octacalcium phosphate combined with collagen orthotopically enhances bone regeneration. J Biomed Mater Res B Appl Biomater 79:210–217

Kaneko H et al (2011) Proteome analysis of rat serum proteins adsorbed onto synthetic octacalcium phosphate crystals. Anal Biochem 418:276–285

Kawai T et al (2009) Synthetic octacalcium phosphate augments bone regeneration correlated with its content in collagen scaffold. Tissue Eng Part A 15:23–32

Kawai T et al (2014) First clinical application of octacalcium phosphate collagen composite in human bone defect. Tissue Eng Part A 20:1336–1341

Kerschnitzki M et al (2016) Bone mineralization pathways during the rapid growth of embryonic chicken long bones. J Struct Biol 195:82–92

Kikawa T et al (2009) Intramembranous bone tissue response to biodegradable octacalcium phosphate implant. Acta Biomater 5:1756–1766

Kobayashi K et al (2014) Osteoconductive property of a mechanical mixture of octacalcium phosphate and amorphous calcium phosphate. ACS Appl Mater Interfaces 6:22602–22611

Kokubo T (1991) Bioactive glass ceramics: properties and applications. Biomaterials 12:155–163

Kong Y et al (1999) OPGL is a key regulator of osteoclastogenesis, lymphocyte development and lymph-node organogenesis. Nature 397:315–323

Kotani S et al (1991) Bone bonding mechanism of beta-tricalcium phosphate. J Biomed Mater Res 25:1303–1315

LeGeros RZ (2002) Properties of osteoconductive biomaterials: calcium phosphates. Clin Orthop Relat Res 395:81–98

LeGeros RZ et al (1989) Solution-mediated transformation of octacalcium phosphate (OCP) to apatite. Scan Electron Microsc 3:129–137 discussion 137–138

Lu X et al (2005) Theoretical analysis of calcium phosphate precipitation in simulated body fluid. Biomaterials 26:1097–1108

Masuda T et al (2017) Application of an indicator-immobilized-gel-sheet for measuring the pH surrounding a calcium phosphate-based biomaterial. J Biomater Appl 31:1296–1304

Meyer JL et al (1978) A thermodynamic analysis of the secondary transition in the spontaneous precipitation of calcium phosphate. Calcif Tissue Res 25:209–216

Miake Y et al (1993) Epitaxial overgrowth of apatite crystals on the thin-ribbon precursor at early stages of porcine enamel mineralization. Calcif Tissue Int 53:249–256

Miyatake N et al (2009) Effect of partial hydrolysis of octacalcium phosphate on its osteoconductive characteristics. Biomaterials 30:1005–1014

Murakami Y et al (2010) Comparative study on bone regeneration by synthetic octacalcium phosphate with various granule sizes. Acta Biomater 6:1542–1548

Onuma K et al (2017) Nanoparticles in β-tricalcium phosphate substrate enhance modulation of structure and composition of an octacalcium phosphate grown layer. CrystEngComm 19:6660–6672

Oyane A et al (2012) Calcium phosphate composite layers for surface-mediated gene transfer. Acta Biomater 8:2034–2046

Rey C et al (2014) What bridges mineral platelets of bone? Bonekey Rep 3:586

Saito K et al (2016) Dose-dependent enhancement of octacalcium phosphate biodegradation with a gelatin matrix during bone regeneration in a rabbit tibial defect model. RSC Adv 6:64165–64174

Sakai S et al (2016) Comparative study on the resorbability and dissolution behavior of octacalcium phosphate, beta-tricalcium phosphate, and hydroxyapatite under physiological conditions. Dent Mater J 35:216–224

Shiraishi N et al (2010) Preparation and characterization of porous alginate scaffolds containing various amounts of octacalcium phosphate (OCP) crystals. J Mater Sci Mater Med 21:907–914

Shiwaku Y et al (2012) Structural, morphological and surface characteristics of two types of octacalcium phosphate-derived fluoride-containing apatitic calcium phosphates. Acta Biomater 8:4417–4425

Suzuki O (2013) Octacalcium phosphate (OCP)-based bone substitute materials. Jpn Dent Sci Rev 49:58–71

Suzuki O et al (1991) Bone formation on synthetic precursors of hydroxyapatite. Tohoku J Exp Med 164:37–50

Suzuki O et al (1993) *Maclura pomifera* agglutinin-binding glycoconjugates on converted apatite from synthetic octacalcium phosphate implanted into subperiosteal region of mouse calvaria. Bone Miner 20:151–166

Suzuki O et al (1995a) Reversible structural changes of octacalcium phosphate and labile acid phosphate. J Dent Res 74:1764–1769

Suzuki O et al (1995b) Adsorption of bovine serum albumin onto octacalcium phosphate and its hydrolyzates. Cell Mater 5:45–54

Suzuki O et al (2006a) Surface chemistry and biological responses to synthetic octacalcium phosphate. J Biomed Mater Res B Appl Biomater 77:201–212

Suzuki O et al (2006b) Bone formation enhanced by implanted octacalcium phosphate involving conversion into Ca-deficient hydroxyapatite. Biomaterials 27:2671–2681

Suzuki O et al (2008) Bone regeneration by synthetic octacalcium phosphate and its role in biological mineralization. Curr Med Chem 15:305–313

Suzuki Y et al (2009) Appositional bone formation by OCP-collagen composite. J Dent Res 88:1107–1112

Suzuki K et al (2014) Effect of addition of hyaluronic acids on the osteoconductivity and biodegradability of synthetic octacalcium phosphate. Acta Biomater 10:531–543

Takami M et al (2009) Osteoclast differentiation induced by synthetic octacalcium phosphate through RANKL expression in osteoblasts. Tissue Eng Part A 15:3991–4000

Tomazic BB et al (1989) Mechanism of hydrolysis of octacalcium phosphate. Scanning Microsc 3:119–127

Yasuda H et al (1999) A novel molecular mechanism modulating osteoclast differentiation and function. Bone 25:109–113

Chapter 21
The Relationship Between the Structure and Calcification of Dentin and the Role of Melatonin

Hiroyuki Mishima, Saki Tanabe, Atsuhiko Hattori, Nobuo Suzuki, Mitsuo Kakei, Takashi Matsumoto, Mika Ikegame, Yasuo Miake, Natsuko Ishikawa, and Yoshiki Matsumoto

Abstract The present study aimed to examine the relationship between the structure and composition of dentin and odontoblasts and the role of melatonin during the calcification process. The expression of MT1 and MT2 melatonin receptor was confirmed in the odontoblasts of the control group. In addition, the expression of MT1 was stronger than that of MT2. A strong expression of MT1 was detected in the odontoblasts in the melatonin-treated groups. MALDI-TOF MS analysis revealed that two peaks of 795 m/z and 818 m/z were found in dentin. These peaks increased commensurately with the amount of melatonin. The number and size of calcospherites in predentin increased in proportion to the concentration of melatonin. The degree of mineralization increased slightly in the melatonin-treated group using CMR analysis. Two peaks could be clearly detected in the melatonin-treated

H. Mishima (✉)
Department of Dental Engineering, Tsurumi University School of Dental Medicine, Yokohama, Japan
e-mail: mishima-h@tsurumi-u.ac.jp

S. Tanabe
Central Clinical Engineering Section, Osaka City General Hospital, Osaka, Japan
e-mail: mrc.skww02@icloud.com

A. Hattori
Department of Biology, College of Liberal Arts and Sciences, Tokyo Medical and Dental University, Ichikawa, Japan
e-mail: ahattori.las@tmd.ac.jp

N. Suzuki
Noto Marine Laboratory, Institute of Nature and Environmental Technology, Kanazawa University, Housu-gun, Japan
e-mail: nobuos@staff.kanazawa-u.ac.jp

M. Kakei
Tokyo Nishinomori Dental Hygienist College, Tokyo, Japan
e-mail: mitsuo-kki@jcom.home.ne.jp

K. Endo et al. (eds.), *Biomineralization*,
https://doi.org/10.1007/978-981-13-1002-7_21

group at nighttime using X-ray diffraction analysis. Melatonin may participate in the dentin composition and the calcification mechanism of dentin.

Keywords Dentin · Melatonin · Melatonin receptor · Calcospherite · Calcification · Circadian rhythm

21.1 Introduction

In the hierarchy of internal biological rhythms, there are the circadian rhythm (circadian cycle: about 24 h), the circalunar rhythm (about 28 days), and the circannual rhythm (about 1 year) (Koukkari and Sothern 2006; Mishima et al. 2013; Pfeffer et al. 2012). There is also circadian rhythm in the concentrations of Ca and P of the blood. It is reported that Ca will deposit on teeth and bones because blood pH tends to be alkaline and blood Ca value decreases at night (Ishida et al. 1983). It became clear that circadian rhythm is shown in oral tissues including salivary glands (Papagerakis et al. 2014).

Melatonin is the synchronization factor of circadian rhythm (Hattori 2017; Koukkari and Sothern 2006). One of the effects of melatonin is the adjustment of circadian rhythm, and it serves as the transmission material of the information at the nighttime. The melatonin synthesis changes between day and night. In the daytime, the melatonin amount decreases (Hattori 2017; Koukkari and Sothern 2006; Pfeffer et al. 2012). Melatonin is also associated with tooth development (Kumasaka et al. 2010; Tachibana et al. 2014). Melatonin may play an essential role in regulating bone growth (Roth et al. 1999; Satomura et al. 2007). When melatonin was administered in aged rats, the bone mass increased, and the internal structure of the bone was reinforced (Tresguerres et al. 2014). Antiaging effect of melatonin is expected (Hattori et al. 2006; Hattori 2017). Many of the physiological functions of melatonin are exerted via two melatonin receptors (MT1 and MT2) of the cell membrane

T. Matsumoto
Department of Laboratory Diagnosis, University Hospital, Nihon University School of Dentistry at Matsudo, Matsudo, Japan
e-mail: matsumoto.takashi@nihon-u.ac.jp

M. Ikegame
Department of Oral Morphology, Science of Functional Recovery and Reconstruction, Graduate School of Medicine, Dentistry and Pharmaceutical Sciences, Advanced Research Center for Oral and Craniofacial Sciences, Okayama University, Okayama, Japan
e-mail: ikegame@md.okayama-u.ac.jp

Y. Miake
Department of Histology and Developmental Biology, Tokyo Dental College, Tokyo, Japan
e-mail: miake@tdc.ac.jp

N. Ishikawa · Y. Matsumoto
Applied Life Science Course, Faculty of Agriculture, Kagawa University, Takamatsu, Japan
e-mail: s18g604@stu.kagawa-u.ac.jp; myoshiki@med.kagawa-u.ac.jp

(Pfeffer et al. 2012; Hattori 2017). MT1 is involved in the transmission of optical information and works on hypnosis, and MT2 is involved in synchronizing the circadian rhythm (Liu et al. 2013). MT1 is also involved in tooth development and formation (Kumasaka et al. 2010; Mishima et al. 2014; Tachibana et al. 2014). Melatonin may regulate various physiological functions in the body and is synchronized with diurnal change (Hattori 2017; Koukkari and Sothern 2006; Shimozuma et al. 2011). We have reported that an increase or decrease in the melatonin secretion influences the incremental line and formation of dentin (Mishima et al. 2013, 2014, 2015). The present study aimed to examine the relationship between the structure and composition of dentin and odontoblasts and the role of melatonin during the calcification process.

21.2 Materials and Methods

21.2.1 Ethics

These animal experiments were conducted with the approval of the animal laboratory ethics committee of the Meikai University School of Dentistry (Approval No. A 1019, A 1105, A 1221, A1525) and Kagawa University (Approval No. 17636). Animal experiments were conducted in compliance with the animal experiment implementation regulations of the Meikai University School of Dentistry and Kagawa University.

21.2.2 Materials

In this experiment, 5-, 6-, and 7-day-old SD rats were used. These rats were divided into three groups: (1) a control group (0.5% alcohol-containing water), (2) a low-concentration group (0.5% alcohol +20 μg/ml melatonin-containing water), and (3) a high-concentration group (0.5% alcohol +100 μg/ml melatonin-containing water). Before and after childbearing, melatonin was administered for 8 days at the 5-day-old rats, 9 days at the 6-day-old rats, and 10 days at the 7-day-old rats. The slaughter was carried out at midday and midnight. The samples taken during the day were classified as daytime specimens, and specimens taken at night were classified as nighttime specimens.

21.2.3 Methods

These samples were removed together with the jaw bones around the incisors. These were fixed in 10% neutral buffered formalin solution. The demineralized specimens were decalcified for 1 week with a 0.5% EDTA decalcification solution. The demineralized specimens were made into the sliced continuous sections with the thickness of about 4 μm with a microtome. The sliced sections were stained with HE staining for the analysis of calcospherites and dentin structure. Immunostaining of the melatonin receptor was performed, and the localization of the melatonin receptor in the tissue was searched. The melatonin receptors were used, the melatonin 1a (MT1, Biorbyt, Cat# orb11085, USA) and melatonin 1b (MT2, LifeSpan BioSciences, Cat# LS-A934, USA). The immunohistochemistry procedure was carried out according to the method of Mishima et al. 2016. The staining sections were observed and analyzed using the light microscopy (ECL-IPSE80i, Nikon, Japan).

On the ground sections, one single-side polishing and double-side polishing were carried out with a grinding stone, a diamond lapping film (final particle size 3 μm), and a diamond paste (final particle size 0.25 μm). These ground sections were observed and analyzed by a light microscopy (Eclipse 80i, Nikon, Japan), a polarizing microscopy (Eclipse LV100N, Nikon), a scanning electron microscope (SEM, JSM-6500F, JEOL, Japan), a contact microradiography (CMR, Softex CMR-K, Japan), an atomic force microscopy (AFM, Nanosurf Easyscan, Nanosurf, AG, Switzerland), X-ray diffraction method (RINT2500, Rigaku, Japan), and a mass spectrometry (matrix-assisted laser desorption ionization time-of-flight mass spectrometer: MALDI-TOF MS, ultrafleXtreme-KG1, Bruker, USA). Measurements of the number of calcospherites in predentin and the expression concentration of melatonin receptor in odontoblasts were performed using image analysis software WinROOF (MITANI, Japan). The measurement and analysis procedure were carried out according to the method of Mishima et al. (2014, 2016). The labial dentin covered the enamel, and lingual dentin covered the thin cementum in incisor. We observed and analyzed both dentins. The statistical significance between the control and melatonin-treated groups was assessed by Bonferroni correction and by Tukey's test. In all cases, the selected significance level was $p < 0.05$ and $p < 0.01$. The Ca, P, and Mg concentrations in blood serum of rats in the control group and melatonin-treated groups were analyzed using a SPOT-Chem blood analysis (SPOTCHEM EZ SP-443, ARKRAY, Japan).

21.3 Results

The number of calcospherites increased in the melatonin-treated group of 6-day-old rats in the nighttime specimens (Fig. 21.1). A significant difference was observed between the control group and the high-concentration group (Fig. 21.1, $^{*}p < 0.05$). However, no clear difference was found between the control group and the

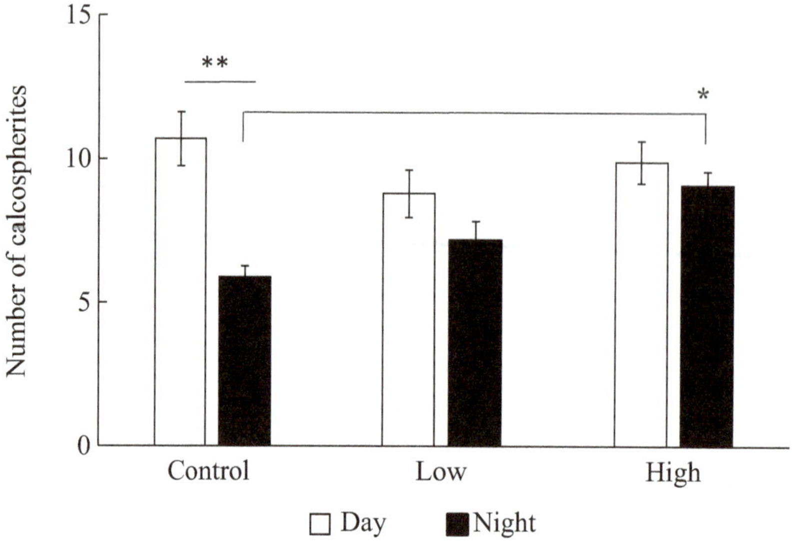

Fig. 21.1 Number of calcospherites in predentin. These data were obtained from the result of HE staining. In the nighttime specimens, calcospherites increased in the melatonin-treated group. 6-days old. Lingual dentin. $*p < 0.05$, $**p < 0.05$

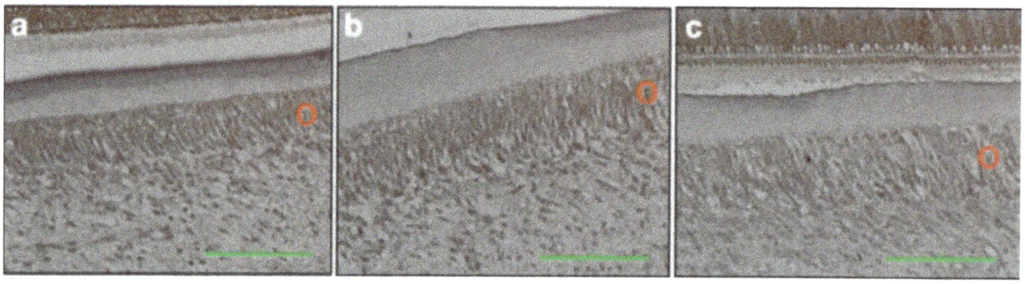

Fig. 21.2 Immunohistochemistry micrographs of the expression of MT1 melatonin receptor at the nighttime. The strong expression of MT1 in odontoblasts was detected in the high groups. 6 days old. Labial dentin. (**a**) High group, (**b**) low group, (**c**) control group. *O* odontoblast. Scale bar, 100 μm

melatonin-treated groups in the daytime specimens. A significant difference was observed between the daytime and nighttime specimens in the control group (Fig. 21.1, $**p < 0.05$). The expression of MT1 and MT2 melatonin receptor was confirmed in the odontoblasts of the control group. In addition, the expression of MT1 was stronger than that of MT2. As compared with the control group (Fig. 21.2c), the strong expression of MT1 was detected in the melatonin-treated groups in the nighttime specimens (Fig. 21.2a, b). A significant difference was observed between the daytime and nighttime specimens in the high-concentration group (Fig. 21.3, $*p < 0.05$). The difference in interference color (arrows) was found for the layers of incremental lines in the high-concentration group in the nighttime specimens (Fig. 21.4a). No change in interference color was observed in the control and low-concentration group (Fig. 21.4b, c). By the backscattered electron image of SEM, the diameter of calcospherites of the control group was 10–18 μm (Fig. 21.5a), and

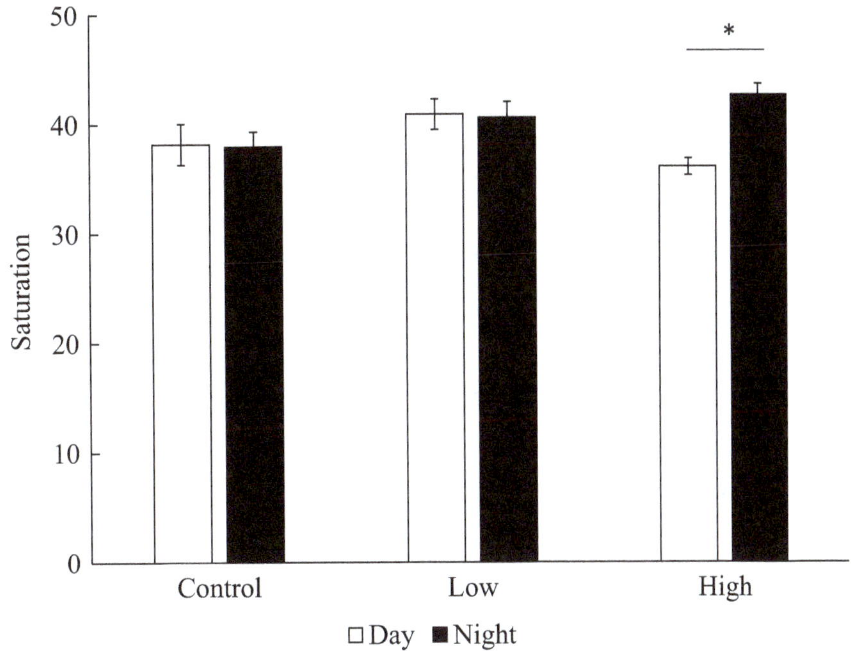

Fig. 21.3 Expression concentration of MT1 melatonin receptor in odontoblasts. The expressions of MT1 of the low and high group were somewhat stronger than that of the control group. The vertical axis represents saturation (range, 0–255). $*p < 0.05$

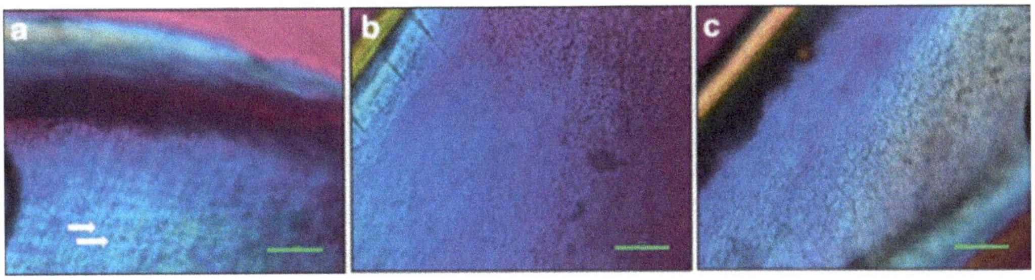

Fig. 21.4 Micrographs of polarizing microscopy of labial ground dentin. The difference in the interference color was found in the layer of incremental lines of the high group (arrows). 6 days old. (**a**) High group, (**b**) low group, (**c**) control group. Scale bar, 100 μm

that of calcospherites of the high group was 13–25 μm (Fig. 21.5b). The size of calcospherites in predentin increased in proportion to the concentration of melatonin. By the CMR images, calcospherites increased in the high-concentration group as compared with the control group (Fig. 21.6, arrow). On the degree of mineralization (mineral-volume %), the control group was 29.00%, the low-concentration group was 32.29%, and the high-concentration group was 32.61%. The degree of mineralization increased slightly in the melatonin-treated group. On the AFM images of ground section, the crystal surfaces of dentin were observed (Fig. 21.7a–c). The crystal surface of dentin regularly arranged with globular uniform size in the high-concentration group (Fig. 21.7c). The diameter on crystal surface in the high-concentration group was 161–258 nm. On the results of X-ray diffraction method,

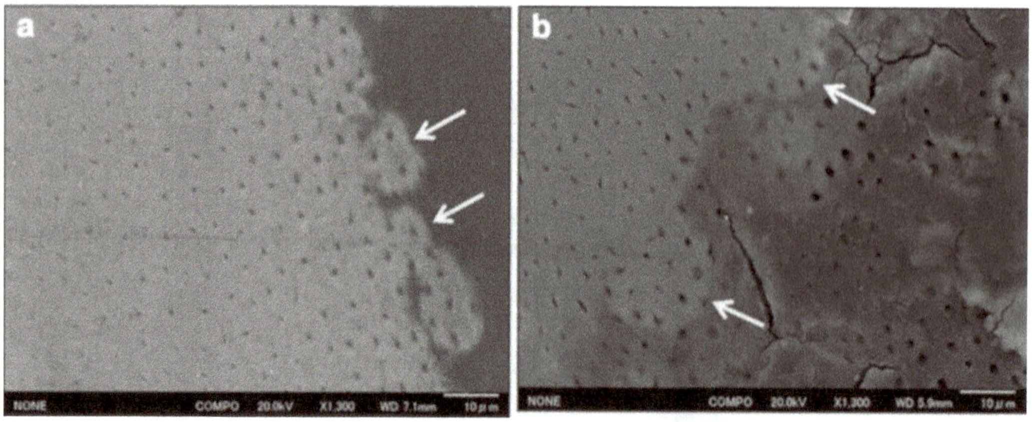

Fig. 21.5 Calcospherites in predentin using the backscattered electron image of SEM. The size of calcospherites in predentin increased in proportion to the concentration of melatonin. 7 days old. (**a**) Control group, (**b**) high group. Arrows: calcospherites. Scale bar, 10 μm

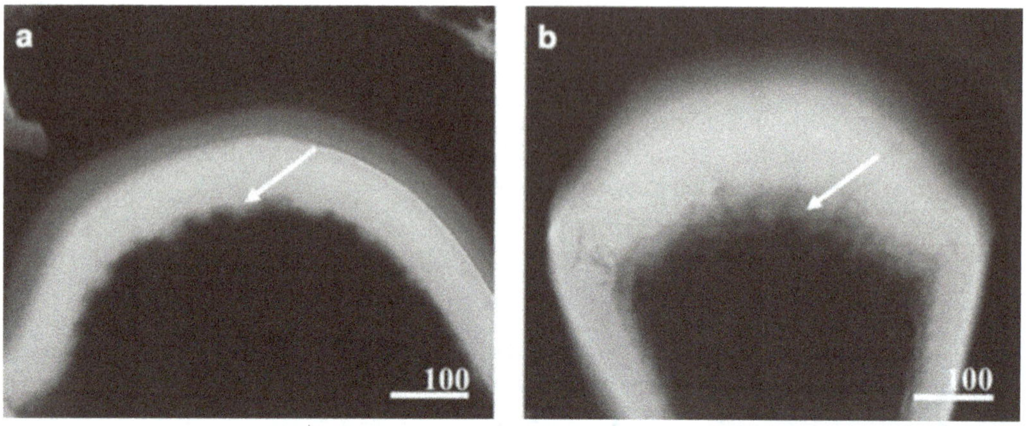

Fig. 21.6 CMR images of the transverse sections of incisor dentin. Calcospherites increased in the high group. The degree of mineralization increased slightly in the high group. The difference in thickness of dentin on (**a**) and (**b**) is due to the difference in the cutting region. 6 days old. (**a**) Control group, (**b**) high group. Arrows show calcospherites. Scale bar, 100 μm

one peak of crystal plane index was detected in the control group (Fig. 21.8a). However, two peaks of crystal plane indices were detected in the high-concentration group in the nighttime specimens (7-days old) (Fig. 21.8b). The low-angle plane index is (002), and the other plane index is one in which three plane indices (211), (112), and (300) overlap.

MALDI-TOF MS analysis of the ground sections revealed that two peaks of 795 m/z and 818 m/z were found in dentin. As the dose of melatonin increased, the detected intensity increased in the nighttime specimens (Fig. 21.9). There was no clear difference in daytime specimens. Figure 21.10 shows the results of Ca, P, and Mg concentration in blood serum using the SPOT-Chem blood analysis. A significant difference was observed between day and night in the control group on the concentration of P (Fig. 21.10, $^{*}p < 0.01$). However, the concentration of P in the melatonin-treated group did not differ between day and night. The difference was

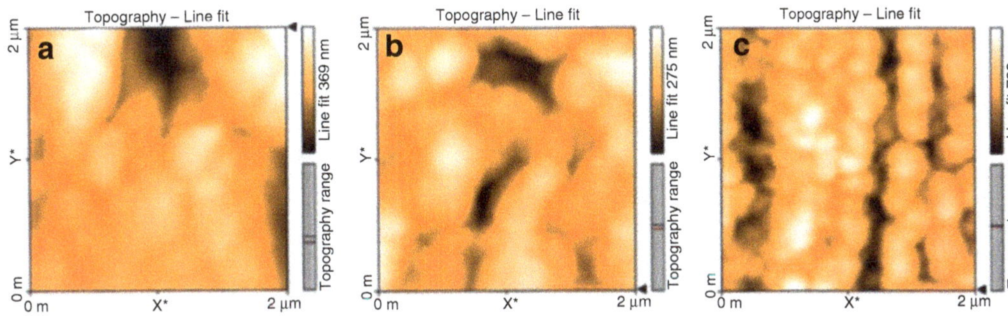

Fig. 21.7 AFM images of longitudinal ground section of dentin. The crystal surface of dentin arranged irregularly both control and low groups. The crystal surface of dentin regularly arranged with uniform size in the high group. 7 days old. (**a**) Control group, (**b**) low group, (**c**) high group. Length of X axis and Y axis, 2 µm

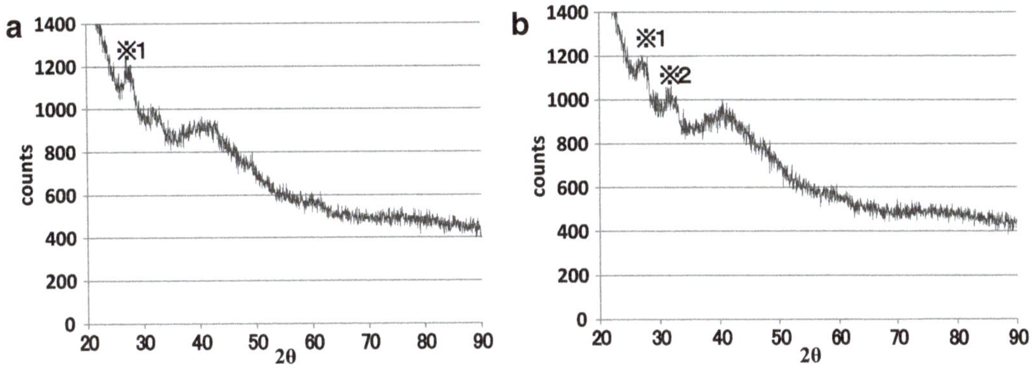

Fig. 21.8 X-ray diffraction patterns of dentin. Two peaks could be clearly detected in the high group at the nighttime. 7 days old. (**a**) Control group, (**b**) high group. ※1 shows (002) and ※2 shows (211), (112), and (300)

observed between day and night in the high-concentration group on the concentration of Ca, but there was no significant difference ($p = 0.08$). The concentration of Ca and P in the blood serum changed by melatonin administration. Regarding the concentration of Mg, there was no change.

21.4 Discussion

From HE staining and SEM observation, the number and size of calcospherites in predentin increased in the melatonin-treated group. By CMR analysis, the calcification was higher in the melatonin-treated groups. Ca and P content of dentin were higher in the melatonin-treated group (Mishima et al. 2013, 2014, 2015). The distribution density of Ca and P was greater in the melatonin-treated group (Mishima et al. 2015). The width of dentinal tubules was narrower than that of the control (Mishima et al. 2015). It is likely that the formation of peritubular dentin was promoted by melatonin (Mishima et al. 2015). From the X-ray diffraction and AFM

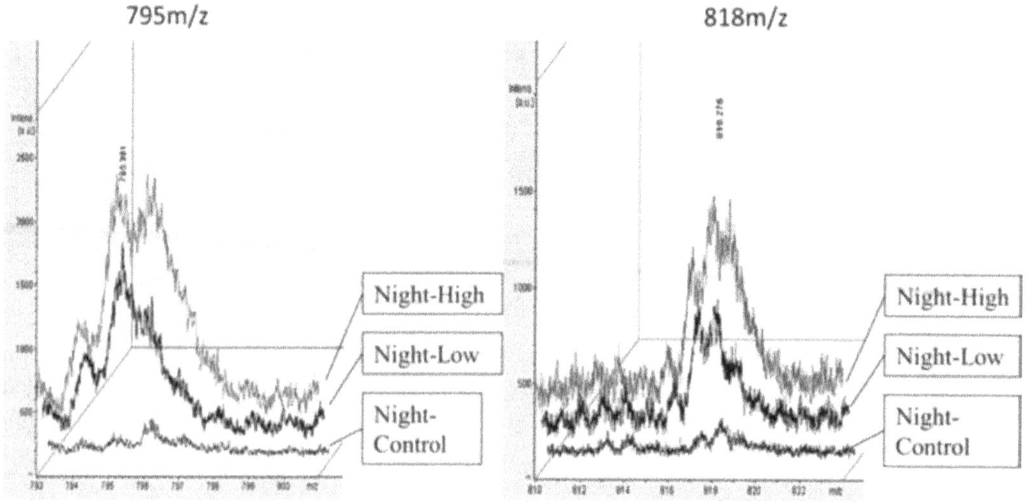

Fig. 21.9 Results of MALDI-TOF MS analysis. Two peaks of 795 m/z and 818 m/z are found in dentin at nighttime. As the dose of melatonin increased, the detected intensity increased. 6 days old. The vertical axis represents intensity (0–2500), and the horizontal axis represents m/z (793–893)

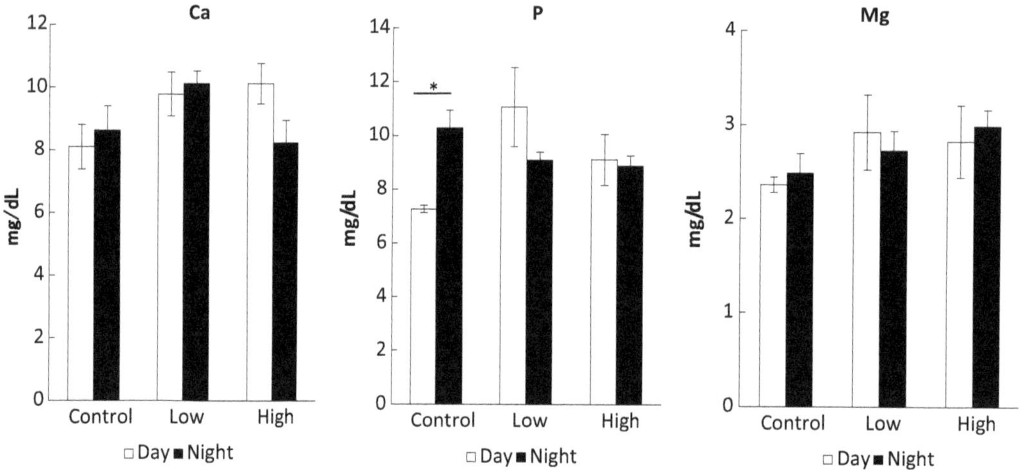

Fig. 21.10 Ca, P, and Mg concentration in blood serum using the SPOT-Chem blood analysis. From the left figure, the results of Ca, P, and Mg are shown. 7 days old. The vertical axis represents mg/dL. $*p < 0.01$

analyses, it was considered that the crystallinity and orientation of the apatite crystal of dentin improved by administration of melatonin. We think that odontoblasts were activated by melatonin administration and promoted the dentin calcification.

From the result of the polarizing microscopy, it is considered that melatonin causes a change in the structure of dentin apatite crystals and collagen fibers. The Korff's fibers were more clearly distributed in the melatonin-treated group of nighttime and daytime specimens (Mishima et al. 2016). It is considered that the odontoblasts were activated by melatonin, and the secretion of collagen fibers was promoted. Mature dentin is made up of approximately 70% inorganic material, 20%

organic material, and 10% water by weight. The organic phase of dentin is composed mainly of type I collagen (Nanci 2003). In mass spectrometry, the peaks of type I collagen are detected at 653–960 m/z in the bone (Schweitzer et al. 2009). The MALDI-TOF MS analysis revealed that two peaks of 795 m/z and 818 m/z were found in dentin. Two peaks are considered to be the peptides in which the type I collagen has been resolved. These detected peaks intensity increased in the melatonin-treated groups. Thus, it is estimated that the peptides which a large amount of collagen was metabolized and resolved increased in the melatonin-treated group. We thought that administration of melatonin promotes collagen secretion of odontoblasts and the collagenation of dentin.

A strong expression of MT1 was detected in the odontoblasts in the melatonin-treated groups. MT1 is considered to be involved in the formation and development of teeth (Mishima et al. 2015). Kumasaka et al. (2010) and Tachibana et al. (2014) report the expression of MT1 in odontoblasts. Melatonin is thought to affect physiological functions of odontoblasts in the daytime and nighttime. It was suggested that the expression of MT1 depends on the amount of melatonin and that melatonin is efficiently incorporated into odontoblasts. Melatonin administration changed the behavior of Ca and P concentration in serum at night. In summary, the present study suggests that melatonin changed the blood composition in the body and influenced the structure, calcification, and crystallinity of dentin.

Acknowledgments The work was supported by JSPS KAKENHI Grant Number15K11034. This study was performed under the cooperative research program of the Center for Advanced Marine Core Research (CMCR), Kochi University (16A006, 16B006, 17A009, 17AB009). Regarding the image of AFM, we were aided by Dr. E. Yoshida of Tsurumi University School of Dental Medicine.

References

Hattori A (2017) Melatonin and aging. Comp Phys Biochem 34:2–11

Hattori A, Suzuki N, Somei M (2006) Melatonin up to date-melatonin effect on bone. Antioquia Med 2:78–86

Ishida M, Yamaoka K, Tanaka Y, Satomura K, Kurose Y, Yabuchi H (1983) The circadian rhythms of blood ionized calcium in humans. Scand J Clin Lab Invest 43:83–86

Koukkari WL, Sothern RB (2006) Introducing biological rhythms. Springer, New York 655 p

Kumasaka S, Shimozuma M, Kawamoto T, Kawamoto T, Mishima K, Tokuyama R, Kamiya Y, Davaadorj P, Saito I, Satomura K (2010) Possible involvement of melatonin in tooth development: expression of melatonin 1a receptor in human and mouse tooth germs. Histochem Cell Biol 133:577–584

Liu R, Fu A, Hoffman AE, Zheng T, Zhu Y (2013) Melatonin enhances DNA repair capacity possibly by affecting genes involved in DNA damage responsive pathways. BMC Cell Biol 14:1. https://doi.org/10.1186/1471-2121/14/1 http://biocellbiol.biomedcentral.com/articles/10.1186/1471-2121-14-1, (cited 2015-11-5)

Mishima H, Inoue M, Kadota R, Hattori A, Suzuki N, Kakei M, Matsumoto T, Satomura K, Miake Y (2013) The connection between the periodicity incremental lines of tooth dentin and the secretion rhythm of melatonin of the signaling molecules of biological clock. J Jpn Assoc Regen Dent 11:27–39

Mishima H, Kadota R, Osaki M, Hattori A, Suzuki N, Kakei M, Matsumoto T, Ikegame M, Miake Y (2014) Analytical and histological studies on the changes of composition and structure of dentin by melatonin medication. J Jpn Assoc Regen Dent 12:11–22

Mishima H, Osaki M, Takeuchi S, Takechi K, Hattori A, Suzuki N, Kakei M, Matsumoto T, Ikegame M, Miake Y (2015) The influence that melatonin gives in dentin histology, the odontoblasts and the period of incremental lines of dentin. J Jpn Assoc Regen Dent 13:2–14

Mishima H, Takeuchi S, Tanabe S, Hattori A, Suzuki N, Kakei M, Matsumoto T, Ikegame M, Takechi K, Miake Y (2016) Effect of biological rhythm synchronous factor melatonin on structure, composition, and calcification of dentin and odontoblasts. J Jpn Assoc Regen Dent 13:2–14

Nanci A (2003) Dentin-pulp complex. In: Nanci A (ed) Ten Cate's oral histology: development, structure, and function. Mosby, St. Louis

Papagerakis S, Zheng L, Schnell S, Sartor MA, Somers E, Marder W, McAlpin B, Kim D, McHugh J, Papagerakis P (2014) The circadian clock in oral health and diseases. J Dent Res 93:27–35

Pfeffer M, Rauch A, Korf HW, von Gall C (2012) The endogenous melatonin (MT) signal facilitates reentrainment of the circadian system to light-induced phase advances by acting upon MT2 receptors. Chronobiol Int 29:415–429

Roth JA, Kim B-C, Lin W-L, Cho M-I (1999) Melatonin promotes osteoblast differentiation and bone formation. J Biol Chem 274:22041–22047

Satomura K, Tobiume S, Tokuyama R, Yamasaki Y, Kudoh K, Maeda E, Nagayama M (2007) Melatonin at pharmacological does enhances human osteoblastic differentiation in vitro and promotes mouse cortical bone formation in vivo. J Pineal Res 42:231–239

Schweitzer MH, Zheng W, Organ CL, Avci R, Suo Z, Freimark LM, Leblue VS, Duncan MB, Heiden MDV, Neveu JM, Lane WS, Cottrell JS, Horner JR, Cantley LC (2009) Biomolecular characterization and protein sequences of the Campanian hadrosaur *B. canadensis*. Science 324:626–631

Shimozuma M, Tokuyama R, Takehara S, Umeki H, Ide S, Mishima K, Saito I, Satomura K (2011) Expression and cellular localization of melatonin-synthesizing enzymes in rat and human salivary glands. Histochem Cell Biol 135:389–396

Tachibana R, Tatehara S, Kumasaka S, Tokuyama R, Satomura K (2014) Effect of melatonin on human dental papilla cells. Int J Mol Sci 15:17304–17317

Tresguerres IF, Tamimi F, Eimar H, Barralet J, Preito S, Torres J, Calvo-Guirado JL, Fernándes-Tresguerres JA (2014) Melatonin dietary supplement as anti-aging therapy for age-related bone loss. Rejuvenation Res 17:341–346

Chapter 22
Fabrication of Hydroxyapatite Nanofibers with High Aspect Ratio *via* Low-Temperature Wet Precipitation Methods Under Acidic Conditions

Masahiro Okada, Emilio Satoshi Hara, and Takuya Matsumoto

Abstract HAp nanofibers (or whiskers) have been attracted considerable attention for their application as adsorbents and reinforcing fillers owing to their unique morphologies. However, fabrication of HAp nanofibers has been limited to high-temperature and/or long-term methods. Herein, we report that HAp nanofibers with more than 5 μm in length (aspect ratio >100) can be easily obtained by a simple wet precipitation method without additives at relatively low temperature (80 °C) under acidic conditions (initial pH of 6.5 and final pH of 3.9), without pH control during the precipitation.

Keywords Hydroxyapatite · Nanofiber · Wet chemical precipitation · Acidic condition · Crystal growth

22.1 Introduction

Hydroxyapatite (HAp) is recognized as a major inorganic component of human hard tissues (bones and teeth). Synthetic HAp, a type of bioceramics, exhibits biocompatibility (i.e., nontoxicity) (Lawton et al. 1989; Abdel-Gawad and Awwad 2010) and excellent cell adhesion properties (Dorozhkin 2010). Therefore, HAp and its composites with polymers or metals have been widely used in orthopedic and dental tissue engineering fields (Choi et al. 2010; Honda et al. 2010; Okada and Matsumoto 2015). Other important applications of HAp include their use as drug delivery carriers (Matsumoto et al. 2004; Bouladjine et al. 2009; Tomoda et al. 2010) and in liquid chromatographic packing materials (Kawasaki 1991) by utilizing the favorable adsorption capacity of the HAp surface for biomolecules, such as

M. Okada (✉) · E. S. Hara · T. Matsumoto
Department of Biomaterials, Graduate School of Medicine, Dentistry and Pharmaceutical Sciences, Okayama University, 2-5-1 Shikata-cho, Kita-ku, Okayama, Japan
e-mail: m_okada@cc.okayama-u.ac.jp; gmd421209@s.okayama-u.ac.jp; tmatsu@md.okayama-u.ac.jp

K. Endo et al. (eds.), *Biomineralization*,
https://doi.org/10.1007/978-981-13-1002-7_22

cell adhesion proteins (Kilpadi et al. 2001; Lee et al. 2010). HAp belongs to a hexagonal crystal system and possesses different properties on its *a* and *c* planes, and hence, its morphology strongly affects protein adsorption properties (Kilpadi et al. 2001; Lee et al. 2010). Therefore, the control of HAp morphology is of fundamental importance to improve its adsorption properties.

HAp nanofibers (or whiskers) have been attracted considerable attention, owing to their unique morphologies, for application as adsorbents and reinforcing components in biomedical composites (Qi et al. 2017). Nevertheless, previous reports have demonstrated the synthesis of HAp nanofibers only at high temperature, during long periods, or by adding additives, such as hydrothermal methods (e.g., 180–200 °C) (Sadat-Shojai et al. 2012; Chen and Zhu 2016), homogeneous precipitation methods (e.g., 72 h) (Aizawa et al. 2005; Zhan et al. 2005), and wet precipitation methods with surfactants (Liu et al. 2002; Chen and Zhu 2016). Therefore, synthesis of HAp nanofibers at mild conditions could reduce costs and enable more diverse applications of HAp. However, the synthesis of HAp nanofibers at low temperature without additives is still challenging.

Herein, we report that HAp nanofibers could be easily obtained by a simple wet precipitation method without additives at relatively low temperature (80 °C) under acidic conditions, without pH control during the precipitation. The formation process of the HAp nanofibers by the simple wet precipitation method was also evaluated.

22.2 Materials and Methods

Unless otherwise mentioned, all materials were of reagent grade and were purchased from Wako Pure Chemical Industries, Ltd. (Osaka, Japan). All materials were used as received. Milli-Q water (Millipore Corp., Bedford, MA, USA) with a specific resistance of 18.2×10^6 Ω·cm was used.

An aqueous solution of $Ca(NO_3)_2 \cdot H_2O$ (10 g/L = 42.3 mM; 160 mL) was poured into a 500-mL conical flask equipped with an inlet for nitrogen and a magnetic stirrer. After the reactor was heated at a predetermined temperature (30, 50, or 80 °C), initial pH of the solution was adjusted to 6.5 (i.e., acidic condition) or 10.0 (i.e., alkaline condition) by adding a 28% ammonia solution. After the temperature and the initial pH were equilibrated for 5 min, an aqueous solution of $(NH_4)_2HPO_4$ (101.6 mM; 40 mL; pH 8.0) was added at a feed rate of 8.0 mL/h into the conical flask, and the resultant mixture was stirred for another 12 h at a constant temperature, with variations within 0.1 °C. During the reaction, although the pH was not controlled, the changes in pH were recorded with a pH meter (HM-31P; pH resolution, 0.01; DKK-TOA Corp., Tokyo, Japan) at a time interval of 2 min. The resulting product was then centrifugally washed three times with distilled water and then dried at room temperature under reduced pressure for 1 day.

The dispersed sample was dried on an aluminum stub and coated using an osmium coater Neoc-Pro (Meiwafosis Co. Ltd., Tokyo, Japan) before particle

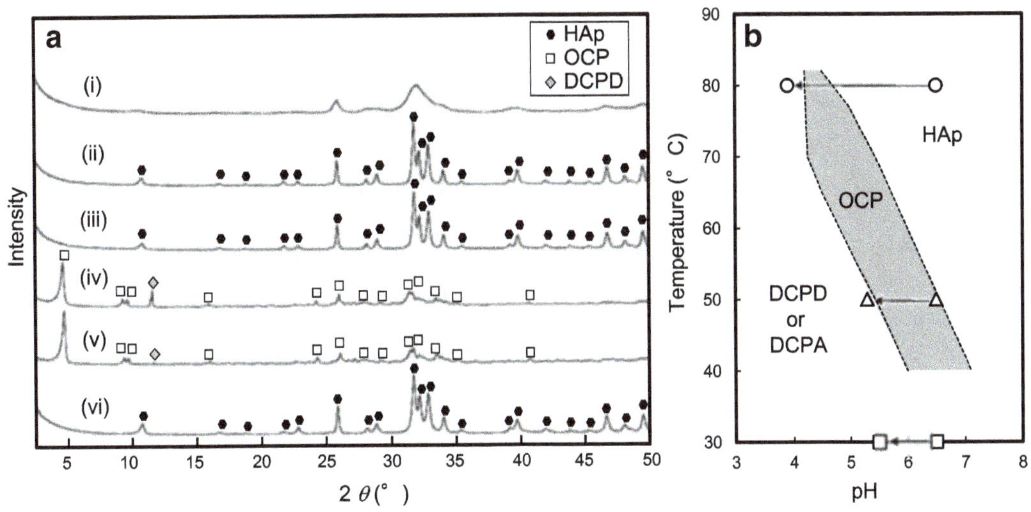

Fig. 22.1 (**a**) XRD patterns of the products synthesized by wet precipitation methods under different initial pH and temperature conditions: (*i*) pH 10.0, 30 °C; (*ii*) pH 10.0, 50 °C; (*iii*) pH 10.0, 80 °C; (*iv*) pH 6.5, 30 °C; (*v*) pH 6.5, 50 °C; (*vi*) pH 6.5, 80 °C. (**b**) A phase diagram of the products after hydrolysis of α-tricalcium phosphates at different pH and temperature conditions (Monma 1980; Monma et al. 1981) and the pH changes during wet precipitation methods at different initial pH and temperature conditions: (open squares) pH 6.5, 30 °C; (open triangles) pH 6.5, 50 °C; (open circles) pH 6.5, 80 °C. *Abbreviations*: *HAp* hydroxyapatite, *OCP* octacalcium phosphate, *DCPD* dicalcium phosphate dihydrate

morphology observation by scanning electron microscopy (SEM) using a JSM-6701F microscope (JEOL Ltd., Tokyo, Japan) operated at 5 kV or the sample was dried on a collodion-coated grid before particle morphology observation and electron diffraction measurement by transmission electron microscopy (TEM) using a JEM-2100F microscope (JEOL Ltd.) operated at 200 kV. The number-averaged size (N = 50) was determined from SEM photographs with image analysis software (Image J; National Institutes of Health, Bethesda, MD, USA). Fourier-transform infrared (FTIR) spectra were obtained using an IRAffinity-1S system (Shimadzu Corp., Kyoto, Japan) with a KBr pellet method at a resolution of 4 cm^{-1} with 32 scans. Product identification was also conducted by X-ray diffraction (XRD) measurements (RINT2500HF; Rigaku Corp., Tokyo, Japan) equipped with a Cu-Kα radiation source.

22.3 Results and Discussion

In the case of alkaline conditions (i.e., initial pH = 10.0), the final pH after the reaction decreased to 8.2–9.3, and HAp crystals were obtained as shown in Fig. 22.1a (i–iii). The crystal morphologies varied by changing the temperature (Fig. 22.2a–c); i.e., more elongated HAp crystals were obtained by increasing the reaction temperature, which is consistent with previous reports (Sadat-Shojai et al. 2013; Okada and Matsumoto 2015). Note that the size distributions of HAp crystals formed in the

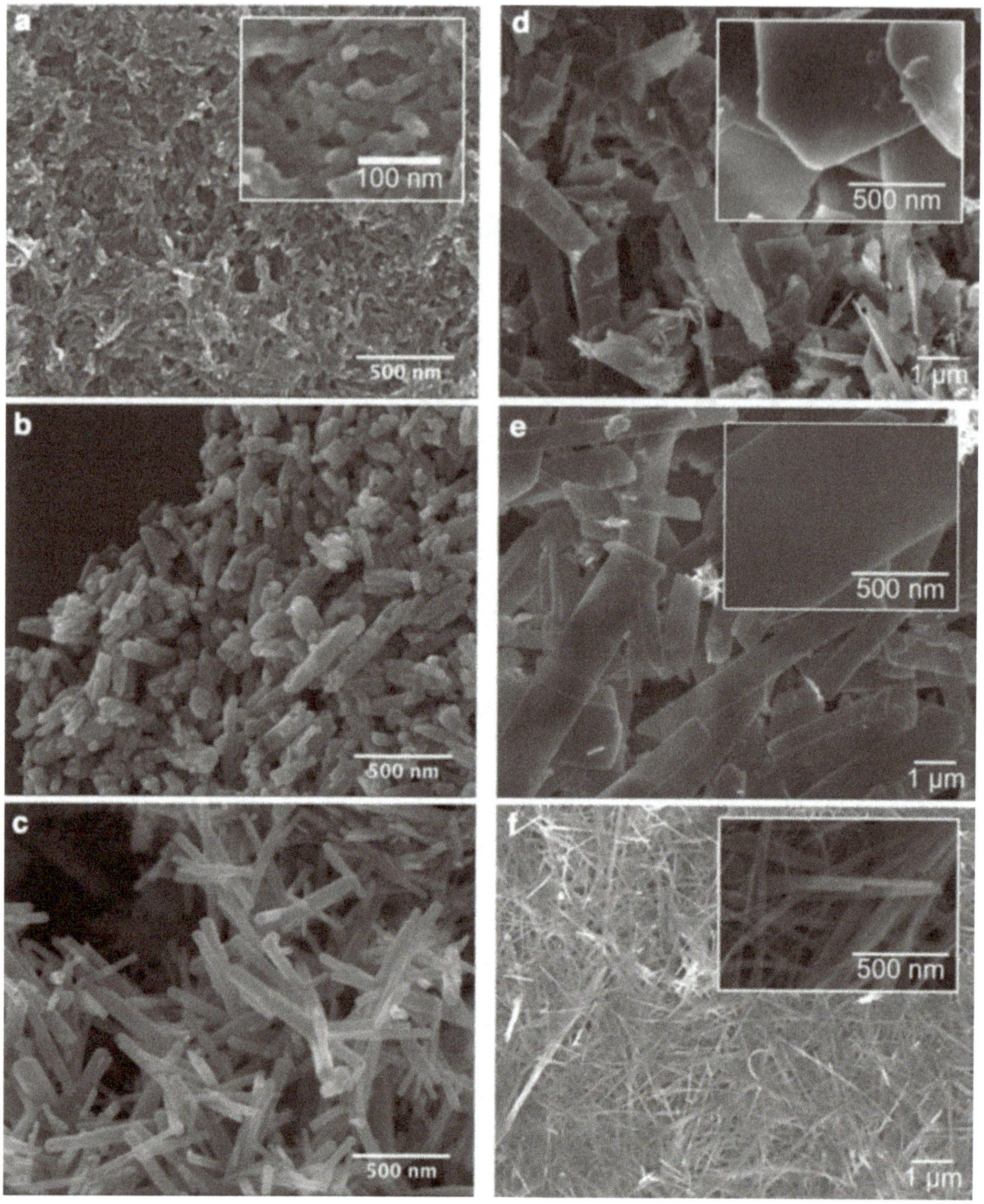

Fig. 22.2 SEM photographs of the products synthesized by wet precipitation methods under different initial pH and temperature conditions: (**a**) pH 10.0, 30 °C; (**b**) pH 10.0, 50 °C; (**c**) pH 10.0, 80 °C; (**d**) pH 6.5, 30 °C; (**e**) pH 6.5, 50 °C; (**f**) pH 6.5, 80 °C. The insets show magnified images

alkaline conditions were broad (i.e., polydispersed), which should be due to long particle nucleation stage. In other words, the saturated solution concentration of HAp is too small at alkaline conditions (Matsumoto et al. 2007), and hence the particle nuclei formed throughout the feeding period (5 h) of phosphate ion solution into the calcium ion solution.

In the case of acidic conditions (i.e., initial pH = 6.5), the final pH significantly dropped to 5.5–3.9 after the reaction, as shown in Fig. 22.1b. Plate-like dicalcium

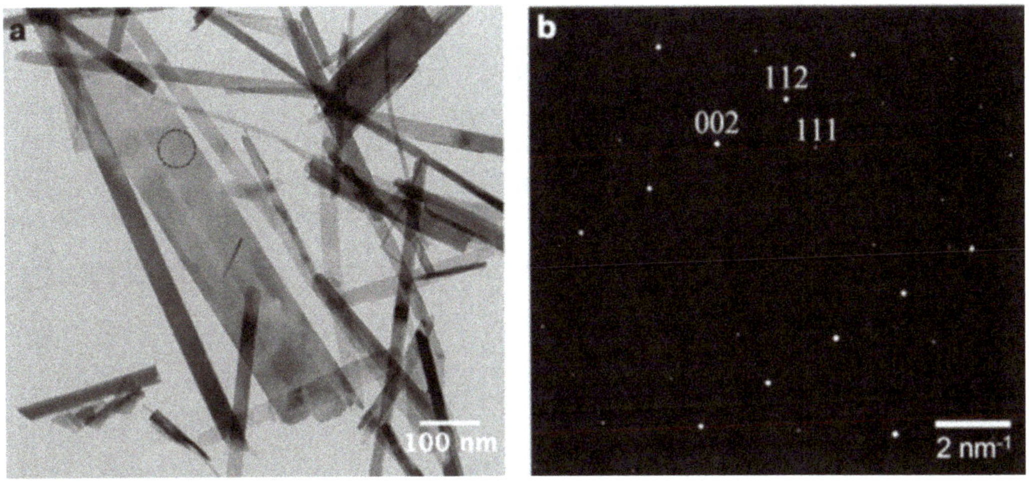

Fig. 22.3 (**a**) TEM image of the product synthesized by the wet precipitation method at initial pH 6.5 and 80 °C and (**b**) electron diffraction pattern of the area highlighted by a dotted circle in the image (**a**). The incident electron beam direction in the diffraction pattern was parallel to [1–10] zone of HAp crystal

phosphate dihydrate (DCPD) and/or octacalcium phosphate (OCP) were formed at lower temperatures of 30 °C and 50 °C (Figs. 22.1a (iv, v) and 22.2d–e), which is almost consistent with the phase diagram (Fig. 22.1b) reported from the data of the hydrolysis products of α-tricalcium phosphate (α-TCP) (Monma 1980; Monma et al. 1981). Interestingly, pure HAp crystals were obtained at 80 °C even in the acidic condition (final pH = 3.9), which is not consistent with the phase diagram for α-TCP hydrolysis (Fig. 22.1b). The HAp crystals formed under the acidic condition at 80 °C showed a fiber-like morphology, with the long axis being parallel to *c* axis of HAp (Fig. 22.3), and were longer than those formed under the alkaline condition at the same temperature.

In order to check the formation process of the HAp nanofibers under the acidic condition at 80 °C, a part of precipitation was collected during the reaction as shown in Fig. 22.4. From the XRD measurements (Fig. 22.4c), only HAp crystals were detected throughout the reaction even at the end of the feeding and ripening periods. From SEM observation (Fig. 22.4b), needle-like crystals of around 500 nm in length were formed at 30 min, and they elongated into fiber-like crystals with more than 10 μm in length and around 50–100 nm in width (i.e., aspect ratio >100) at 1300 min.

Taken together, these results indicate that needle-like HAp was firstly precipitated at the initial pH of 6.5 at 80 °C, which is consistent with the phase diagram (Fig. 22.1b). The firstly formed HAp acted as a seed crystal during the following feeding and ripening periods even at acidic conditions. The unexpected stability of enamel apatite (i.e., ribbon-like apatite crystal elongated extremely in its *c*-axis direction) at acidic conditions has been also reported; that is, enamel apatite did not transformed to DCPD or other calcium phosphates even at pH 4 for 2 months due to a decrease in the ion product of enamel apatite with the decrease in pH (Larsen and Jensen 1989). The acidic condition would be preferable for preventing both secondary nuclei formation (due to an increase in the saturated solubility of HAp

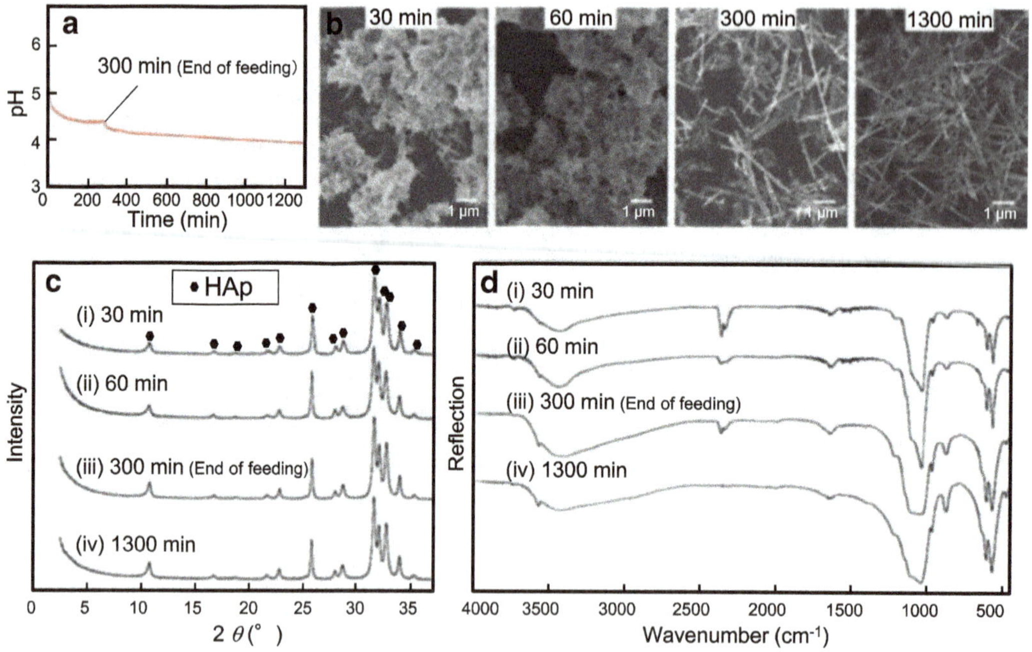

Fig. 22.4 (**a**) A variation of pH during the wet precipitation method at initial pH of 6.5 and 80 °C. (**b**) SEM photographs, (**c**) XRD patterns, and (**d**) FTIR spectra of the part of precipitation collected during the wet precipitation method at 30, 60, 300 (end of feeding), and 1300 min

(Matsumoto et al. 2007) and CO_3^{2-} contamination (due to a decrease in the saturated solubility of CO_2), which are known to inhibit HAp crystal growth (i.e., elongation).

The HAp nanofibers prepared by the simple wet precipitation method without additives at relatively low temperature (80 °C) have potential applications as adsorbents and reinforcing components in biomedical composites because of their unique morphologies (Qi et al. 2017). The preparation method described here accompanies with the crystal growth of HAp (without secondary nuclei formation, under appropriate conditions). Further optimization of this low-temperature wet precipitation method could enable (1) the preparation of more uniform size distribution of HAp nanocrystals for the pre-prepared seed crystals with controlled initial size and number of seeds (or by developing a modified wet precipitation method with a stepwise pH control from alkaline to acidic condition during the reaction) and (2) the development of brush-like HAp coating for the substrates pre-coated with HAp seed crystals. Note that brush-like HAp coating of titanium substrate showed superior osteoconductivity compared with other morphologies (i.e., needle-like, plate-like, net-like, and spherical) of HAp (Kuroda and Okido 2012). Nevertheless, brush-like HAp coating has been limited to some metallic substrates because the previously developed methods require electroconductive and thermally stable substrates due to their coating conditions [e.g., electrochemical and/or high temperature conditions such as above 140 °C (Kuroda and Okido 2012) for wet methods and above 300 °C (Teshima et al. 2012) for dry methods]. The fabrication of brush-like HAp coated substrate at low temperature and its application will be reported in the near future.

Acknowledgments This work was supported partly by the Japan Society for the Promotion of Science KAKENHI (grant numbers: JP16H05533, JP15K1572307, and JP25220912), the Matching Planner Program (MP27115663113) from Japan Science and Technology Agency, and the Cooperative Research Project of Research Center for Biomedical Engineering, Ministry of Education, Culture, Sports, Science and Technology of Japan.

References

Abdel-Gawad EI, Awwad SA (2010) Biocompatibility of intravenous nano hydroxyapatite in male rats. Nat Sci 8:60–68

Aizawa M, Porter AE, Best SM, Bonfield W (2005) Ultrastructural observation of single-crystal apatite fibres. Biomaterials 26:3427–3433

Bouladjine A, Al-Kattan A, Dufour P, Drouet C (2009) New advances in nanocrystalline apatite colloids intended for cellular drug delivery. Langmuir 25:12256–12265

Chen F, Zhu YJ (2016) Large-scale automated production of highly ordered ultralong hydroxyapatite nanowires and construction of various fire-resistant flexible ordered architectures. ACS Nano 10:11483–11495

Choi S-W, Zhang Y, Thomopoulos S, Xia Y (2010) In vitro mineralization by preosteoblasts in poly(DL-lactide-co-glycolide) inverse opal scaffolds reinforced with hydroxyapatite nanoparticles. Langmuir 26:12126–12131

Dorozhkin SV (2010) Nanosized and nanocrystalline calcium orthophosphates. Acta Biomater 6:715–734

Honda M, Fujimi TJ, Izumi S, Izawa K, Aizawa M, Morisue H, Tsuchiya T, Kanzawa N (2010) Topographical analyses of proliferation and differentiation of osteoblasts in micro- and macropores of apatite-fiber scaffold. J Biomed Mater Res A 94:937–944

Kawasaki T (1991) Hydroxyapatite as a liquid chromatographic packing. J Chromatogr 544:147–184

Kilpadi KL, Chang PL, Bellis SL (2001) Hydroxylapatite binds more serum proteins, purified integrins, and osteoblast precursor cells than titanium or steel. J Biomed Mater Res 57:258–267

Kuroda K, Okido M (2012) Hydroxyapatite coating of titanium implants using hydroprocessing and evaluation of their osteoconductivity. Bioinorg Chem Appl 2012:730693 7 pages

Larsen MJ, Jensen SJ (1989) Stability and mutual conversion of enamel apatite and brushite at 20 °C as a function of pH of the aqueous phase. Arch Oral Biol 34:963–968

Lawton DM, Lamaletie MDJ, Gardner DL (1989) Biocompatibility of hydroxyapatite ceramic: response of chondrocytes in a test system using low temperature scanning electron microscopy. J Dent 17:21–27

Lee JS, Wagoner Johnson AJ, Murphy WL (2010) A modular, hydroxyapatite-binding version of vascular endothelial growth factor. Adv Mater 22:5494–5498

Liu Y, Wang W, Zhan Y, Zheng C, Wang G (2002) A simple route to hydroxyapatite nanofibers. Mater Lett 56:496–501

Matsumoto T, Okazaki M, Inoue M, Yamaguchi S, Kusunose T, Toyonaga T, Hamada Y, Takahashi J (2004) Hydroxyapatite particles as a controlled release carrier of protein. Biomaterials 25:3807–3812

Matsumoto T, Okazaki M, Nakahira A, Sasaki J, Egusa H, Sohmura T (2007) Modification of apatite materials for bone tissue engineering and drug delivery carriers. Curr Med Chem 14:2726–2733

Monma H (1980) Preparation of octacalcium phosphate by the hydrolysis of α-tricalcium phosphate. J Mater Sci 15:2428–2434

Monma H, Ueno S, Kanazawa T (1981) Properties of hydroxyapatite prepared by the hydrolysis of tricalcium phosphate. J Chem Technol Biotechnol 31:15–24

Okada M, Matsumoto T (2015) Synthesis and modification of apatite nanoparticles for use in dental and medical applications. Jpn Dent Sci Rev 51:85–95

Qi M-L, He K, Huang Z-N, Shahbazian-Yassar R, Xiao G-Y, Lu Y-P, Shokuhfar T (2017) Hydroxyapatite fibers: a review of synthesis methods. JOM 69:1354–1360

Sadat-Shojai M, Khorasani MT, Jamshidi A (2012) Hydrothermal processing of hydroxyapatite nanoparticles – a Taguchi experimental design approach. J Cryst Growth 361:73–84

Sadat-Shojai M, Khorasani MT, Dinpanah-Khoshdargi E, Jamshidi A (2013) Synthesis methods for nanosized hydroxyapatite with diverse structures. Acta Biomater 9:7591–7621

Teshima K, Wagata H, Sakurai K, Enomoto H, Mori S, Yubuta K, Shishido T, Oishi S (2012) High-quality ultralong hydroxyapatite nanowhiskers grown directly on titanium surfaces by novel low-temperature flux coating method. Cryst Growth Des 12:4890–4896

Tomoda K, Ariizumi H, Nakaji T, Makino K (2010) Hydroxyapatite particles as drug carriers for proteins. Colloids Surf B Biointerfaces 76:226–235

Zhan J, Tseng YH, Chan JCC, Mou CY (2005) Biomimetic formation of hydroxyapatite nanorods by a single-crystal-to- single-crystal transformation. Adv Funct Mater 15:2005–2010

Chapter 23
Physico-chemical Characterisation of the Processes Involved in Enamel Remineralisation by CPP-ACP

Keith J. Cross, N. Laila Huq, Boon Loh, Li-Ming Bhutta, Bill Madytianos, Sarah Peterson, David P. Stanton, Yi Yuan, Coralie Reynolds, Glen Walker, Peiyan Shen, and Eric C. Reynolds

Abstract Casein phosphopeptides derived from tryptic digests of milk caseins spontaneously assemble with calcium and phosphate ions at high pH to form casein phosphopeptide-amorphous calcium phosphate complexes (CPP-ACP). These complexes have been shown to be able to repair lesions in tooth enamel (biohydroxyapatite – HA) both *in vitro* and *in vivo* (specifically white spot lesions in the early stages of tooth decay). In order to better understand the processes involved in enamel remineralisation, the chemical equilibria between the CPP and calcium and phosphate ions as a function of pH were investigated. Furthermore, a thin-enamel slab technique was developed with enhanced sensitivity to monitor the diffusion of radio-opaque ions into individual lesions over a period of days to weeks.

Keywords Enamel · CPP-ACP · Remineralisation · Hydroxyapatite · Diffusion · NMR · Model

23.1 Introduction

Dental caries is initiated by the action of plaque odontopathogenic bacteria that ferment dietary sugars and starches, thus producing organic acids that demineralise the subsurface of enamel hydroxyapatite (Robinson et al. 2000). Since enamel caries is

---

K. J. Cross · N. L. Huq · B. Loh · L.-M. Bhutta · B. Madytianos · S. Peterson · D. P. Stanton
Y. Yuan · C. Reynolds · G. Walker · P. Shen · E. C. Reynolds (✉)
Oral Health Cooperative Research Centre, Melbourne Dental School,
Bio21 Institute of Molecular Science and Biotechnology, The University of Melbourne,
Melbourne, VIC, Australia
e-mail: keith.cross@unimelb.edu.au; laila@unimelb.edu.au; billym@student.unimelb.edu.au; speterson1@student.unimelb.edu.au; dstanton@unimelb.edu.au; yuay@unimelb.edu.au; coralie@unimelb.edu.au; gdwalker@unimelb.edu.au; peiyan@unimelb.edu.au; e.reynolds@unimelb.edu.au

K. Endo et al. (eds.), *Biomineralization*,
https://doi.org/10.1007/978-981-13-1002-7_23

[1]	Arg^{1}-Glu-Leu-Glu-Glu-Leu-Asn-Val-Pro-Gly-Glu-Ile-Val-Glu-Ser(*P*)-Leu-(Ser(*P*)-)$_3$(Glu-)$_2$-Ser-Ile-Thr-Arg^{25} β-CN(1-25)
[2]	Gln^{59}-Met-Glu-Ala-Glu-Ser(*P*)-Ile-(Ser(*P*)-)$_3$(Glu-)$_2$-Ile-Val-Pro-Asn-Ser(*P*)-Val-Glu-Gln-Lys^{79} α_{S1}-CN(59-79)
[3]	Asn^{46}-Ala-Asn-Glu-Glu-Glu-Tyr-Ser-Ile-Gly-(Ser(*P*)-)$_3$(Glu-)$_2$-Ser(*P*)-Ala-Glu-Val-Ala-Thr-Glu-Glu-Val-Lys^{70} α_{S2}-CN(46-70)
[4]	Lys^{1}-Asn-Thr-Met-Glu-His-Val-(Ser(*P*)-)$_3$(Glu-)$_2$-Ser-Ile-Ile-Ser(*P*)-Gln-Glu-Thr-Tyr-Lys^{21} α_{S2}-CN(1-21)

Fig. 23.1 Sequences of the predominant tryptic phosphopeptides of CPP-ACP in three-letter code. The cluster sequence motif critical to calcium and phosphate binding is highlighted in red

essentially a chemical process, at early stages of dental caries, the hydroxyapatite mineral loss is reversible. Any products that prevent enamel demineralisation and promote remineralisation are described as exhibiting anticaries activity. The principal components of dairy products associated with their anticariogenic activity are multi-phosphorylated caseins complexed with calcium and phosphate. Enzymic hydrolysis of caseins yields phosphopeptides known as casein phosphopeptides (CPP). These peptides, with their multiple phosphoseryl residues, bind relatively large quantities of calcium and phosphate ions in an amorphous, bioavailable form (Reynolds et al. 1995). The resulting complexes are known as casein phosphopeptide-amorphous calcium phosphate (CPP-ACP). The two dominant, self-assembling peptides are β-CN(1-25) and α_{S1}-CN(59-79) forming 20–30% by mass of the total CPP (Fig. 23.1). These bovine casein-derived peptides all contain the cluster sequence motif -(Ser(*P*)-)$_3$(Glu-)$_2$.

The aim of this study was to investigate the interactions between the peptides and crystalline and non-crystalline mineral components during the remineralisation process.

23.2 Materials and Methods

23.2.1 Materials

Extracted human third molars were obtained from patients attending the Melbourne Dental School with ethics approval (1340048). Enamel slices (~300 μ thick) were prepared from these teeth for examination.

23.2.2 Ion-Binding Studies

To evaluate the influence of pH on the calcium and phosphate ion equilibria, solutions of CPP-ACP, α_{S1}-CN(59-79)-ACP, and β-CN(1-25) were subjected to pH titrations. Calcium and phosphate ion concentrations were determined using microfiltration using previously described protocols, (Cross et al. 2005) modified to use a Dionex ion analyser.

23.2.3 Nuclear Magnetic Resonance Studies

NMR spectra were acquired at 599.741 MHz on a Varian Unity Inova spectrometer as described previously (Cross et al. 2016). Solution-phase diffusion measurements were performed using the sLED experiment as described previously (Altieri et al. 1995).The amplitude of the NMR signal is a function of the applied magnetic field gradient and the Stokes-Einstein radius of the diffusing species ($S \propto \exp(-\alpha DG^2)$,where D is the diffusion coefficient, G is the magnetic field gradient, and α depends on experimental values. The diffusion coefficient is related to the hydrodynamic radius by $D = k_BT/6\pi\rho R$ where k_B is the Boltzmann constant, T the absolute temperature, ρ the solution viscosity, and R the hydrodynamic radius of the spherical particles.

23.2.4 Remineralisation Studies

The novel technique utilised thin slabs of enamel (~300 μ thick) cut from human third molars that allowed sound mineral portions of the slabs to be used as controls in measuring the time course of remineralisation of artificial lesions. The technique is an extension of that previously described (Cochrane et al. 2008), with remineralisation of individual slabs being assessed after 0, 2, 3, 6, 12, 15, and 20 days immersion in a remineralisation solution at either pH 5·5 or pH 7·0. Diffusion of radio-opaque ions into the artificially prepared lesions was monitored by TWIM (Thomas et al. 2006). Acid-resistant nail polish was used to define the remineralisation zone and applied three times to prevent leakage during the soaking in the remineralisation solutions. Remineralising solutions consisted of 1% solutions of either CPP-ACP or β-CN(1-25)-ACP prepared at either pH 7.0 or 5.5 to compare the effects of neutral and acidic pH.

Lesion-sections were subjected to transversal wavelength-independent microradiography (TWIM) at days 0, 2, 3, 6, 12, 15, and 20 to visualise the time dependence of mineral ion uptake during enamel remineralisation. Microradiographs acquired on day 0 were used as control images for each lesion-section. The lesion-sections remained soaked in the remineralisation solutions except when being X-rayed.

DOSY experiments were performed using the sLED technique to determine the relative rates of diffusion of the complexes using either the integrated aromatic or aliphatic signals of a β-CN(1-25)-ACP sample.

SDS-PAGE of CPP cross-linked using glutaraldehyde was conducted to analyse the multimerisation of CPP as described previously (Cross et al. 2016).

23.3 Results

23.3.1 *The CPP-ACP Complexes Exist in Equilibria with Both Bound and Free Calcium and Phosphate Ions*

When prepared at pH 9, the CPP-ACP complexes have most of the calcium and phosphate peptide bound. However, these complexes exist in solution in equilibrium with free ionic calcium and phosphate. Figure 23.2 shows sigmoidal pH titration curves for β-CN(1-25)-ACP representative of results obtained in this study. The pK_a values for Ca^{2+} and Pi binding are 5.983 ± 0.038 and 6.302 ± 0.067, respectively.

Further pH titrations were performed on 1% and 2% β-CN(1-25)-ACP complexes prepared with varying Ca/Pi ratio and varying peptide:Ca ratio. Plots of the bound calcium and phosphate concentrations against pH revealed sigmoidal curves whose shape remained independent of the Ca/Pi ratio. For the complexes prepared at ratios of Ca/Pi ranging from 1.6 to 1.51, and 12–15 Ca/peptide, the pH dependence

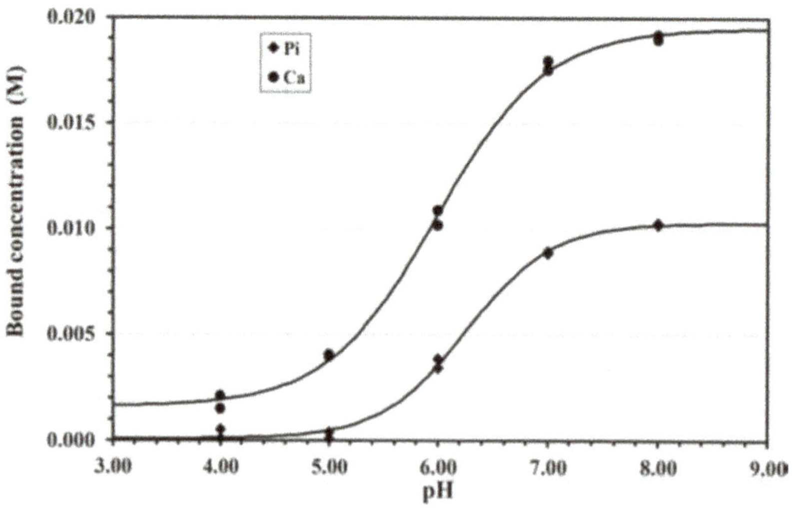

Fig. 23.2 Representative pH titration curves for a laboratory-prepared sample of β-CN(1-25)-ACP. The solid-line curves are fit to the Henderson-Hasselbalch formula yielding effective pK_a values of 6.302 ± 0.067 for the phosphate ion curve and 5.983 ± 0.038 for the calcium ion curve. Note that at low pH, the peptides bind residual calcium ions but no phosphate ions

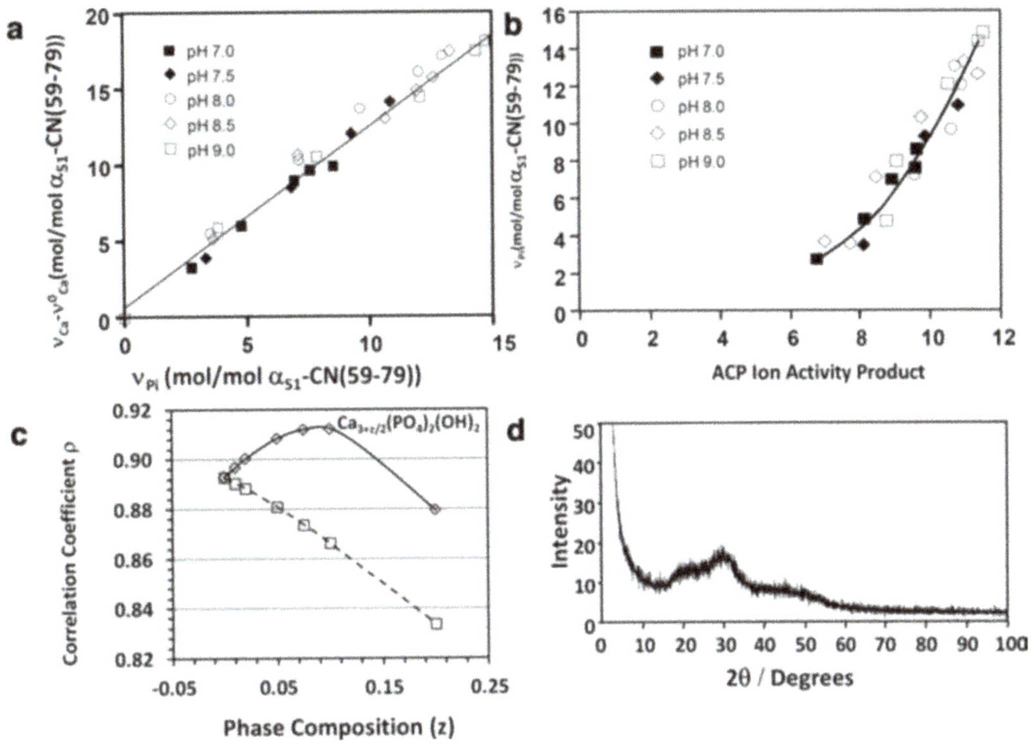

Fig. 23.3 (**a**) A plot illustrating the linear relationship between CPP-bound inorganic phosphate and CPP-bound calcium in excess of that bound at low pH (denoted by $\nu^0{}_{Ca}$). (**b**) A plot of CPP-bound inorganic phosphate against ACP ion activity product. This illustrates that only an amorphous calcium phosphate phase predicts a one-to-one functional dependence of calcium phosphate ion activity product and the activity of phosphate (shown here) or calcium. (**c**) A plot illustrating that the best fit between the ion activity product and the phosphate (or calcium) activity occurs with a slightly calcium-rich, non-stoichiometric ACP phase having the formula $Ca_{3.0425}(PO_4)_2(OH)_{0.085}$. The lower curve is for calcium-deficient ACP phases and does not have a maximum at realistically achievable compositions. (**d**) X-ray powder diffraction image of a CPP-ACP sample demonstrating the broad peaks expected from an amorphous solid

of the bound calcium and phosphate were similar. Further analysis using α_{S1}-CN(59-79)-ACP revealed a well-defined phase of ACP stabilised by the CPP (Fig. 23.3a–c). Figure 23.3d shows a representative powder X-ray diffraction pattern of CPP-ACP that is consistent with an amorphous phase of calcium phosphate.

23.3.2 The CPP-ACP Complexes Are Small Readily Diffusible Species

The sLED experiment yields a diffusion-dependent signal whose functional dependence on the applied, magnetic-field gradient is dependent on the hydrodynamic radius of the molecule being studied. Figure 23.4a shows a plot of sLED signal intensity against the applied magnetic field gradient. This provides the ratio of hydrodynamic radii of the β-CN(1-25)-ACP complex relative to that of water. The

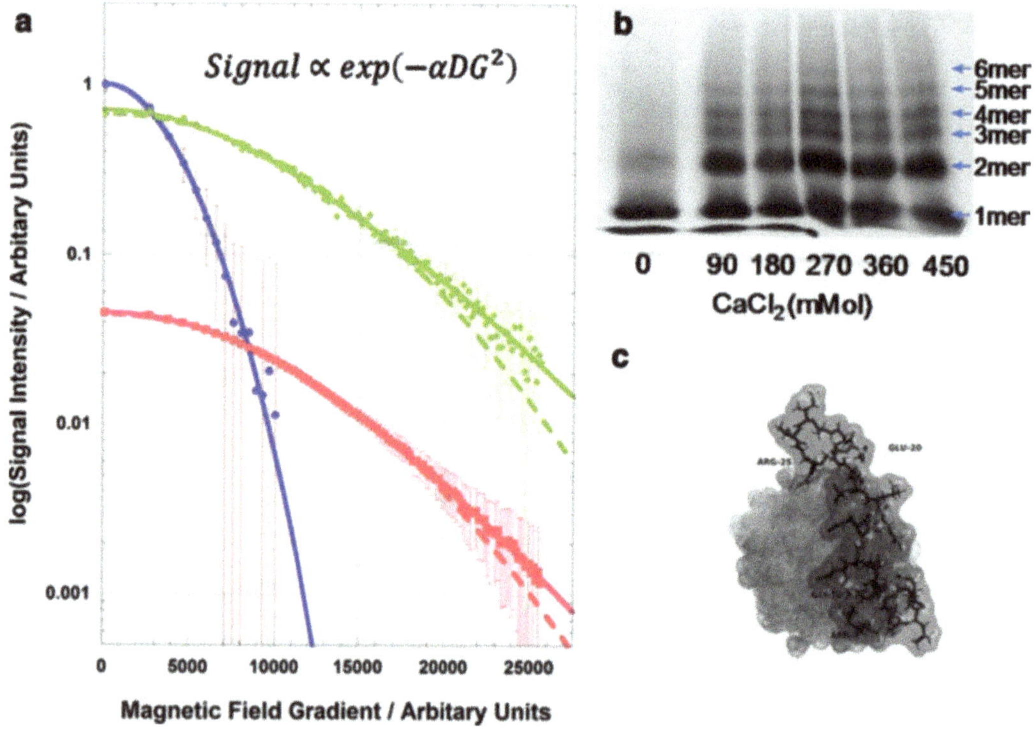

Fig. 23.4 (**a**) A representative plot of data from the sLED NMR experiment (Altieri et al. 1995) that uses magnetic field gradients to measure the relative rates of diffusion of various protonated species. The water signal (blue) can be compared with either the integrated aromatic (green) or aliphatic (red) signals of a CPP-ACP sample. The data from both peptide curves provided an internal consistency check. The Stokes-Einstein equation relates the hydrodynamic radius of a particle and its diffusion constant, allowing the determination of the hydrodynamic radius of the complexes given the known radius of water. The calculated hydrodynamic radii of the CPP-ACP complexes ranged from 1.53 ± 0.03 nm at pH 6 to 1.92 ± 0.08 nm at pH 9. The deviation from the fitted curves at high-magnetic-field-gradient values fits a two-component model consistent with the formation of aggregates. (**b**) A representative SDS-PAGE gel featuring the cross linking of the CPP using glutaraldehyde, observed in the presence of calcium ions. The multimerisation was also observed in the presence of calcium and phosphate ions suggesting that the complexes contain up to six CPP peptides. (**c**) A model of the CPP-ACP complex consistent with these and various other experiments. The peptide is depicted as sticks within a translucent van der Waals surface, and the ACP is shown as a pale grey van der Waals surface

measured hydrodynamic radii of the β-CN(1-25)-ACP complex range from 1.53 ± 0.03 nm at pH 6 to 1.92 ± 0.08 nm at pH 9. The deviation from the fitted curves at high-magnetic-field-gradient values fits a two-component model that is consistent with the formation of aggregates.

SDS-PAGE of CPP cross-linked using glutaraldehyde, in the presence of either calcium ions (Fig. 23.4b) or calcium and phosphate ions (Cross et al. 2016), suggests that the complexes contain up to six CPP peptides. Figure 23.4c shows a model of the CPP-ACP complex consistent with the results of these experiments.

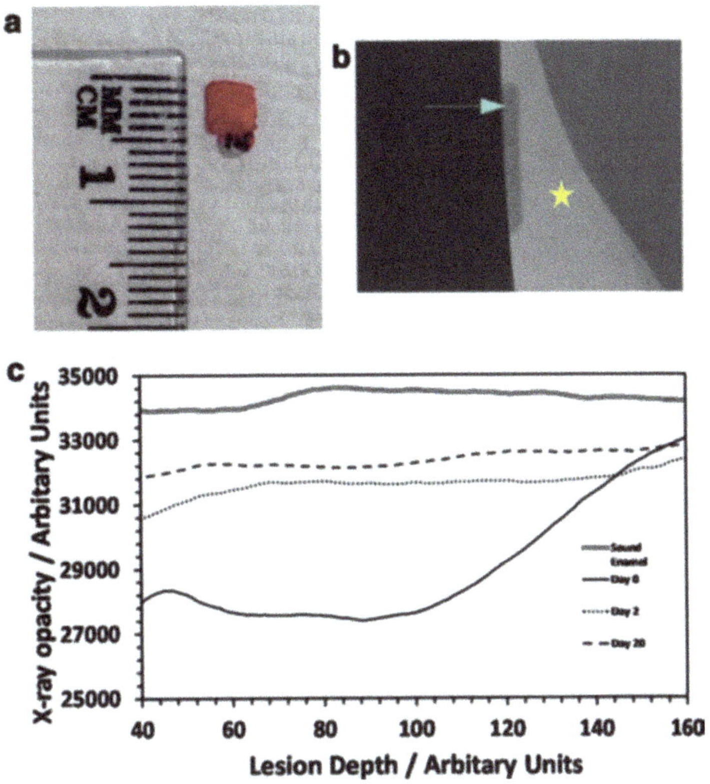

Fig. 23.5 Key features of the developed method to study the time dependence of remineralisation of enamel using thin slabs of enamel (~300 μ) cut from human third molars. The sound enamel regions provide the experimental control regions for the experiments. (**a**) Thin slab of enamel cut from human third molar and prepared with acid-resistant nail polish defining the remineralisation zone. (**b**) X-ray micrograph showing demineralised zone (arrow) and adjacent sound enamel (star). (**c**) Time-dependent, X-ray opacity of a specific enamel slab demonstrating diffusion of mineral ions into the lesion. Remineralisation occurs within a few days. This plot of X-ray opacity against lesion depth enables the calculation of A_s being the area under the sound enamel curve, A_m representing the areas under the individual 'remineralised' enamel curves, and A_d being the area under the 'demineralised' enamel curve (day 0) to determine extent of remineralisation (see Fig. 23.6)

23.3.3 *Both CPP-ACP and β-CN(1-25)-ACP Complexes Release Mineral Ions that Remineralise Demineralised Enamel Lesions*

Blocks of enamel from third molars with demineralised lesions were prepared that yielded multiple uniformly demineralised lesion-sections that would enable inter-tooth and intra-tooth comparisons (Fig. 23.5a). The sound enamel regions provided the experimental control regions for the experiments. Acid-resistant nail polish was used to define the remineralisation zone. Microradiography was used to visualise the time dependence of mineral ion uptake, in enamel remineralisation experiments. Figure 23.5b shows a sample X-ray micrograph with the demineralised zone (arrow) and the adjacent sound enamel (star).

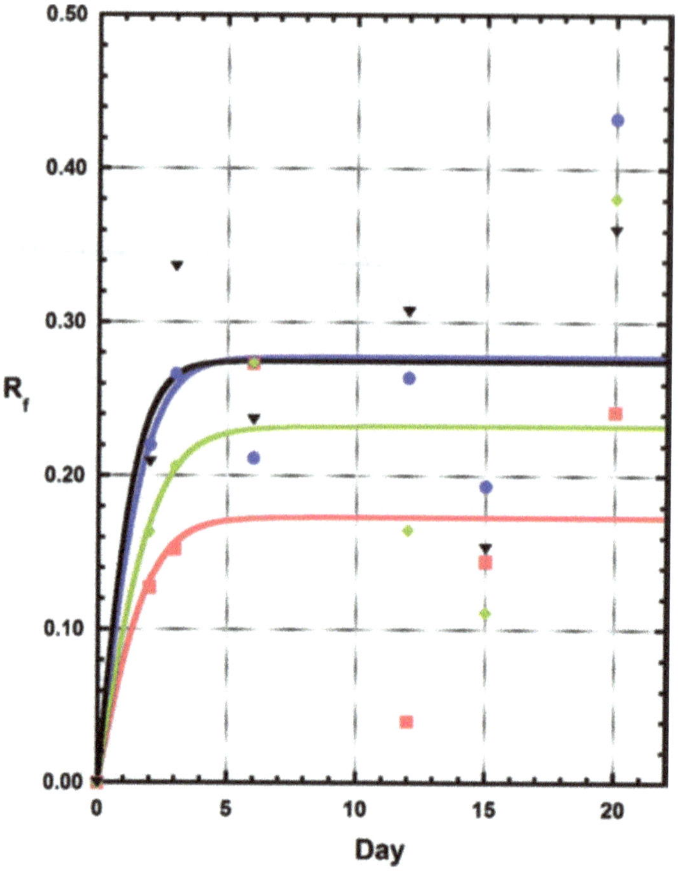

Fig. 23.6 Plot of time-dependent remineralisation for four lesion-sections. Each data point represents the extent of remineralisation calculated by the ratio $R_f = \frac{A_m - A_d}{A_s - A_d}$, where A_m is the area under the 'remineralised' enamel curve, A_d is the area under the 'demineralised' enamel curve (day 0), and A_s is the area under the sound enamel curve. Statistically significant differences in the extent of remineralisation are observed between different samples and may be due to biological differences: the lowest R_f of 0.17 ± 0.04 (in the graph above) differs significantly from the maximum R_f of 0.28 ± 0.04 at a $p = 0.025$

Figure 23.5c shows a plot of the time-dependent, X-ray opacity of a specific enamel slab after demineralisation at day 0 and following remineralisation until day 20. The X-ray data showed a diffusion-dependent increase in electron density, interpreted as mineralisation.

A time-dependent uptake of mineral was observed in the presence of both CPP-ACP and β-CN(1-25)-ACP at both pH values. The calculated data from each sample was fitted to the time-dependent part of a diffusion equation of the form

$$R_f = R_{f_{\max}} \times \tanh(kt)$$

where 'k' represents the rate constant for diffusion and 't' represents the elapsed time taken in days. The Pearson correlation coefficients for the non-linear curve fit confirmed that the data were consistent with a simple diffusion model for remineralisation. Figure 23.6 illustrates time-dependent plots of the calculated extent of remineralisation (R_f) for four representative sections. The data is consistent with mineral ions from CPP-ACP and β-CN(1-25)-ACP diffusing into and interacting with the enamel crystals. A recent study of the interaction of CPP-ACP with either enamel or saliva-coated enamel (Huq et al. 2018) indicates that chemical equilibrium is established within a few hours; thus, the rate-limiting step for enamel remineralisation is the rate of diffusion of ions into the subsurface enamel.

23.4 Discussion

In this study, a variety of methods have been used to characterise the complexes formed by the casein phosphopeptides with calcium and phosphate ions. CPP bind calcium and phosphate to form stable CPP-ACP complexes in alkaline solution. These studies show that the ratio of bound calcium to bound phosphate is constant and independent of pH in the range of pH 7–9. Furthermore, the ion activity product fits a single curve for a calcium-rich, non-stoichiometric calcium phosphate phase. DOSY experiments using the sLED sequence demonstrated that the complex has a small but significant variation in size with pH. These experiments further revealed the ability of the small complexes to aggregate as concentrations were increased. The model of the CPP-ACP complex with all amino acids in the peptides interacting with the ACP surface is consistent with earlier findings that the peptide length influences the extent of binding to calcium and phosphate ions (Cross et al. 2005).

The importance of small readily diffusible CPP-ACP complexes is confirmed by the experiments using thin slabs of human enamel with artificial lesions that mimic early carious lesions. To enable the time-dependent monitoring, the current remineralisation procedures (Shen et al. 2011) required extensive improvements. The use of the single section for all-time points required a thicker section to withstand repeated handling. To accommodate the increased thickness, TWIM was used instead of the commonly used transverse microradiography (TMR) technique, both methods being validated techniques for monitoring carious lesions (Thomas et al. 2006). In addition, the acid-resistant nail varnish was reapplied three times to prevent leakage during the soaking in remineralisation solutions. To improve the signal-to-noise ratio, an additional 500-μ-thick aluminium filter was used with an optimal X-ray tube voltage of 30 kV.

We observed statistically significant differences in the extent of remineralisation within the multiple lesion-sections derived from the same individual tooth. These differences were attributed to varying microporosities of the demineralised lesion-sections of each individual tooth.

In conclusion, the CPP-ACP complexes were characterised to be a small readily diffusible species that can release the mineral ions on contact with demineralised enamel lesions. Furthermore both CPP-ACP and β-CN(1-25) complexes were able to remineralise within a few days in in vitro experiments.

Acknowledgements This study was funded by the Oral Health Cooperative Research Centre and NHMRC. Extracted human third molars were obtained from patients attending the Melbourne Dental School with ethics approval (1340048).

References

Altieri AS, Hinton DP, Byrd RA (1995) Association of biomolecular systems via pulsed field gradient NMR self-diffusion measurements. J Am Chem Soc 117(28):7566–7567

Cochrane NJ, Saranathan S, Cai F, Cross KJ, Reynolds EC (2008) Enamel subsurface lesion remineralisation with casein phosphopeptide stabilised solutions of calcium, phosphate and fluoride. Caries Res 42(2):88–97. https://doi.org/10.1159/000113161

Cross KJ, Huq NL, Palamara J, Perich JW, Reynolds EC (2005) Physicochemical characterization of casein phosphopeptide-amorphous calcium phosphate nanocomplexes. J Biol Chem 280(15):15362–15369

Cross KJ, Huq NL, Reynolds EC (2016) Casein phosphopeptide-amorphous calcium phosphate nanocomplexes: a structural model. Biochemistry 55(31):4316–4325. https://doi.org/10.1021/acs.biochem.6b00522

Huq NL, Cross KJ, Myroforidis H, Stanton DP, Chen YY, Ward BR, Reynolds EC (2018) Molecular interactions of peptide encapsulated calcium phosphate delivery vehicle at enamel surfaces. Proc BIOMIN XIV

Reynolds EC, Cain CJ, Webber FL, Black CL, Riley PF, Johnson IH, Perich JW (1995) Anticariogenicity of calcium phosphate complexes of tryptic casein phosphopeptides in the rat. J Dent Res 74(6):1272–1279

Robinson C, Shore RC, Brookes SJ, Strafford S, Wood SR, Kirkham J (2000) The chemistry of enamel caries. Crit Rev Oral Biol Med 11(4):481–495

Shen P, Manton DJ, Cochrane NJ, Walker GD, Yuan Y, Reynolds C, Reynolds EC (2011) Effect of added calcium phosphate on enamel remineralization by fluoride in a randomized controlled in situ trial. J Dent 39(7):518–525. https://doi.org/10.1016/j.jdent.2011.05.002

Thomas RZ, Ruben JL, de Vries J, ten Bosch JJ, Huysmans MC (2006) Transversal wavelength-independent microradiography, a method for monitoring caries lesions over time, validated with transversal microradiography. Caries Res 40(4):281–291

Chapter 24
Molecular Interactions of Peptide Encapsulated Calcium Phosphate Delivery Vehicle at Enamel Surfaces

Noorjahan Laila Huq, Keith John Cross, Helen Myroforidis, David Phillip Stanton, Yu-Yen Chen, Brent Robert Ward, and Eric Charles Reynolds

Abstract Phosphorylated peptides derived from milk caseins, known as casein phosphopeptides (CPP), self-assemble and encapsulate the calcium and phosphate mineral in the form of amorphous calcium phosphate (ACP), thus forming CPP-ACP nanocomplexes that are nontoxic and biocompatible. The biomedical application is the repair of tooth surfaces (enamel) at early stages of tooth decay. These nanocomplexes release calcium and phosphate ions to rebuild demineralised HA crystals in enamel subsurface lesions. The topical application of CPP-ACP at the tooth surface initiates a series of interactions at the enamel mineral hydroxyapatite surface and at the enamel salivary pellicle that are not well understood. In this study, we have shown that the β-casein (1-25) peptide binds reversibly to Ca^{2+}, Mg^{2+}, Mn^{2+}, La^{2+}, Ni^{2+}, and Cd^{2+} metal ions. In contrast, binding to Sn^{2+}, Fe^{2+}, and Fe^{3+} ions resulted in ion-induced aggregation. The casein peptides as well as the mineral ions dissociate from the CPP-ACP complexes to adsorb to both the uncoated and saliva-coated mineral surface with the mineralisation increasing monotonically with increasing pH. Furthermore, SEM of the CPP-ACP revealed images of spherical particles surrounded by ACP mineral. In conclusion, the enamel remineralisation process involves an array of interactions between the peptide and mineral ions of the CPP-ACP delivery vehicle and the tooth enamel mineral with its salivary pellicle.

Keywords Enamel · CPP-ACP · Saliva · SEM · Hydroxyapatite · Mineralisation

N. L. Huq · K. J. Cross · H. Myroforidis · D. P. Stanton · Y.-Y. Chen · B. R. Ward
E. C. Reynolds (✉)
Oral Health Cooperative Research Centre, Melbourne Dental School, Bio21 Institute of Molecular Science and Biotechnology, The University of Melbourne, Melbourne, Victoria, Australia
e-mail: laila@unimelb.edu.au; keith.cross@unimelb.edu.au; dstanton@unimelb.edu.au; yyyc@unimelb.edu.au; brentrw@unimelb.edu.au; e.reynolds@unimelb.edu.au

K. Endo et al. (eds.), *Biomineralization*,
https://doi.org/10.1007/978-981-13-1002-7_24

24.1 Introduction

Dental caries is the destruction of tooth surfaces by acid generated by plaque odontopathogenic in a complex chemical process (Robinson et al. 2000). The reversibility of enamel hydroxyapatite mineral loss at early stages of dental caries has led to the development of various anticariogenic approaches to repair enamel lesions (Cochrane et al. 2010). One oral therapeutic consists of phosphorylated peptides derived from milk caseins, known as casein phosphopeptides (CPP) that self-assemble and encapsulate the calcium and phosphate mineral in the form of amorphous calcium phosphate (ACP) (Reynolds et al. 1995).

At the tooth surface, the mechanism of the remineralisation process by CPP-ACP including the changes in the chemical equilibria of the complexes and the enamel lesions is unclear. Above the enamel hydroxyapatite are further zones of chemical complexity, including the layer of salivary proteins known as the acquired enamel pellicle and the outermost layer of oral biofilm. Our long-term goal has been to study the molecular interactions between CPP-ACP complexes (Cross et al. 2016) and enamel hydroxyapatite, salivary proteins (Huq et al. 2016), and the oral biofilm (Dashper et al. 2016) that would occur during topical application of CPP-ACP in the oral cavity. In this study, we investigate the interactions between peptide and crystalline and non-crystalline mineral components during the remineralisation process by the peptide encapsulated delivery vehicle CPP-ACP.

24.2 Materials and Methods

The sequences of four bovine casein-derived tryptic phosphopeptides containing the cluster sequence motif -(Ser(*P*)-)$_3$(Glu-)$_2$ are shown in Fig. 24.1. The two dominant, self-assembling peptides are β-CN(1-25) and α_{S1}-CN(59-79) forming 20–30% by mass of the total CPP (Fig. 24.1).

[1] Arg^{1}-Glu-Leu-Glu-Glu-Leu-Asn-Val-Pro-Gly-Glu-Ile-Val-Glu-Ser(*P*)-Leu-<u>(Ser(*P*)-)$_3$(Glu-)$_2$</u>-Ser-Ile-Thr-Arg^{25} β-CN(1-25)

[2] Gln^{59}-Met-Glu-Ala-Glu-Ser(*P*)-Ile-<u>(Ser(*P*)-)$_3$(Glu-)$_2$</u>-Ile-Val-Pro-Asn-Ser(*P*)-Val-Glu-Gln-Lys^{79} α_{S1}-CN(59-79)

[3] Asn^{46}-Ala-Asn-Glu-Glu-Glu-Tyr-Ser-Ile-Gly-<u>(Ser(*P*)-)$_3$(Glu-)$_2$</u>-Ser(*P*)-Ala-Glu-Val-Ala-Thr-Glu-Glu-Val-Lys^{70} α_{S2}-CN(46-70)

[4] Lys^{1}-Asn-Thr-Met-Glu-His-Val-<u>(Ser(*P*)-)$_3$(Glu-)$_2$</u>-Ser-Ile-Ile-Ser(*P*)-Gln-Glu-Thr-Tyr-Lys^{21} α_{S2}-CN(1-21)

Fig. 24.1 The sequences of the four major casein tryptic phosphopeptides are depicted using the three-letter code with the motif <u>-(Ser(*P*)-)3(Glu-)2</u> underlined

24.2.1 Adsorption Studies

An assay was developed to determine the binding of the CPP-ACP components **1** and **2** (Fig. 24.1) to enamel using an in vitro model with synthetic HA used as a substitute for dental enamel (Huq et al. 2016). The standard curve was derived from peak heights of the RP-HPLC profiles of purified peptides with concentrations ranging from 10 to 1000 μg/ml in 25 mM NaCl and 25 mM imidazole buffer (pH 7). CPP of the same concentrations were incubated with end-over-end rotation for 1–4 h at 37 °C with 2 mg of HA. The samples were centrifuged at 10,000 *g* for 15 min to pellet peptide bound to HA. The supernatants analysed by RP-HPLC provided the unbound peptide concentration. The partitioning of the free and peptide-bound ions was determined followed by measurements of calcium and phosphate ions (Cross et al. 2005). The saliva collection procedures and approval were as recently described (Huq et al. 2016).

24.2.2 Chemical Equilibria Studies

Test and control solutions were added to 2 mg HA. After mixing thoroughly, the samples were incubated for 2 h at RT with end-over-end rotation. To remove the HA crystals, the samples were centrifuged at 10,000 g. The HA crystal-free supernatants as well as the original solutions were subjected to ion quantitation for the ions in both peptide-free and peptide-bound states. In a second study, the HA crystals were pre-equilibrated with water at the 3 pH values. Following centrifugation, the calcium, phosphate, H^+, and OH^- ions released from the uncoated and saliva-coated HA crystals into the supernatants were measured. These supernatants were used to prepare the 0.2% CPP-ACP solutions. The partitioning of the ions associated with the peptide complexes and those free in solution was determined. These supernatants were then added to the pre-equilibrated HA. The concentrations of total, free, and CPP-bound calcium and phosphate ions and pH values of the 0.2% CPP-ACP solutions prepared at pH 5.5, 7.0, and 8.5 before and after incubation with crystalline-uncoated HA and saliva-coated HA were measured.

The dissociation study was performed by adding varying amounts of HA to 1% CPP-ACP solution at pH 7 and 5.5 and monitoring the supernatant profile by RP-HPLC.

24.2.3 SEM Studies

SEM of a 5% CPP-ACP solution was performed using 1 kV with 25 pA current with a T1 detector in a Teneo VS instrument (FEI). Images at 10^4, 5×10^4, and 8×10^4 magnification were obtained.

24.3 Results

24.3.1 *β-Casein (1-25) Peptide Demonstrates a Range of Interactions with Metal Ions*

We selected one of the principal components of CPP β-CN(1-25) (**1**, Fig. 24.1) for exposure to different metal ions to examine the recovery of peptide **1** by RP-HPLC at pH 2. A single peak with identical retention times on the chromatogram (Fig. 24.2) was observed for peptide **1** incubated with Ca^{2+}, Mg^{2+}, Mn^{2+}, La^{2+}, Ni^{2+}, and Cd^{2+} ions. This was indicative of reversible ion binding. However, peptide **1** incubated with Sn^{2+}, Fe^{2+}, and Fe^{3+} ions, eluted as multiple broadened peaks indicative of ion-induced aggregation. This study confirms that β-CN(1-25) is capable of releasing the bound calcium ions at low pH without experiencing permanent aggregation.

24.3.2 *The Predominant Peptides of the CPP-ACP Complex Bind to Uncoated HA and Saliva-Coated HA*

To determine if the pure peptides derived from CPP directly interact with enamel, adsorption studies were performed with enamel substitute HA and saliva-coated HA. We analysed the individual adsorption patterns of the two peptides **1** and **2** with

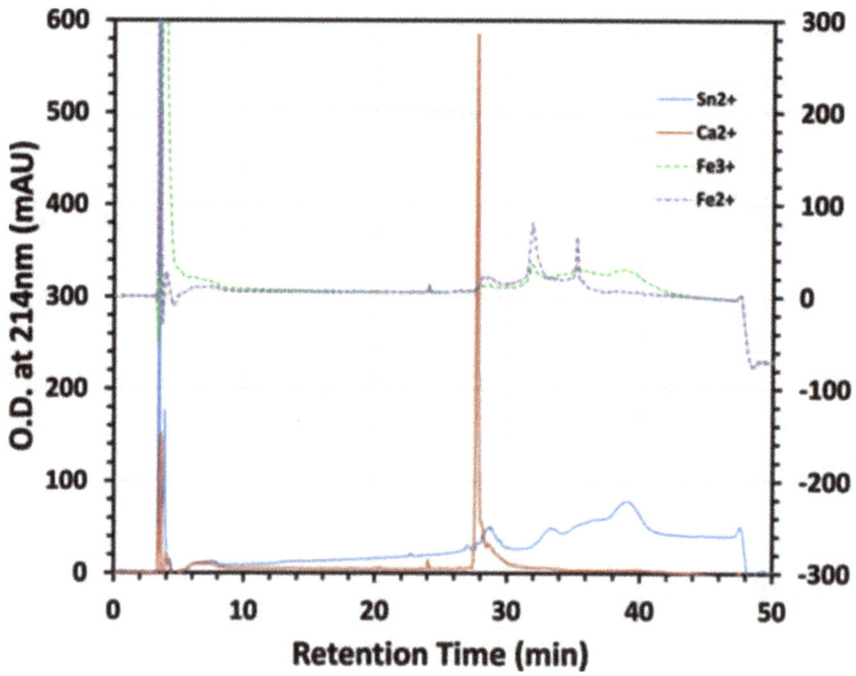

Fig. 24.2 RP-HPLC chromatogram depicting the recovery elution profiles of β-CN(1-25) incubated with Ca^{2+}, Sn^{2+}, Fe^{2+}, and Fe^{3+} ions. The binding to Ca^{2+} ions by β-CN(1-25) is reversible; this is pivotal to the delivery of mineral by CPP-ACP to the enamel

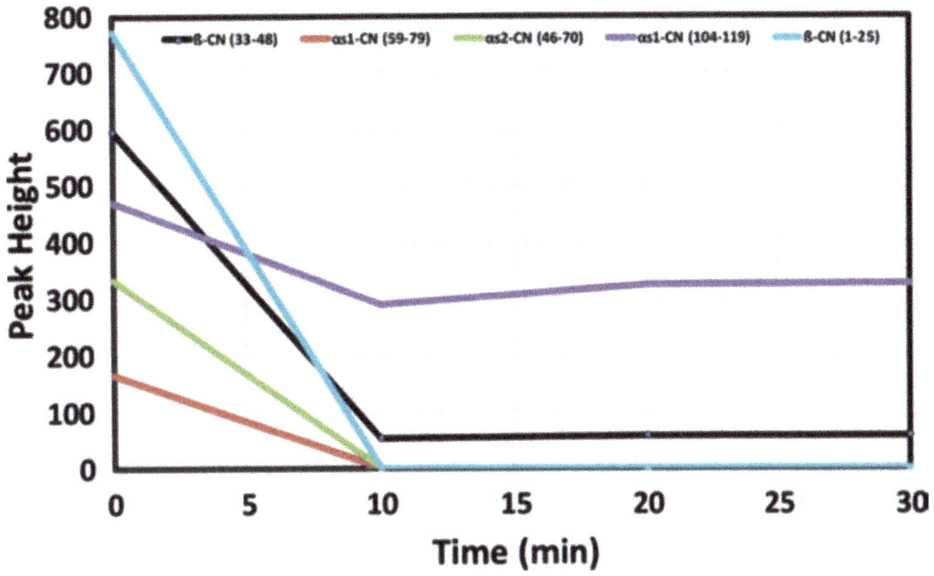

Fig. 24.3 RP-HPLC analysed loss of soluble casein phosphopeptides from CPP-ACP at pH 5.5 after addition of HA at 0 min. The multi-phosphorylated [**1-4**] and mono-phosphorylated β-CN(33-48) peptides dissociate from the ACP to adsorb onto the crystalline HA

HA for Langmuir and Freund-type binding. Both peptides bound to HA surfaces according to a Langmuir-type adsorption model with peptide **1** ($K = 323 \pm 149$ ml/μmol) having a higher affinity for HA than peptide **2** ($K = 49 \pm 22$ ml/μmol). The adsorption profile of bound versus total showed an intermediate and final plateau indicating biphasic processes. At lower peptide concentrations, both peptide **1** ($K = 463 \pm 200$ ml/μmol) and peptide **2** ($K = 194 \pm 122$ ml/μmol) had a greater affinity for the saliva-coated HA surface, than their respective affinities for an uncoated HA surface.

24.3.3 *Casein Peptides Dissociate from the CPP-ACP Complex to Bind to HA*

The levels of soluble peptides from the CPP-ACP complexes at pH values 7.0 and 5.5 were monitored by RP-HPLC. Addition of HA caused a reduction of the soluble levels of peptides confirming that the multi-phosphorylated [**1-4**] and mono-phosphorylated peptide β-CN(33-48) dissociate from the ACP to adsorb onto HA. Figure 24.3 shows a representative time-dependent loss by 1% CPP-ACP at pH 5.5.

24.3.4 The Chemical Equilibria of HA Surfaces Is Altered by the Addition of the Individual Peptides and Peptide-ACP Complexes

The changes in chemical equilibria of HA surfaces were monitored during binding studies of crystalline HA exposed to pure peptides **1** or **2** (both without Ca^{2+}) or β-CN(1-25)-ACP. The addition of HA to a solution of either of the two pure peptides **1** or **2** dissolved at 120 mg/l concentrations resulted in the post-addition measurement of 244 ± 11 mM and 124 ± 5 mM calcium, respectively, in the peptide solutions. This was interpreted as a peptide adsorption-mediated release of calcium ions from the crystalline HA into the solution (Misra 1997). In contrast, albumin (120 mg/l), used as a control, elicited a much lower adsorption-mediated release of 57 ± 16 mM calcium from HA. The initial Ca^{2+} concentration in a 240 mg/l solution of the β-CN(1-25)-ACP complex was reduced after the addition of HA. The Ca^{2+} reduction from 355 ± 67 to 246 ± 68 mM was attributed to the calcium ions in the amorphous phase previously associated with the peptide **1** now binding to or precipitating with crystalline HA.

24.3.5 The CPP-ACP Complexes Exhibit a pH-Dependent Release of Mineral Ions to Uncoated and Saliva-Coated HA Crystals

The movement of calcium, phosphate, and hydroxyl ions to and from the uncoated and saliva-coated HA crystals during exposure to CPP-ACP was monitored during binding studies (Table 24.1). Table 24.1 shows a net loss of total calcium and phosphate ions from the CPP-ACP on binding to HA at pH 5.5, 7.0, and 8.5. This loss represented transfer of mineral from the amorphous phase of ACP to the crystalline HA. The net transfer was greatest at the highest pH 8.5.

While the CPP-ACP complexes prepared at pH 9 have most of the calcium and phosphate peptide bound, these complexes exist in solution in equilibrium with free ionic calcium and phosphate (Cross et al. 2005). The values in brackets indicate the proportion of free ions (Table 24.1). The proportion of mineral ions bound within complexes was reduced after incubation with both uncoated and saliva-coated HA. This was attributed to the dissociation of peptides from the complexes to remain free in solution and/or to adsorb to HA. The reductions in pH experienced by the CPP-ACP solutions following exposure to HA were attenuated in the presence of saliva-coated HA (Table 24.1).

The degree of saturation of the calcium phosphate solutions was calculated using the solubility products at 37 °C of hydroxyapatite (HA) (K_{sp}~10^{-117}), octacalcium phosphate (OCP) (K_{sp}~10^{-96}), dicalcium phosphate dihydrate (DCPD) (K_{sp}~10^{-6}), and ACP (K_{sp}~10^{-25}) (Cross et al. 2005). The calcium and phosphate ions were

Table 24.1 Summary of the concentrations of total, free, and CPP-bound calcium and phosphate ions and pH values of the 0.2% CPP-ACP solutions prepared at pH 5.5, 7.0, and 8.5 before and after incubation with crystalline HA and saliva-coated HA

Solution [calcium] (μM) before incubation with HA			
Total	5261 ± 32	5285 ± 17	5225 ± 9
Free	4801 ± 50 (91%)	1847 ± 49.12 (35%)	365 ± 9 (7%)
CPP-bound	460 ± 60	3438 ± 52	4860 ± 13
Initial pH	pH 5.55	pH 6.99	pH 8.5
Supernatant after incubation with HA			
Total	5001 ± 43	4201 ± 105	3573 ± 128
Free	4807 ± 92 (96%)	2066 ± 36 (49%)	524 ± 35 (15%)
CPP-bound	194 ± 102	2134 ± 111	3049 ± 133
HA-bound	260 ± 54	1084 ± 106	1652 ± 128
Final pH	pH 5.32	pH 6.85	pH 7.89
Supernatant after incubation with saliva-coated HA			
Total	5042 ± 51	4224 ± 51	3620 ± 52
Free	4908 ± 169 (97%)	2058 ± 50 (49%)	527 ± 21 (15%)
CPP-bound	134 ± 177	2166 ± 72	3093 ± 56
HA-bound	219 ± 60	1061 ± 54	1605 ± 53
Final pH	pH 5.55	pH 6.88	pH 8.04
Solution [phosphate] (μM) before incubation with HA			
Total	3699 ± 6	3744 ± 21	3739 ± 16
Free	3354 ± 184 (91%)	1420 ± 73 (38%)	386 ± 3 (10%)
CPP-bound	346 ± 185	2324 ± 76	3353 ± 15
Initial pH	pH 5.55	pH 6.99	pH 8.5
Supernatant after incubation with HA			
Total	3461 ± 35	2930 ± 42	2485 ± 89
Free	3223 ± 175 (93%)	1599 ± 44 (55%)	627 ± 29 (25%)
CPP-bound	238 ± 179	1331 ± 61	1858 ± 94
HA-bound	238 ± 36	814 ± 47	1254 ± 90
Final pH	pH 5.32	pH 6.85	pH 7.89
Supernatant after incubation with saliva-coated HA			
Total	3427 ± 37	2757 ± 53	2443 ± 50
Free	3191 ± 50 (93%)	1475 ± 59 (54%)	518 ± 41 (21%)
CPP-bound	236 ± 62	1281 ± 79	1925 ± 65
HA-bound	272 ± 37	987 ± 57	1296 ± 53
Final pH	pH 5.55	pH 6.88	pH 8.04

saturated with respect to the HA phase for both total and unbound fractions at all pH values (Table 24.2). In summary, these studies have confirmed that mineral ions are released from CPP-ACP that adsorb onto the crystalline HA and that mineralisation increases monotonically with increasing pH.

Table 24.2 Degree of saturation of calcium phosphate solutions before and after incubation of 0.2% CPP-ACP at different pH with HA or saliva-coated HA

A	Total fraction: total calcium and phosphate in 0.2% CPP-ACP						
		Mineral					
Original pH	Final pH	HA	DCPD	TCP	OCP	Acid ACP	Basic ACP
pH 5.55	pH 5.55	**4.05**	0.92	0.465	**1.41**	0.21	0.07
pH 6.99	pH 6.99	**36.40**	**2.86**	**4.21**	**7.45**	**1.78**	0.65
pH 8.5	pH 8.5	**152.45**	**2.67**	**15.07**	**16.23**	**5.94**	**2.43**
After incubation with HA							
pH 5.55	pH 5.32	**2.60**	0.68	0.29	0.99	0.13	0.05
pH 6.99	pH 6.85	**26.20**	**2.27**	**2.99**	**5.67**	**1.27**	0.46
pH 8.5	pH 7.89	**74.96**	**2.43**	**7.81**	**10.52**	**3.17**	**1.24**
After incubation with saliva-coated HA							
pH 5.55	pH 5.55	**3.89**	0.87	0.44	1.36	0.20	0.07
pH 6.99	pH 6.88	**26.90**	**2.25**	**3.06**	**5.74**	**1.30**	0.47
pH 8.5	pH 8.04	**86.06**	**2.38**	**8.81**	**11.28**	**3.55**	**1.41**
B	Unbound fraction: calcium and phosphate in 0.2% CPP-ACP not associated with peptide complex						
		Mineral					
Original pH	Final pH	HA	DCPD	TCP	OCP	Acid ACP	Basic ACP
pH 5.55	pH 5.55	**3.78**	0.85	0.43	1.32	0.19	0.07
pH 6.99	pH 6.99	**18.48**	**1.35**	**1.97**	**3.83**	0.83	0.31
pH 8.5	pH 8.5	**31.80**	0.50	**2.63**	**3.59**	**1.04**	0.45
After incubation with HA							
pH 5.55	pH 5.32	**2.50**	0.65	0.28	0.95	0.13	0.04
pH 6.99	pH 6.85	**16.62**	**1.37**	**1.795**	**3.637**	0.76	0.28
pH 8.5	pH 7.89	**23.81**	0.73	**2.19**	**3.514**	0.89	0.36
After incubation with saliva-coated HA							
pH 5.55	pH 5.55	**3.76**	0.836	0.427	**1.309**	0.19	0.07
pH 6.99	pH 6.88	**16.91**	**1.34**	**1.82**	**3.64**	0.77	0.29
pH 8.5	pH 8.04	**26.56**	0.68	**2.38**	**3.64**	0.96	0.40

(A) Calcium and phosphate in total fraction; (B) calcium and phosphate in unbound fraction. Values in bold indicate saturation with respect to the phase

24.3.6 SEM Reveals Images of Non-crystalline Morphology for CPP-ACP Complexes

Preliminary SEM images of 5% CPP-ACP solution show areas with a non-crystalline morphology expected for colloidal complexes (Fig. 24.4).

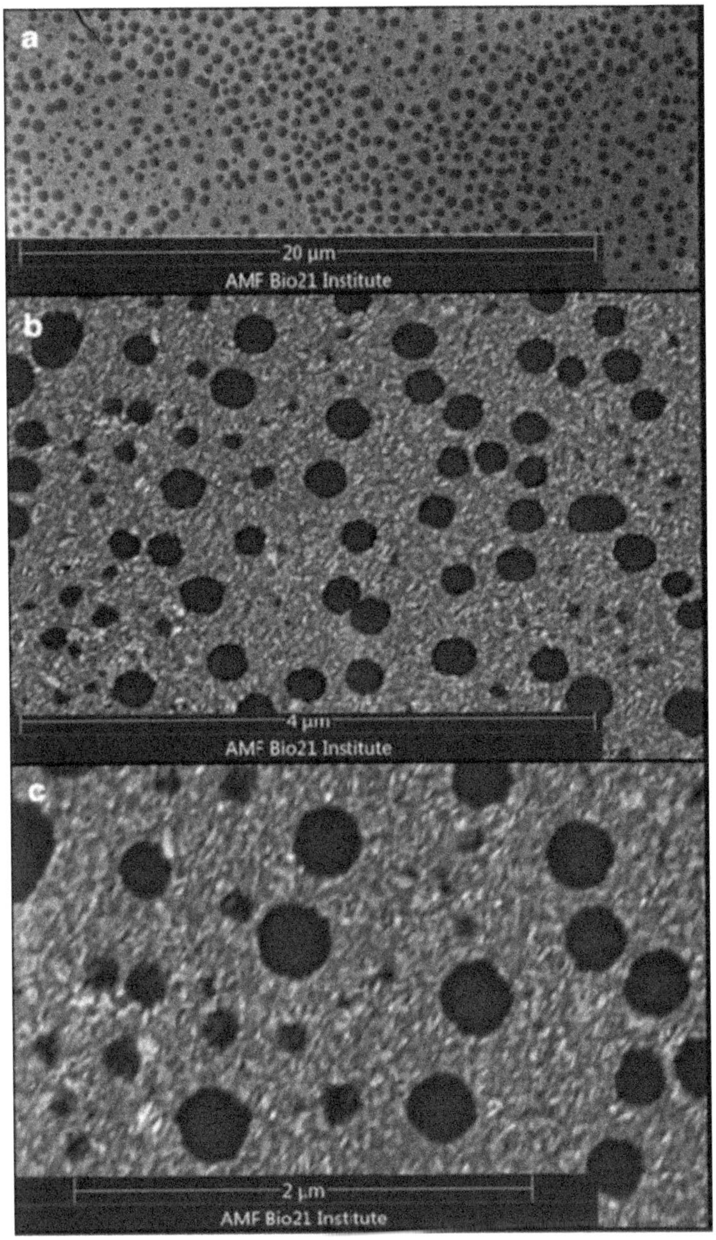

Fig. 24.4 SEM images of CPP-ACP at increasing magnification, taken using a T1 (BSE) detector with beam deceleration in a Teneo VS Instrument (FEI) for enhanced surface details. Two µl of 5% CPP-ACP, pH 7.24, was deposited onto a silicon substrate on an aluminium stub, and the excess liquid was removed after 1 min. CPP appeared to have formed spherical particles that were surrounded by ACP. Landing energy, 1 keV; stage bias, −2 kV

24.4 Discussion

The observed biomimicry of CPP that spontaneously self-assemble at pH 9 forming complexes with calcium phosphate ions offers a functional advantage for the stable storage and delivery of mineral ions. This paper describes interactions of the peptide and mineral components of this delivery vehicle with enamel substitute HA.

In addition to the adsorption of purified casein phosphopeptides onto uncoated HA, these studies confirmed that casein phosphopeptides also adsorbed onto the saliva-coated HA being a mimic of the enamel salivary pellicle. Previously, we have demonstrated that the casein phosphopeptides interact with salivary proteins including those forming the enamel pellicle (Huq et al. 2016). Collectively, these studies confirm that during topical application of a formulation with CPP-ACP complexes, the peptides are not simply inert carriers of mineral. Instead, they are capable of adsorbing to the crystalline enamel surface that has been recently brushed as well as interacting with the salivary pellicle that forms on the enamel surface.

Since HA is not an inert material, the molecular events at the HA surface are of interest. The casein phosphopeptides elicited an adsorption-mediated release of calcium ions from HA into the solution. This is consistent with previous studies documenting the release of ions from HA during adsorption of proteins and amino acids (Misra 1997; Pearce 1981). In contrast when HA was introduced to the peptide-ACP complexes in solution, there was a net loss of calcium and phosphate ions from the solution indicating a net gain of calcium and phosphate ions by the crystalline HA. These studies confirm that the mineral ions of the amorphous phase of ACP that is stabilised by the peptides transfer to the crystalline HA monotonically with increasing pH. Furthermore, during topical application, the dissociation of the CPP-ACP complexes and the subsequent migration of ions to the enamel surface are not hindered by the enamel salivary pellicle.

In conclusion, within the oral environment, the enamel remineralisation process involves a complex interplay between the peptide and mineral ions of the CPP-ACP delivery vehicle and the tooth enamel mineral with its salivary pellicle.

Acknowledgements We would like to thank Mr. Roger Curtain from the Bio21 Advanced Microscopy Facility, the University of Melbourne for his assistance in SEM imaging.

References

Cochrane NJ, Cai F, Huq NL, Burrow MF, Reynolds EC (2010) New approaches to enhanced remineralization of tooth enamel. J Dent Res 89:1187–1197

Cross KJ, Huq NL, Palamara JE, Perich JW, Reynolds EC (2005) Physicochemical characterization of casein phosphopeptide-amorphous calcium phosphate nanocomplexes. J Biol Chem 280:15362–15369

Cross KJ, Huq NL, Reynolds EC (2016) Casein phosphopeptide-amorphous calcium phosphate nanocomplexes: a structural model. Biochemistry 55:4316–4325

Dashper SG, Catmull DV, Liu SW, Myroforidis H, Zalizniak I, Palamara JE, Huq NL, Reynolds EC (2016) Casein phosphopeptide-amorphous calcium phosphate reduces streptococcus mutans biofilm development on glass ionomer cement and disrupts established biofilms. PLoS One 11:e0162322

Huq NL, Myroforidis H, Cross KJ, Stanton DP, Veith PD, Ward BR, Reynolds EC (2016) The interactions of CPP-ACP with saliva. Int J Mol Sci 17:915

Misra DN (1997) Interaction of ortho-phospho-l-serine with hydroxyapatite: formation of a surface complex. J Colloid Interface Sci 194:249–255

Pearce EI (1981) Ion displacement following the adsorption of anionic macromolecules on hydroxyapatite. Calcif Tissue Int 33:395–402

Reynolds EC, Cain CJ, Webber FL, Black CL, Riley PF, Johnson IH, Perich JW (1995) Anticariogenicity of calcium phosphate complexes of tryptic casein phosphopeptides in the rat. J Dent Res 74:1272–1279

Robinson C, Shore RC, Brookes SJ, Strafford S, Wood SR, Kirkham J (2000) The chemistry of enamel caries. Crit Rev Oral Biol Med 11:481–495

Chapter 25
Preparation of Random and Aligned Polycaprolactone Fiber as Template for Classical Calcium Oxalate Through Electrocrystallization

Lazy Farias, Nicole Butto, and Andrónico Neira-Carrillo

Abstract The aim of this study was to evaluate the effect of random and oriented electrospun polycaprolactone (PCL) fiber meshes on conductive indium tin oxide (ITO) electrode on the in vitro electrocrystallization (EC) of calcium oxalate (CaOx). For that, random and aligned PCL fibers were prepared through flat and rotating collectors and directly collected on conductive ITO support that was used as organic solid template for controlling the in vitro EC of CaOx. Our findings revealed that electrospun PCL surface topology induced preferentially the nucleation and crystal growth of CaOx along on individual aligned PCL fibers during the EC of CaOx. Scanning electron microscopy (SEM), energy dispersive X-ray spectroscopy (EDX), chronoamperometry, and X-ray diffraction (XRD) spectroscopy of CaOx crystals show that the morphological orientation of PCL fiber meshes acted as selective good nucleation site at PCL surface controlling their CaOx crystal morphologies and the crystallographic orientation of crystals inducing the coexistence of dehydrated CaOx (COD) and monohydrated CaOx (COM) crystals as the unique polymorphism.

Keywords Electrospun fibers · Electrocrystallization · Calcium oxalate (CaOx) · Indium zinc oxide (ITO) · Polycaprolactone (PCL) · Dehydrated CaOx (COD) · Monohydrated CaOx (COM)

L. Farias · N. Butto · A. Neira-Carrillo (✉)
Department of Biological and Animal Sciences, School of Veterinary and Animal Sciences, University of Chile, Santiago, Chile
e-mail: nbutto@veterinaria.uchile.cl; aneira@uchile.cl

K. Endo et al. (eds.), *Biomineralization*,
https://doi.org/10.1007/978-981-13-1002-7_25

25.1 Introduction

Biological crystallization or biomineralization is the process by which living organisms from bacteria to eukaryotes cells form hierarchical hybrid biogenic minerals (Lowenstam and Weiner 1989; Estroff 2008). Its role in nature is diverse such as protection, motion, storage, optical and gravity sensing, defense, detoxification, etc. (Mann 2000). They are highly organized from molecular level to the nano- and macroscale, with intricate nano-architectures that ultimately make up a myriad and remarkable properties and complex shape of different functional soft and hard tissues (Sumper and Brunner 2006; Guru and Dash 2014; Neira-Carrillo et al. 2015a, b). These properties can inspire mimetic strategies intending to design nanomaterials based on mineral controlled crystallization concept. Biological crystallization, however, also occurs in a pathological manner in nature, e.g., concretions, gallstones (Wang et al. 2006; Xie et al. 2015), and the mineralization of CaOx within the urinary tract often called urolithiasis (Khan and Canales 2009). Therefore, biominerals are outstanding materials not only for understanding the biomineralization concept but also for novel confined-materials synthesis and design, avoiding undesirable pathological biomineralization. Composite biogenic nanomaterials are also of increasing interest to materials scientists who seek novel materials syntheses such as fibrillary hydrogel, platelet or fiber structures, and crystalline matrices and/or interfaces with similar crystalline forms to those produced by nature. There is an abundant diversity of chemical compositions and structures for minerals such as carbonates, silicates, phosphates, oxalate, oxides, etc. (Pai and Pillai 2008; Neira-Carrillo et al. 2010, 2015a, b). In general, in vitro study of inorganic minerals can be performed by using additives or organic substrates through different experimental methodologies.

With this in mind, random and oriented electrospun polycaprolactone (PCL) fiber meshes on indium tin oxide (ITO) support were prepared through electrospinning and used as an organic template for controlling the in vitro electrocrystallization (EC) of CaOx. Electrospinning is a nanofabrication technique, in which the organic polymer fibers orientation can be topologically controlled at the surface of PCL meshes. Electrospinning involves the application of an electric field to a drop of polymer solution that is deformed and forced to be ejected to a metallic plate collector in which the arrangement of fibers can be controlled with random (Kishan and Cosgriff-Hernandez 2017) or aligned (Lee et al. 2017) fibers orientation.

Therefore, in order to study the effect of PCL surface topology as organic solid template for controlling the in vitro EC of CaOx, random and aligned PCL fibers were directly collected on ITO glass electrode by using flat and rotating collectors. The use of EC has been documented for CaOx (Neira-Carrillo et al. 2015a, b) and for other inorganic minerals such as calcium carbonate crystals (Pavez et al. 2004; Buttlo et al. 2017; Sanchez et al. 2017).

25.2 Materials and Methods

The in vitro EC of CaOx on PCL electrospun fiber meshes was carried out onto conductive ITO electrode at 9 mA using 18% PCL solution (Mw, 80,000, Sigma-Aldrich) in organic ethyl acetone/acetate 3:1 (v:v) solvents in an electrospinning instrument (Fluidnatek® LE-10). Random and aligned PCL fiber meshes were spun on a fixed metal flat (30 × 30 cm) and rotary (10 cm in diameter) collectors, respectively. The control of PCL surface topology was achieved by using the following parameters: 16 kV, solution flow rate of 1200 μl/h, 15 min, nozzle-collector distance from between 15 and 18 cm, and rotating speed of 2000 rpm. The modified ITO-containing PCL fiber meshes were immersed in an electrocrystallization solution composed of sodium oxalate (Sigma-Aldrich®), calcium nitrate (MERCK®), and ethylenediaminetetraacetic acid tetrasodium salt (Sigma-Aldrich®) and put into an electrochemical cell. The potenciostat-galvanostat (Epsilon-BASi) instrument and the Epsilon EC-USB program were used for performing all the EC of CaOx assays. The SEM-EDX surface morphology of the resultant CaOx crystals was examined using a scanning electron microscope (Jeol JSM-IT300LV, JEOL USA Inc., USA) connected to an energy dispersive X-ray detector for elemental analysis with computer-controlled software, the Aztec EDX system (Oxford Instruments, Abingdon, UK). Powder X-ray diffraction (PXRD) was performed by using a Siemens D-5000X X-ray diffractometer with Cu-*K*a radiation (graphite monochromator) and an ENRAF Nonius FR 590. The crystal structure of CaOx was determined by using Cu-*K*a radiation (40 kV), steps of 0.2°, and the geometric Bragg-Brentano (θ–θ) scanning mode with an angle (2θ) range of 5–70°. The DiffracPlus program was used as a data control software.

25.3 Results

25.3.1 *Preparation of PCL Fibers and Chronopotentiometric Curve of CaOx*

Random and oriented electrospun polycaprolactone (PCL) fiber meshes were prepared by using electrospinning directly deposited on ITO support as working electrode for conducting the in vitro EC of CaOx. Therefore, EC of CaOx using surface-modified ITO PCL fiber meshes with controlled topology was used as solid template, and their electrochemical potentiometric behavior follows at room temperature for 5 min. We observed a notorious difference in the behavior of electrochemical curves during the EC of CaOx when both surface-modified ITO PCL fiber meshes were used indicating a different mechanism of CaOx crystallization

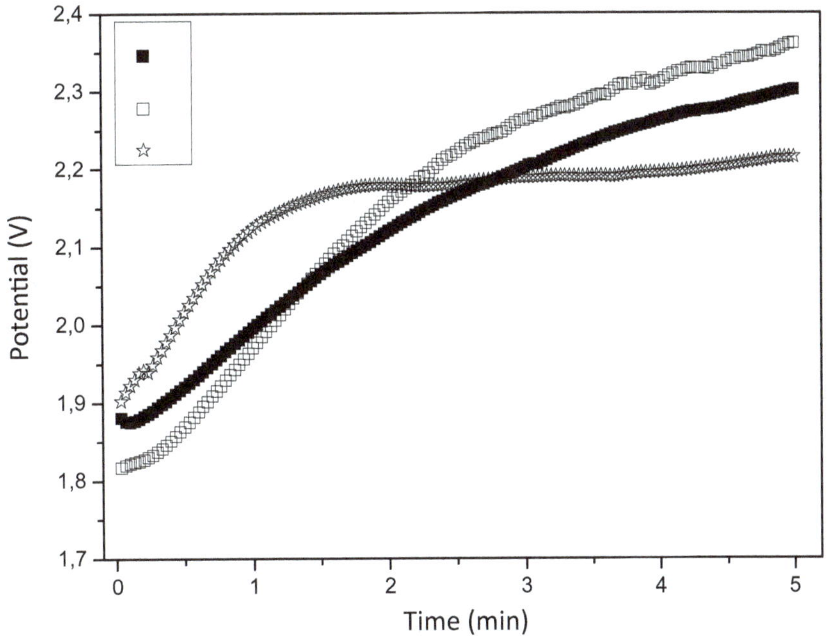

Fig. 25.1 Chronopotentiometric curves for EC of CaOx crystals on ITO electrode substrate. Without additive as control (■) and in the presence of random PCL fiber (□) and aligned PCL fiber (☆) meshes

(Fig. 25.1). This can be rationalized by increasing the formed CaOx material when the EC was performed at constant applied current of 9 mA. Thus, when the in vitro EC of CaOx in the presence of aligned PCL fiber mesh was performed (Fig. 25.1☆), the electrochemical potential reached a maximum value of 2.2 V at 1.5 min, keeping this constant value until the end of the test. Meanwhile when the PCL fiber meshes with random distribution were used as template (Fig. 25.1□), the potential (V) showed a progressive increase behavior of 2.35 V until the end of the experiment. The same potentiometric curve was also observed in absence of surface-modified ITO as control essays reaching ca. of 2.30 V until the end of the experiment.

25.3.2 SEM, EDX, and XRD Characterization of CaOx Obtained by EC Method

The morphological aspect and distribution of CaOx crystals grown on modified-ITO support were carried out by scanning electron microscopy (SEM). SEM analysis showed that crystals grown on surface-modified ITO with randomly PCL fibers were found into network-PCL fiber mesh forming conglomerate crystalline particles. Here, classic bypyramidal morphology of COD crystals was observed (Fig. 25.2a). On the other hand, CaOx crystals formed on surface-modified ITO with aligned PCL fibers grown along and surrounding on PCL fibers (inset, Fig. 25.2b). Here, we also observed several COD crystals with distinct

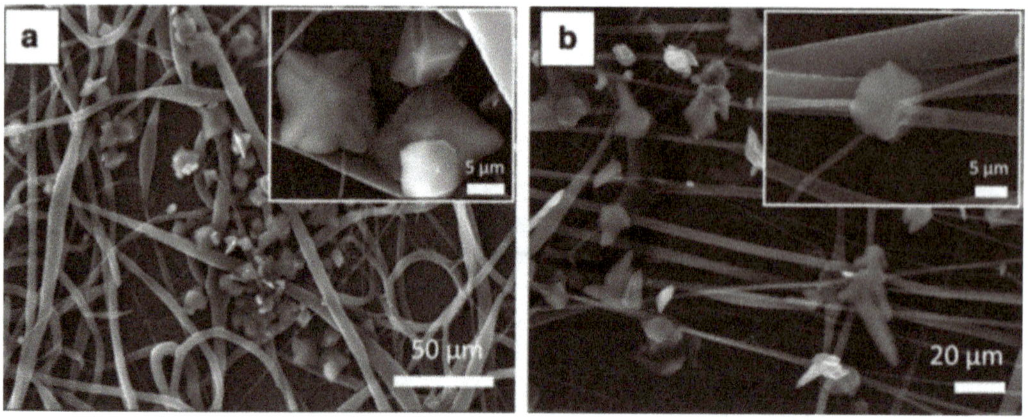

Fig. 25.2 SEM images of CaOx crystals obtained through EC method on surface-modified ITO with (**a**) random PCL fiber and (**b**) with aligned PCL fibers meshes

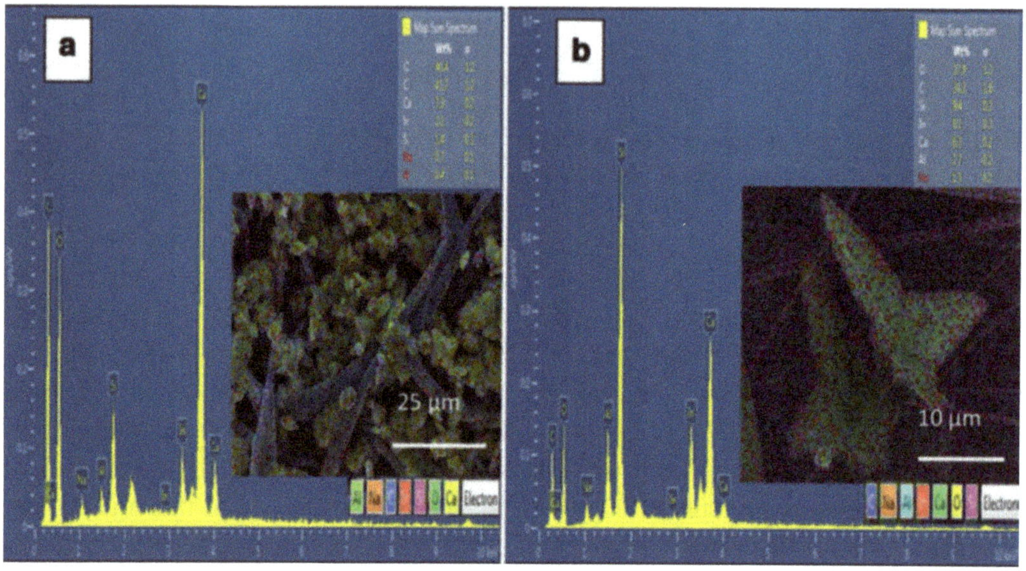

Fig. 25.3 EDX measurements of CaOx crystals obtained through EC method on surface-modified ITO with (**a**) random PCL fiber and (**b**) aligned PCL fiber meshes. The colors assigned to each element were arbitrarily selected in the EDX measurements

morphological COD with slight crystalline shape of CaOx crystals (Fig. 25.2b). Regular and flower-like COD crystals morphologies were also observed in other part deposited on aligned PCL fiber samples. This result indicated that the growth of crystal faces normal to the [100] direction was selectively inhibited by changing the topological surface of PCL fibers as template on the surface-modified ITO support.

The energy dispersive X-ray spectroscopy (EDX) detector on CaOx crystals was also used, demonstrating the characteristic elemental and chemical composition of CaOx crystals (Fig. 25.3) and to the conductive ITO support. The SEM and EDX studies of CaOx were carried out by using "analysis" as observation condition and the "charge-up reduction mode" as observation mode. The weight percent (wt.-%) concentration of elements at the crystal surface was automatically calculated

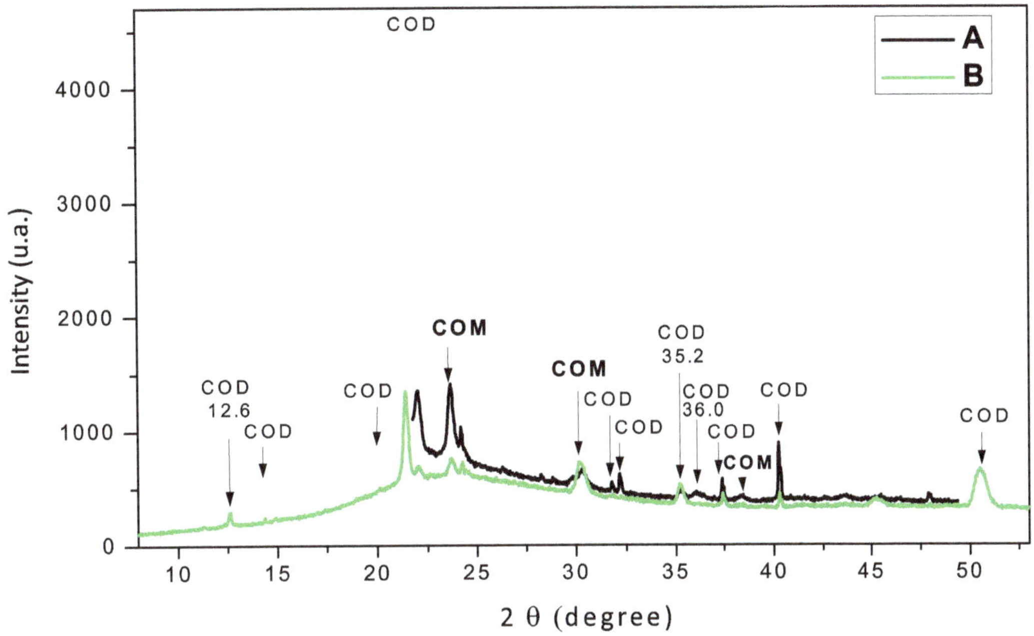

Fig. 25.4 XRD spectra of CaOx crystals obtained through EC on surface-modified ITO with (**a**) random PCL fibers mesh, black line, and (**b**) aligned PCL fibers mesh, green line. Diffraction peaks show crystalline polymorphs of monohydrate (COM) and dihydrate (COD) CaOx

through EDX software. In order to determine the internal lattice of crystalline CaOx products, X-ray diffraction (XRD) analysis was also performed. Figure 25.4 shows XRD pattern of CaOx crystals obtained by EC in the presence of surface-modified ITO with random PCL fibers (Fig. 25.4a) and surface-modified ITO with aligned PCL fibers (Fig. 25.4b). In general, the XRD spectra demonstrated the coexistence of COD and COM polymorphism; the crystalline peaks showed slight difference in the intensity of the main reflections of COD and COM, which are ascribed at $2\theta = 14.3°, 20.0°, 21.3°, 32.2°, 37.2°, 40.2°$, and $50.7°$ and $2\theta = 15.0°, 23.0°, 67.0°$, and $30.2°$, respectively. It was noted that the portion of COD crystals in the resultant product on surface-modified ITO became dominant. The current type of CaOx polymorphism designations is in agreement with COM and COD crystals obtained by using acid-rich biopolymers as additive (Jung et al. 2005).

25.4 Discussion

In vitro electrocrystallization on controlled surface-modified ITO with PCL fiber meshes as classical crystallization of CaOx was performed. Thus, EC of CaOx on ITO working electrode with random and aligned electrospun PCL fibers was used as solid template to evaluate the topology effect onto ITO electrode on the morphology, distribution, and polymorphism of the CaOx crystals. Random and aligned

PCL fibers were obtained by using flat and rotary collectors through electrospinning technique, respectively. In summary, CaOx crystals were effectively electrodeposited, and a clear difference in the distribution, morphology, and crystal growth of CaOx crystals was observed. We suggest that the active surface topology of PCL fiber meshes can act as good nucleation point and in particular on the aligned surface of each PCL fibers inducing a favorable site for the in vitro crystallization of CaOx. In addition, polymorphism of CaOx can be selectively controlled onto surface-modified ITO, although the absence of chemical functionality on PCL fiber as template. Here, we observed a coexistence in the polymorphism of calcium oxalate; however, the COD crystals were the predominant particles on the surface of the ITO substrates.

Acknowledgments The authors are grateful to Project Fondecyt 1171520 and 1140660, Program U-Redes, Vice-Presidency of Research and Development, University of Chile.

References

Buttlo N, Cabreras-Barjas G, Neira-Carrillo A (2017) Electrocrystallization of $CaCO_3$ crystals obtained through phosphorylated chitin. Crystals. Submitted_ID: Crystals-260718

Estroff LA (2008) Introduction: on biomineralization. Chem Rev 108:4329–4331

Guru PS, Dash S (2014) Sorption on eggshell waste-a review on ultrastructure, biomineralization and other applications. Adv Colloid Interf Sci 209:49–67

Jung T, Kim WS, Choi CK (2005) Crystal structure and morphology control of calcium oxalate using biopolymeric additives in crystallization. J Cryst Growth 279:154–162

Khan S, Canales B (2009) Genetic basis of renal cellular dysfunction and the formation of kidney stones. Urol Res 37:169–180

Kishan AP, Cosgriff-Hernandez EM (2017) Recent advancements in electrospinning design for tissue engineering applications: a review. J Biomed Mater Res A 105:2892–2905

Lee SJ, Heo M, Lee D, Heo DN, Lim HN, Kwon IK (2017) Fabrication and design of bioactive agent coated, highly-aligned electrospun matrices for nerve tissue engineering: preparation, characterization and application. Appl Surf Sci 424:359–367

Lowenstam HA, Weiner S (1989) On biomineralization. Oxford University Press, New York

Mann S (2000) The chemistry of form. Angew Chem Int Ed 39:3392–3406

Neira-Carrillo A, Yazdani-Pedram P, Vasquez-Quitral P, Arias JL (2010) Selective calcium oxalate crystallization induced by monomethylitaconate grafted polymethylsiloxane. Mol Cryst Liq Cryst 522:307–317

Neira-Carrillo A, Vásquez-Quitral P, Fernández MS, Luengo-Ponce F, Yazdani-Pedram M, Cölfen H, Arias JL (2015a) Sulfonated polymethylsiloxane as an additive for selective calcium oxalate crystallization. Eur J Inorg Chem 2015(7):1167–1177

Neira-Carrillo A, Vásquez-Quitral P, Sánchez M, Vargas-Fernández A, Silva F (2015b) Control of calcium oxalate morphology through electrocrystallization as an electrochemical approach for preventing pathological disease. Ionics 21:3141–3149

Pai R, Pillai S (2008) Divalent cation-induced variations in polyelectrolyte conformation and controlling calcite morphologies: direct observation of the phase transition by atomic force microscopy. J Am Chem Soc 130:13074–13078

Pavez J, Silva J, Melo F (2004) Homogeneous calcium carbonate coating obtained by electrodeposition: in situ atomic force microscope observations. Electrochim Acta 50:3488–3494

Sánchez M, Vásquez-Quitral P, Butto N, Díaz-Soler F, Yazdani-Pedram M, Silva JF, Neira-Carrillo A (2017) Effect of alginate from Chilean *Lessonia nigrescens* and MWCNTs on $CaCO_3$ crystallization by classical and non-classical methods. Crystals, Submitted_ID: Crystals-260775

Sumper M, Brunner E (2006) Learning from diatoms: nature's tools for the production of nanostructured silica. Adv Funct Mater 16:17–26

Wang L, Qiu SR, Zachowicz W, Guan XY, DeYoreo JJ, Nancollas GH, Hoyer JR (2006) Modulation of calcium oxalate crystallization by linear aspartic acid-rich peptides. Langmuir 22:7279–7285

Xie B, Halter TJ, Borah BM, Nancollas GH (2015) Aggregation of calcium phosphate and oxalate phases in the formation of renal stones. Cryst Growth Des 15:204–211

Part VI
Bio-inspired Materials Science and Engineering

Chapter 26
Dysprosium Biomineralization by *Penidiella* sp. Strain T9

Takumi Horiike, Hajime Kiyono, and Mitsuo Yamashita

Abstract Biomineralization approaches have gained significant attention as a means to recover rare earth elements from acidic mine drainage and industrial liquid wastes. We isolated an acidophilic fungus, *Penidiella* sp. strain T9, that accumulates dysprosium (Dy) from acidic model drainage during growth. To develop the application of biomineralization by the strain T9, we elucidated the localization and the chemical structure of biomineralized Dy and performed to establish the labo-scale bioprocess for selective recovery of Dy. High-magnification scanning electron microscopic analysis showed that the strain T9 formed a mineralized Dy (T9-Dy) layer with 1.0 μm thickness over the cell surface, along with some intracellular nano-micro meter-sized Dy particles. X-ray photoelectron spectrometry and X-ray absorption fine structure analyses showed that the chemical composition of T9-Dy corresponded to $DyPO_4$. X-ray diffraction analysis did not yield any spectrum from T9-Dy. Therefore, we concluded that the strain T9 accumulates and mineralizes Dy as an amorphous $DyPO_4$. Dysprosium desorption rate from T9-Dy was 100% using 0.3 M hydrochloric acid. Furthermore, after desorption process, the strain T9 grows again in the new medium and retains the Dy accumulation ability. Thus, the strain T9 has a potential as a bioaccumulator for Dy recovery from acidic drainage through biomineralization.

Keywords Biomineralization · Bioaccumulation · Drainage · Dysprosium · Acidophilic microorganism · Metal-biotechnology

T. Horiike · M. Yamashita (✉)
Shibaura Institute of Technology, Saitama, Japan
e-mail: i030589@shibaura-it.ac.jp; yamashi@shibaura-it.ac.jp

H. Kiyono
Shibaura Institute of Technology, Tokyo, Japan
e-mail: h-kiyono@shibaura-it.ac.jp

K. Endo et al. (eds.), *Biomineralization*,
https://doi.org/10.1007/978-981-13-1002-7_26

26.1 Introduction

Rare earth elements (REE) are indispensable ingredients in the manufacturing of high-tech products (US Geological Survey 2015). In particular, dysprosium (Dy) has increased its global demand because to use in making heat resistant magnets for high-tech products; nevertheless, the supply of Dy is limited. Acidic mine drainage and industrial liquid waste containing low concentration of Dy have attracted attention as a new Dy resource (Protano and Riccobono 2002). Therefore, it is important to develop new recovery techniques from Dy-containing drainage using as a new resource.

Recently, biotechnological approaches for metal resource recycling have been emphasized (Zhuang et al. 2015). Biomineralization and bioaccumulation are studied for recovering targeting metal from mine drainage and industrial waste (Nancharaiah et al. 2016). An REE-bioaccumulating acidophilic fungus, *Penidiella* sp. strain T9 was isolated and able to recover approximately 50% (w/v) soluble Dy from acidic model drainage during growth (Horiike and Yamashita 2015). To exploit this capability on an industrial scale, the rate of accumulation and reaction time must be improved. To start addressing these issues, we have explored the localization and the chemical structure of Dy-containing compounds following their biogenetic solidification by the strain T9. To develop the application of biomineralization by the strain T9, we elucidated the localization and the chemical structure of biomineralized Dy and performed to establish the labo-scale bioprocess for selective recovery of Dy.

26.2 Materials and Methods

26.2.1 Media and Cultivation Conditions

The Basal salt medium (BSM) was prepared in accordance with a recent study (Horiike and Yamashita 2015). For Dy bioaccumulation tests, BSM was prepared at pH 2.5 with 20 mM potassium hydrogen phthalate-hydrochloric acid (HCl) buffer. Cultivation was carried out at 30 °C on a rotary shaker at 120 rpm.

26.2.2 Dy Bioaccumulation by Strain T9

The Dy accumulation test was performed in accordance with a recent study (Horiike and Yamashita 2015). The strain T9 was cultivated in 50 mL of BSM containing 100 mg/L Dy (as $DyCl_3$) and cultivated on a rotary shaker at 120 rpm at 30 °C for 7 days. After 7 days of cultivation, the strain T9 cells were centrifuged (15,900× *g*, 20 min, 4 °C) and then collected by filtration using an Omnipore membrane filter

(0.2-μm pore size; Merck Millipore, MA, USA). The cell pellet on the filter was washed twice with sterile saline water (isotonic solution).

26.2.3 Analytical Methods

To characterize Dy precipitate prepared by the strain T9, scanning electron microscopy-energy dispersive X-ray spectroscopy (SEM-EDX), X-ray absorption fine structure (XAFS) analyses, and X-ray diffractometry (XRD) were conducted with the detail procedure and the standard materials prepared according to reference (Horiike et al. 2016).

26.2.4 Purification of Dy from Dy Precipitate

Dy precipitate prepared by the strain T9 after 3 days cultivation was used. Each of HCl and ethylenediamine-*N, N, N′, N′*-tetraacetic acid (EDTA), as solubilizing reagents of Dy-precipitated compounds in the strain T9, was prepared at 300 mM, 30 mM, and 3.0 mM, respectively. The final concentration of Dy in the solution containing HCl or EDTA was 500 mg/l (3.0 mM Dy) from Dy precipitate, and then the mixture was reacted at 30 °C on a rotary shaker at 120 rpm for 3 h. The concentration of Dy in the solution was determined using inductively coupled plasma-atomic emission spectrometry (ICP-AES).

26.3 Results and Discussion

26.3.1 Localization of Dy-Precipitated Compounds in Penidiella *sp. Strain T9*

To clarify the localization of Dy-precipitated compounds in the strain T9, sections of T9 cells were observed using SEM-EDX after the Dy bioaccumulation test (Fig. 26.1). Bright dots and bright regions were observed in the cell (1.0 μm diameter) and on the cell surface (1.0 μm thickness), respectively. Three points, bright dot (Spot 1), bright region (Spot 2), and cytoplasm as background (Area 3), were further analyzed using EDX (Fig. 26.1b–d). Specific high peaks corresponding to Dy, P, and O at spots 1 and 2 were observed; these peaks were absented from area 3 (background). Peaks of C and N were found at all three points. From these results, we conclude that the strain T9 mainly incorporates a layer of Dy on the cell surface and nano-micro sized particles (bright dots) of Dy in the cytoplasm. Furthermore, since P and O were also detected in Dy-precipitated material, we infer that the Dy

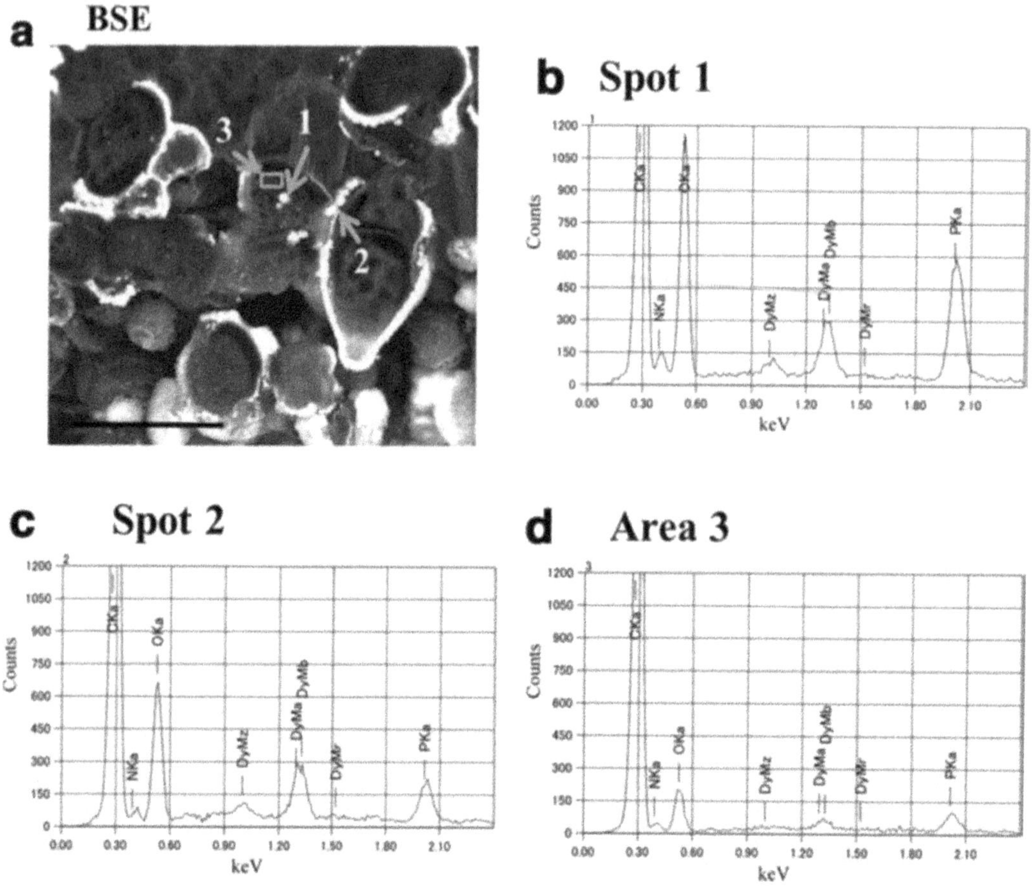

Fig. 26.1 SEM-EDX analyses of a cross section of the Dy compounds from the strain T9. (**a**) Back scattered electron (BSE) image of a cross section of strain T9 with Dy. The image reveals nanoparticles and precipitates in cytoplasmic regions (i.e., Spot 1) and the cell wall (i.e., Spot 2), respectively. Bar, 10 μm. EDX spectra in (**b**) Spot 1, (**c**) Spot 2, and (**d**) Area 3. Area 3 corresponds to a background cytoplasmic region. (Horiike et al. 2016)

compounds also contain phosphate. High-magnification SEM-EDX analysis showed that the strain T9 formed a precipitated Dy (T9-Dy) layer with 1.0-μm thickness over the cell surface and some nanometer-sized particles of Dy in the cytoplasm (data not shown). The T9-Dy layer consisted of coagulated nanometer-sized particles.

26.3.2 Chemical Structure of Dy-Precipitated Compounds

To determine the chemical state of T9-Dy, Dy L_{III}-edge spectrum in XANES of T9-Dy, $DyPO_4$ (chemical precipitate), CMC-Dy (Dy-binding carboxymethyl cellulose), and CP-Dy (Dy-binding cellulose phosphate) was carried out (Horiike et al. 2016). The strength of the peak across the samples was as follows: $DyPO_4 \leqq$ T9-Dy < CMC-Dy $\leqq$ CP-Dy. This indicates that the strength of peak depends on both the ligand and structure around Dy. The Dy L_I-edge spectrum in XANES is shown (Horiike et al. 2016). The full width at half maximum values of Peak B was as follows: $DyPO_4$ ≒ T9-Dy < CMC-Dy ≒ CP-Dy. A shoulder (C) of Peak B (at ~9072 eV) was observed in the spectra of T9-Dy and $DyPO_4$. From the results, we conclude that the chemical bond and the local structure around Dy in the T9-Dy are closer to that of $DyPO_4$ than that of either CMC-Dy or CP-Dy. To identify the ligand-bonding environment in T9-Dy, Dy L_{III}-edge spectrum in FT-EXAFS was carried out (Horiike et al. 2016). Peak E corresponds to P and C, and Peak F corresponds to Dy or P around Dy. From the FT-EXAFS results, the ligand-bonding environment in the T9-Dy appears to be very similar to that observed in $DyPO_4$.

To characterize the crystalline phase of T9-Dy, XRD analysis was performed. XRD patterns of wet and dry T9-Dy indicated a halo peak at 30° and indistinct peaks, respectively (data not shown), showing that they are amorphous. The positions of the distinct peaks are the same as those reported for $DyPO_4 \cdot 1.5H_2O$ (ICDD 20-0385). Taken together, these data indicate that the crystalline phase of the T9-Dy is clearly different from that of chemically precipitated $DyPO_4$.

The acidophilic fungus *Penidiella* sp. strain T9 accumulates and incorporates Dy in a form that corresponds to $DyPO_4$. The precipitated Dy formed from nano- to micro-meter sized particles in the cytoplasm and aggregates on the cell surface. Therefore, we suggest that the strain T9 must have an active uptake mechanism for Dy into the cells and an ability to sorb Dy into phosphate groups present in the cell wall. These findings highlight the importance of phosphoric acid to improve Dy recovery by the strain T9, which has the available capacity in the cells to accumulate Dy.

26.3.3 Purification of Dy from Dy-Precipitated Compounds

To purify Dy from T9-Dy, an examination of Dy solubilization from T9-Dy prepared by 3 days cultivation was performed using a mineral acid (HCl) or EDTA (Fig. 26.2). One hundred percent of Dy contained in T9-Dy was dissolved by 300 mM HCl at 30 min incubation, but 26% and 5% of Dy were dissolved by 30 mM and 3.0 mM HCl, respectively, at 3 h. The results suggested that the purification of Dy from microbial Dy precipitant using the strain T9 was easier than chemical Dy precipitant, which was not dissolved by HCl. Ninety six percent, 100%, and 95% of Dy from T9-Dy were dissolved in 300 mM, 30 mM, and 3.0 mM of EDTA, respectively, at 3 h. Thus, 300 mM HCl and 30 mM EDTA were more effective chemicals to purify Dy from T9-Dy.

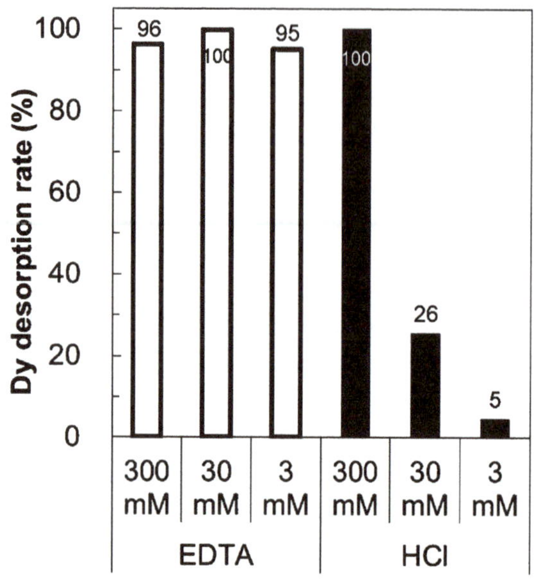

Fig. 26.2 Dy desorption rate from T9-Dy using EDTA or HCl. White bars, using EDTA; black bars, using HCl

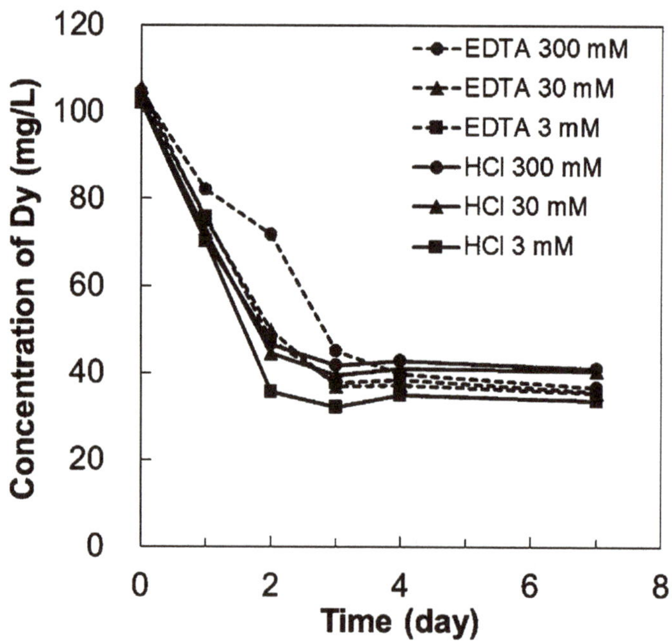

Fig. 26.3 Time course of the Dy concentration during cultivation in BSM using the strain T9 after desorption. Broken lines, cells after desorption using EDTA; solid lines, cells after desorption using HCl. Concentrations of desorption reagents; 300 mM (solid circle), 30 mM (solid triangle), 3.0 mM (solid square)

26.3.4 Reuse of the Strain T9 to Recover Dissolved Dy

The reusability of the strain T9 in the REE accumulation-desorption cycle is important to develop an economical REE recovery process. The cells of T9 strain after the Dy desorption were cultivated in a new BSM, and then Dy accumulation test was carried out reusing the T9 cells. The dissolved Dy in the culture were decreased less than 50% after 3 days of cultivation using the cells treated with EDTA or HCl in desorption (Fig. 26.3). These results indicated that the cells of the strain T9 grew again in the new medium and retained the Dy accumulation ability after desorption process using HCl or EDTA. Taken together, the strain T9 has a great potential as a bioaccumulator to develop a continuous recycling system of Dy. Mineral acids, such as HCl, HNO_3, and H_2SO_4, and chelating agents, such as EDTA and NTA (nitrilotriacetic acid), have lethal effects on most of microbial cells (Tsezos 1984). Since the strain T9 has ability to tolerate chemicals like HCl and EDTA, the strain has strong potential to be developed as the REE-accumulator for REE recovery cycle.

Acknowledgments XAFS analysis was performed under the approval of the Photon Factory Program Advisory Committee. This study was supported partially by the Japan Oil, Gas and Metals National Corporation and the Kurita Water and Environment Foundation.

References

Horiike T, Yamashita Y (2015) A new fungal isolate, *Penidiella* sp. strain T9, accumulates the rare earth element dysprosium. Appl Environ Microbiol 81:3062–3068

Horiike T, Kiyono H, Yamashita M (2016) *Penidiella* sp. strain T9 is an effective dysprosium accumulator, incorporating dysprosium dysprosium phosphate compounds. Hydrometallurgy 166:260–265

Nancharaiah YV, Mohan SV, Lens PNL (2016) Biological and bioelectrochemical recovery of critical and scarce metals. Trends Biotechnol 34:137–155

Protano G, Riccobono F (2002) High contents of rare earth elements (REEs) in stream waters of a Cu–Pb–Zn mining area. Environ Pollut 117:499–514

Tsezos M (1984) Recovery of uranium from biological adsorbents-desorption equilibrium. Biotechnol Bioeng 26:973–981

U. S. Geological Survey (2015) Mineral commodity summaries 2015. U.S. Geological Survey, Virginia

Zhuang WQ, Fitts JP, Ajo-Franklin CM, Maes S, Alvarez-Cohen L, Hennebel T (2015) Recovery of critical metals using biometallurgy. Curr Opin Biotechnol 33:327–335

Chapter 27
Various Shapes of Gold Nanoparticles Synthesized by Glycolipids Extracted from *Lactobacillus casei*

Yugo Kato, Fumiya Kikuchi, Yuki Imura, Etsuro Yoshimura, and Michio Suzuki

Abstract Gold nanoparticles have particular properties distinct from bulk gold crystals. The gold nanoparticles are used in various applications in optics, catalysis, and drug delivery. Although many reports on microbial synthesis of gold nanoparticles have appeared, the molecular mechanism of gold nanoparticle synthesis in microorganisms is unclear. Previously we reported that the amounts of diglycosyl diacylglycerol (DGDG) and triglycosyldiacylglycerol (TGDG) bearing unsaturated fatty acids were much reduced after formation of gold nanoparticles. DGDG purified from *L. casei* induced the synthesis of gold nanoparticles in vitro. These results suggested that glycolipids, such as DGDG, play important roles in reducing Au(III) to Au(0). In this paper, we reported that the concentration change of DGDG induced various shapes of gold nanoparticles in vitro. Our work will lead to the development of novel and efficient methods to synthesize metal nanoparticles using microorganisms.

Keywords Gold nanoparticle · *Lactobacillus casei* · Glycolipid

Y. Kato · F. Kikuchi · Y. Imura · M. Suzuki (✉)
Department of Applied Biological Chemistry, Graduate School of Agricultural and Life Sciences, The University of Tokyo, Bunkyo-ku, Tokyo, Japan
e-mail: amichiwo@mail.ecc.u-tokyo.ac.jp

E. Yoshimura
Department of Applied Biological Chemistry, Graduate School of Agricultural and Life Sciences, The University of Tokyo, Bunkyo-ku, Tokyo, Japan

Department of Liberal Arts, The Open University of Japan, Chiba, Japan
e-mail: ayoshim@mail.ecc.u-tokyo.ac.jp

K. Endo et al. (eds.), *Biomineralization*,
https://doi.org/10.1007/978-981-13-1002-7_27

27.1 Introduction

Gold nanoparticles (containing a few tens of gold atoms) have various unique properties. A gold nanoparticle solution is wine-red in color, because of surface plasmon resonance (SPR) (Jin 2010; Zhang et al. 2010). Over the past two decades, such nanoparticles have found novel applications in general industry, chemistry, biology, and medicine. Antibody-bearing nanoparticles are useful labeling agents in electron microscopy and can reveal the detailed locations of organic molecules within cell organelles (Bendayan and Garzon 1988). Gold nanoparticles attached to DNA fragments can detect DNA-DNA interactions (which trigger color changes) (Storhoff et al. 2000). This technology is used to diagnose viral infections (Wang et al. 2001; Cao et al. 2002). When synthesizing gold nanoparticles, the appropriate selections of reducing agents active on gold ions, and dispersing agents that hold the particle size in the nanometer range, are important. Industrially, large amounts of gold nanoparticles are synthesized in the reaction of gold with citric acid under conditions of high temperature and pressure (Frens 1973). Novel methods using macromolecular polymers or biomacromolecules, such as proteins and DNA, have been used to develop more functional gold nanoparticles (controlled in terms of shape) at low financial and energy costs, in the absence of unwanted by-products (Selvakannan et al. 2004; Xie et al. 2009; Liu et al. 2011). Recently, many methods using microorganisms to synthesize metallic nanoparticles have been reported. For example, some previous works about synthesize gold nanoparticles using by *Rhodobacter capsulatus* (Feng et al. 2008), silver nanoparticles using by *Fusarium oxysporum* (Ahmad et al. 2003), CdS quantum dots using by *Escherichia coli* (Sweeney et al. 2004) were reported. In such processes, the microorganisms are cultured at normal temperature under normal pressure and do not produce any toxic by-product. Such benefits suggest that the use of microorganisms to synthesize gold nanoparticles will be important in the future. To improve the efficiency of such synthesis, it is essential to clarify the molecular mechanisms involved. Recently, we reported that diglycosyl diacylglycerol (DGDG) plays important roles in reducing Au(III) to Au(0) by *Lactobacillus casei* (Kikuchi et al. 2016). This report shows the function of DGDG for the synthesis of gold nanoparticles.

27.2 Materials and Methods

We extracted lipid from *L. casei* (strain JCM1134, purchased from RIKEN Microbe Division) according to the Bligh and Dyer method (Bligh and Dyer 1959). We extracted thin layer chromatography (TLC) analysis. After spotting of samples in the origin point, plates were transferred to TLC chambers saturated with the chromatographic solvent (chloroform/methanol/acetic acid, 65:25:10). DGDG was extracted from TLC plate and dissolved in ethanol. To confirm DGDG, we measured mass spectra on a matrix-assisted laser-desorption ionization–time-of-flight mass spectrometer (ultraflex MALDI-TOF/TOF, Bruker). The sample solution was mixed with 500 mM 2, 5-dihydroxybenzoic acid in chloroform/methanol (1:1) solution as the matrix and dried on the plate.

DGDG extraction from the TLC plate dissolved in 40 μL ethanol was applied to 960 μL of auric acid solution (final concentration of $K[AuCl_4]$: 250 μM). The mixture solution was incubated at 37 °C for 24 h. Forty microliters of ethanol without DGDG was mixed with 960 μL of auric acid solution (final concentration of $K[AuCl_4]$: 250 μM) as a negative control experiment. UV/VIS spectra of the supernatant were measured using UV/VIS spectroscopy photometer (V-550 spectrophotometer, JASCO). To examine the formation of gold nanoparticles, we used transmission electron microscopies (TEM) observation and energy dispersive X-ray spectrometry (EDS). TEM analyses were performed using a JEOL JEM-2000EX TEM operated at 200 kV, and EDS analyses were performed using a JEOL EX-24025JGT.

27.3 Results

27.3.1 Extraction of DGDG from L. casei

L. casei cells were suspended in chloroform/methanol solution to extract lipids, and these extracts were subjected to TLC. The extracted sample separated from the TLC was analyzed by MALDI-TOF MS. The spectrum of MALDI-TOF MS showed four major peaks at 939.6, 953.6, 967.6, and 981.6 (*m/z*) and certain isotope peaks (Fig. 27.1a). These peaks showed the different chain length of the unsaturated fatty acids in DGDG. The chemical structure of DGDG was shown in Fig. 27.1b. R_1 and R_2 mean the alkyl chains containing one double bond in each chain.

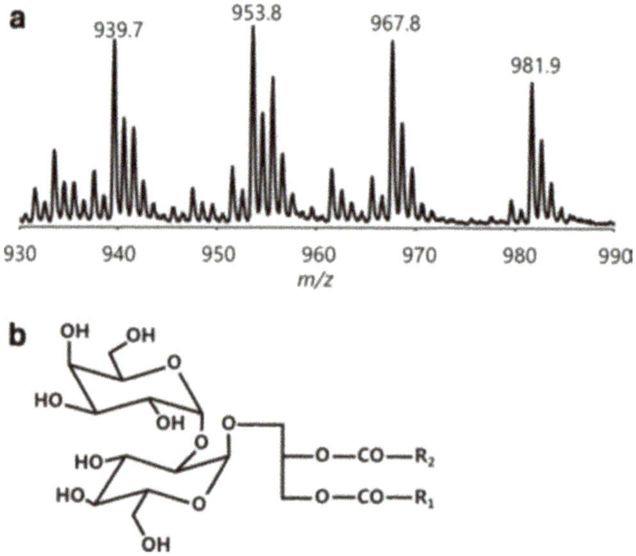

Fig. 27.1 (**a**) MALDI-TOF-MS spectrum of the extract from TLC. (**b**) The schematic structure of DGDG. R_1 and R_2 showed the alkyl chains of with one double bonding

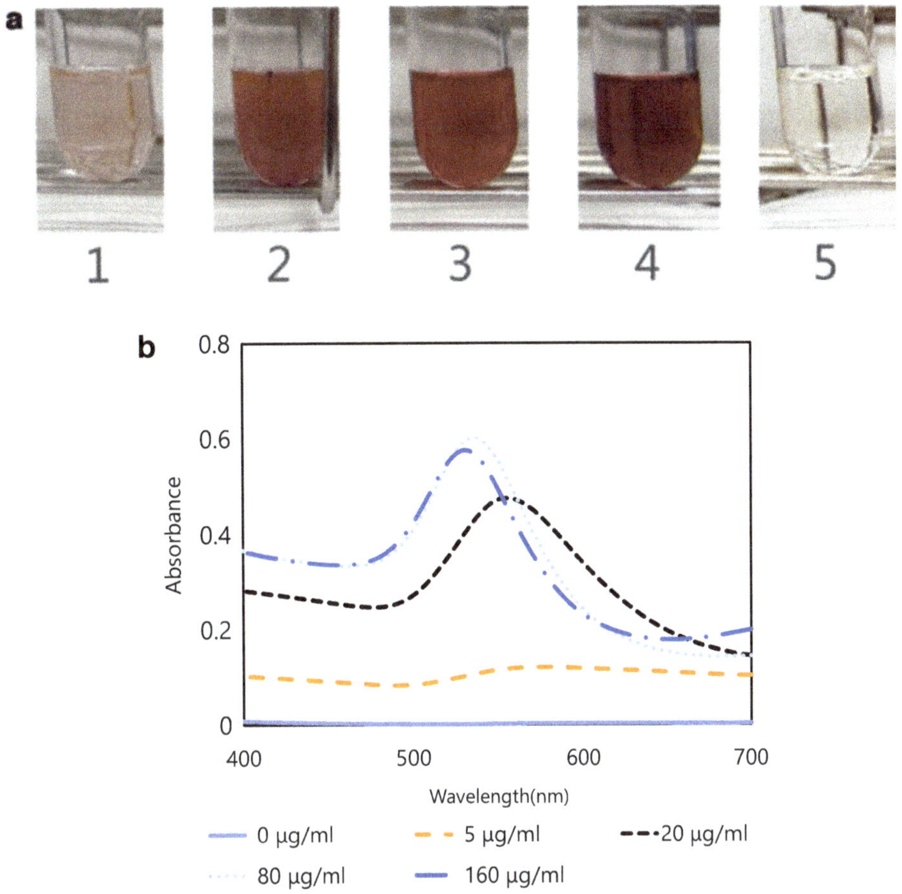

Fig. 27.2 (**a**) Auric acid solution (0.25 mM $K[AuCl_4]$) with DGDG purified from the TLC plate (1) 5.0 µg/mL, (2) 20 µg/mL, (3) 80 µg/mL, (4) 160 µg/mL, (5) 0 µg/mL), (**b**) UV/VIS spectra after 24 h. Light blue line, 0 µg/mL; orange break line, 5.0 µg/mL; black break line, 20 µg/mL; light blue dotted line, 80 µg/mL; dark blue dotted and break line, 160 µg/mL

27.3.2 Reaction of Auric Acid Solution with DGDG

Purified DGDG from *L. casei* was solubilized in ethanol to mix with auric acid. Then, the solution was incubated at 37 °C for 24 h. The colors of auric acid solution without DGDG kept the transparent yellow. On the other hand, the color of auric acid solution with DGDG became violet (Fig. 27.2a). The absorbance spectrum of each solution at wavelengths from 400 to 700 nm was measured (Fig. 27.2b). The intensity and wavelength of peak top varied by the DGDG concentration. The high concentration of DGDG showed the smaller wavelength indicating that the high concentration of DGDG synthesize the small nanoparticles. On the other hand, the low concentration of DGDG induced the bathochromic shift indicating that low concentration of DGDG induced the bigger nanoparticles.

27.3.3 Observation Nanoparticles by TEM

To investigate morphology of nanoparticles, the sample of each solution was subjected to TEM (Fig. 27.3a). TEM observations showed that black dots corresponding to gold nanoparticles were synthesized in all conditions. TEM observation of the condition with 5.0 μg/mL DGDG showed sphere shape of nanoparticles (Fig. 27.3a-1). 20 μg/mL DGDG synthesized small nanoparticles and rod shape of gold (Fig. 27.3a-2). 80 μg/mL DGDG induced the small and triangle shape of gold (Fig. 27.3a-3). 160 μg/mL DGDG synthesized the hexagonal shape of gold (Fig. 27.3a-4). EDS showed that the various shapes of nanoparticles were composed of Au (sphere shape (Fig. 27.3b-1), rod shape (Fig. 27.3b-2), triangle shape (Fig. 27.3b-3), and hexagonal shape (Fig. 27.3b-4).

27.4 Discussion

In the present study, incubation of DGDG with auric acid in vitro succeeded to produce gold nanoparticles, suggesting that DGDG has a function of both reducing and dispersing agents. The carboxylic groups of citric acid bind to the surface of Au(0) to create nanoparticles (Frens 1973). The degradation products of DGDG may interact with the Au(0) surface to stabilize nanoparticles. On the other hand, the size of particles synthesized by *L. casei* was 30 nm on average (Kikuchi et al. 2016). The gold nanoparticles synthesized by DGDG were slightly larger than those synthesized by *L. casei* cells, suggesting that the ability of dispersing capacity of DGDG is not enough to make the 30 nm nanoparticles. The high concentration of DGDG induced the various shape of gold crystals suggesting that DGDG also affected the crystal growth of gold. However, the other dispersing agents within *L. casei* cells may also play roles in inhibiting Au(0) aggregation and crystal growth. Further work is thus needed to reveal exactly how *L. casei* forms gold nanoparticles. Identification of the key organic molecules may allow modification of *L. casei* genes, permitting such recombinants to promote the synthesis of gold nanoparticles more effectively. In the future, the modified recombinant *L. casei* strains may be used for the applications in metal recycling and phytoremediation.

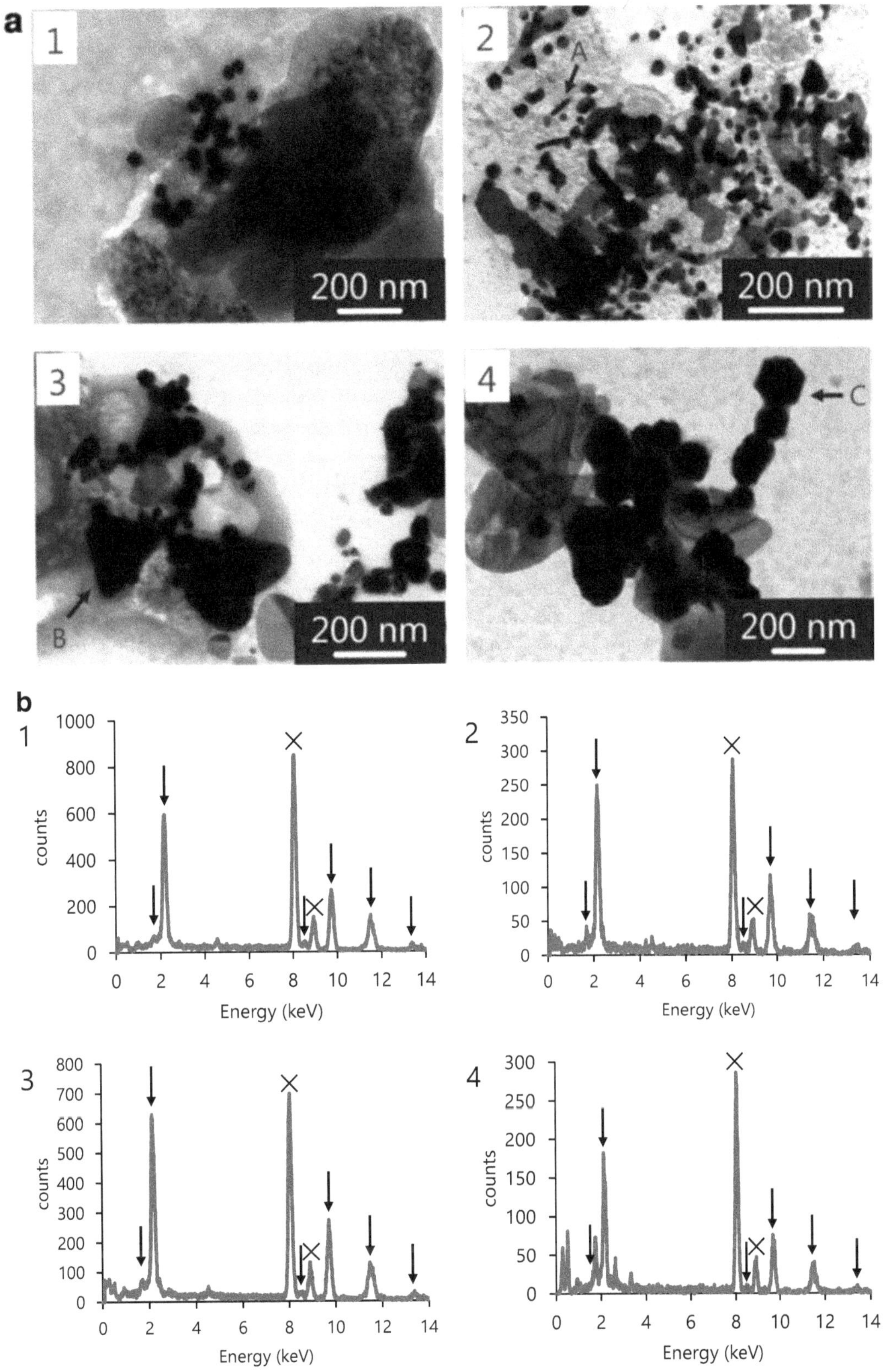

Fig. 27.3 (**a**) TEM image of gold nanoparticles synthesized by DGDG (*1*, 5.0 μg/mL; *2*, 20 μg/mL; *3*, 80 μg/mL; *4*, 160 μg/mL; DGDG). Arrow A indicates the rod shape of gold, arrow B indicates the triangle shape of gold, arrow C indicates the hexagonal shape of gold. (**b**) EDS spectra of nanoparticles of (**a**) (*1*, sphere shape; *2*, rod shape; *3*, triangle shape; *4*, hexagonal shape). The arrows showed the characteristic X-ray peaks of Au. X showed the peak of Cu from the copper grid

References

Ahmad A et al (2003) Extracellular biosynthesis of silver nanoparticles using the fungus Fusarium oxysporum. Colloids Surf B Biointerfaces 28:313–318

Bendayan M, Garzon S (1988) Protein G-gold complex: comparative evaluation with protein A-gold for high-resolution immunocytochemistry. J Histochem Cytochem 36:597–607

Bligh EG, Dyer WJ (1959) A rapid method of total lipid extraction and purification. Can J Biochem Physiol 37:911–917

Cao YC, Jin R, Mirkin CA (2002) Nanoparticles with Raman spectroscopic 21 fingerprints for DNA and RNA detection. Science 297:1536–1540

Feng Y et al (2008) Diversity of aurum bioreduction by Rhodobacter capsulatus. Mater Lett 62:4299–4302

Frens G (1973) Controlled nucleation for the regulation of the particle size in monodisperse gold suspensions. Nature Phys Sci 241:20–21

Jin R (2010) Quantum sized, thiolate-protected gold nanoclusters. Nano 2:343–362

Kikuchi F et al (2016) Formation of gold nanoparticles by glycolipids of *Lactobacillus casei*. Sci Rep 6:34626

Liu CL et al (2011) Insulin-directed synthesis of fluorescent gold nanoclusters: preservation of insulin bioactivity and versatility in cell imaging. Angew Chem Int Ed Eng 50:7056–7060

Selvakannan P et al (2004) Water-dispersible tryptophan-protected gold nanoparticles prepared by the spontaneous reduction of aqueous chloroaurate ions by the amino acid. J Colloid Interface Sci 269:97–102

Storhoff JJ et al (2000) What controls the optical properties of DNA-linked gold nanoparticle assemblies? J Am Chem Soc 122:4640–4650

Sweeney R et al (2004) Bacterial biosynthesis of cadmium sulfide nanocrystals. Chem Biol 11:1553–1559

Wang J, Xu D, Kawde AN, Polsky R (2001) Metal nanoparticle-based electrochemical stripping potentiometric detection of DNA hybridization. Anal Chem 73:5576–5581

Xie J, Zheng Y, Ying JY (2009) Protein-directed synthesis of highly fluorescent gold nanoclusters. J Am Chem Soc 131:888–889

Zhang Q, Xie J, Yu Y, Lee JY (2010) Monodispersity control in the synthesis of monometallic and bimetallic quasi-spherical gold and silver nanoparticles. Nanoscale 2:1962–1975

Chapter 28
Octacalcium Phosphate Overgrowth on β-Tricalcium Phosphate Substrate in Metastable Calcium Phosphate Solution

Mayumi Iijima and Kazuo Onuma

Abstract The effects of the particle size of β-tricalcium phosphate (β-$Ca_3(PO_4)_2$; β-TCP) on octacalcium phosphate ($Ca_8(HPO_4)_2(PO_4)_4 \cdot 5H_2O$; OCP) overgrowth on a β-TCP substrate were evaluated under physiological conditions by using two types of substrate; one composed of micrometer-sized particles (micro-TCP substrate) and one composed of nanometer-sized particles (nano-TCP substrate). When the β-TCP substrate was immersed in a simple calcium phosphate solution, it was quickly covered with OCP. The morphology and size of the OCP crystals, as well as the structure, thickness, and crystal density of the overgrown OCP layer, depended on the β-TCP particle size. In case of the micro-TCP substrate, OCP crystals grew directly on the micrometer-sized particles. In case of the nano-TCP substrate, string-like (S) precipitates initially deposited, and then flake-like (F) crystals formed on them. Plate-like (PL) OCP crystals grew on the flake-like crystals; as a result, a three-layer structure (S-layer/F-layer/PL-layer) was formed. Small amounts of tiny OCP crystals and HAp-nanofibers precipitated in the micro-TCP substrate, whereas only HAp-nanofibers precipitated in the nano-TCP substrate. Thus, various types of OCP-overgrown layers were fabricated on β-TCP scaffold. These findings will facilitate the structural design of OCP-coating layers on a β-TCP scaffold.

Keywords Octacalcium phosphate · Coating · Wet chemical method · Overgrowth · β-tricalcium phosphate · Scaffold · Particle size

28.1 Introduction

Both β-TCP and OCP have been proven to have promising osteoconductive characteristics. β-TCP has been applied in the form of granules and three-dimensional (3D) scaffolds (Hench and Polak 2002; Karageogiou and Kaplan 2005; Wang et al.

M. Iijima · K. Onuma (✉)
Biomaterial Research Group, Health Research Institute Central 6, National Institute of Advanced Industrial Science and Technology, Tsukuba, Ibaraki, Japan
e-mail: mayumi-iijima@aist.go.jp; k.onuma@aist.go.jp

K. Endo et al. (eds.), *Biomineralization*,
https://doi.org/10.1007/978-981-13-1002-7_28

2015). The biocompatibility and degradability of conventional micrometer-sized β-TCP powder have been improved by the use of nanometer-sized β-TCP (Zhang et al. 2008; Kato et al. 2016). On the other hand, OCP is a metastable phase of HAp and tends to transform into HAp spontaneously (Brown et al. 1962). The intrinsic properties of OCP are hypothesized to be responsible for its excellent performance in vivo; moreover, implanted OCP granules have provided cores for nucleating multiple osteogenic sites (Suzuki et al. 1991, 2006). The combined usage of β-TCP with its better formability and OCP with its better osteoconductivity would boost the potential of both materials as a bone graft substitute. A practical way to achieve this is coating β-TCP scaffolds with OCP.

The purpose of the present study was to examine OCP formation on a β-TCP substrate in a simple calcium phosphate solution and to evaluate the effect of the particle size of the β-TCP substrate on the overgrowth of OCP under physiological conditions. To achieve this, micrometer- and nanometer-sized β-TCP particles were used to form β-TCP substrate.

28.2 Materials and Methods

Reagent-grade β-TCP powder (Wako, Ltd.) and atomized powder were molded into substrate composed with micrometer-sized particles (0.5–3 μm) (micro-TCP substrate, Fig. 28.1a) and with nanometer-sized particles (<100 nm) (nano-TCP substrate, Fig. 28.1b).

Each substrate section was immersed in a calcifying solution (5 mM $CaCl_2$, 5 mM K_2HPO_4+KH_2PO_4, 50 mM CH_3COONa, pH 6.2, 37±0.5 °C) for required

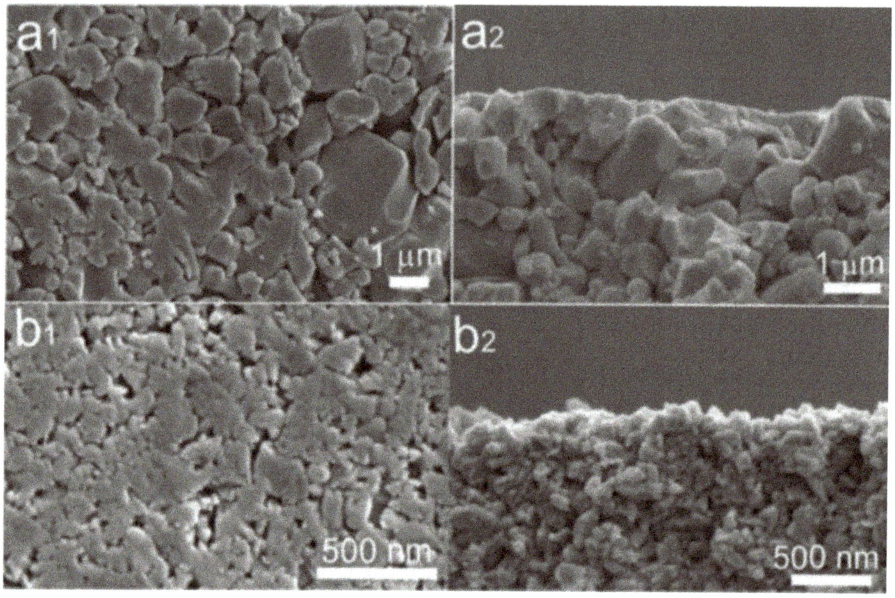

Fig. 28.1 SEM images of the surfaces (a1, b1) and cross sections (a2, b2) of (**a**) micro-TCP substrate and (**b**) nano-TCP substrate before immersion

periods. After the reaction terminated, the substrate was rinsed in Mill-Q water and in 99.5% ethanol and dried in air. The crystals in the overgrown layer and inside the substrate were characterized using powder XRD, microbeam XRD, thin-film in-plane XRD, FE-SEM, and TEM.

28.3 Results and Discussion

28.3.1 Early Stage of Overgrowth

On the micro-TCP substrate (Fig. 28.2), crystal growth started with the formation of sparse island-like aggregates of string-like precipitates, which gradually grew into small flakes (1–10 min) and subsequently increased in size (–30 min). Plate-like OCP crystals grew directly on the β-TCP particles and completely covered the substrate surface after 40 min. Thin-film in-plane XRD of the 40 min overgrown layer exhibits a shoulder peak at 4.7° (2θ), which corresponds to the (100) peak of OCP. It became strong after 60 min. On the nano-TCP substrate (Fig. 28.2), particles with a size of 10–20 nm precipitated after 1 min. These particles fused into strings (3 min), which subsequently formed root-like structure (5 min). The top part of the root-like deposits grew into small flakes (10 min), which completely covered the substrate surface. Thirty minutes overgrown layer exhibits a shoulder peak at 4.7° (2θ). Subsequently, plate-like OCP crystals grew on the thin layer of the flakes (60 min).

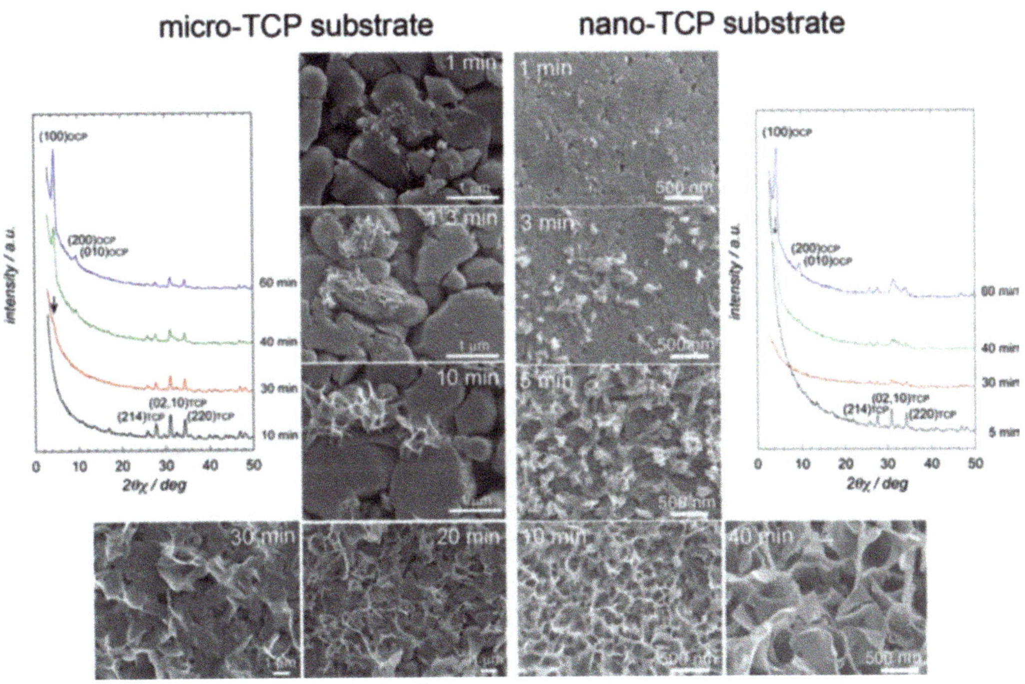

Fig. 28.2 Time-resolved SEM observations and thin-film in-plane XRD measurements of TCP substrate after 1–60 min immersion. Characteristic XRD peaks of OCP (JCPDF 26-1056) and β-TCP (JCPDF 09-0169) are labeled. An arrow indicates shoulder peak of $(100)_{OCP}$ at 4.7° (2θ)

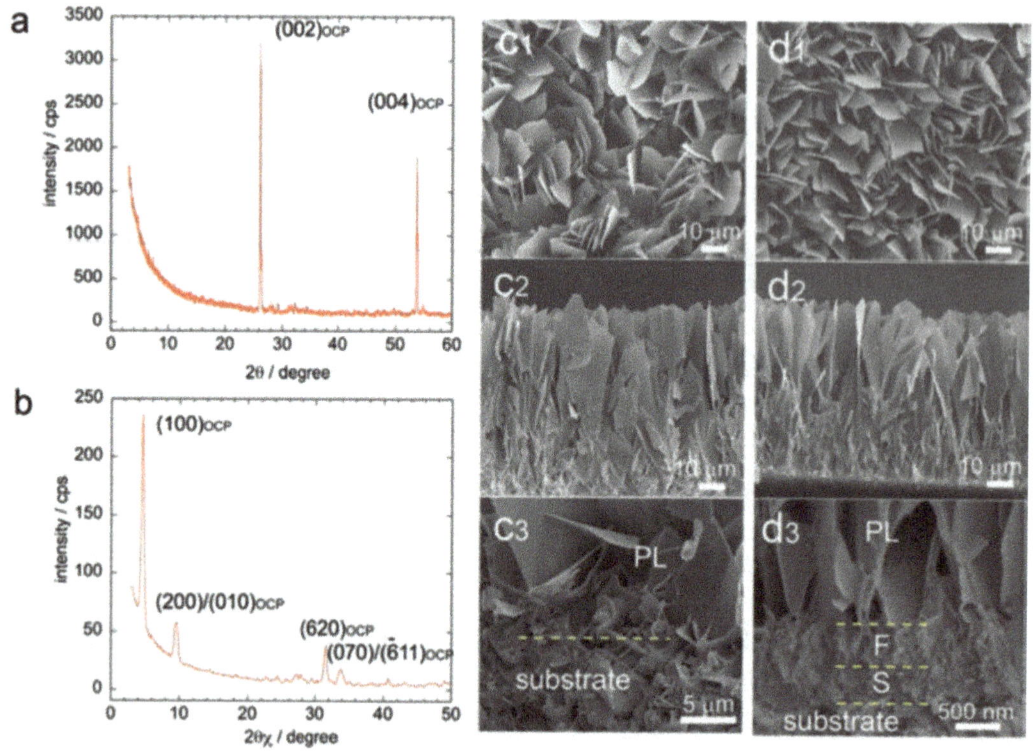

Fig. 28.3 (**a**) Powder XRD, (**b**) thin-film in-plane XRD profiles of micro-TCP substrate and SEM images of (**c**) micro-TCP substrate and (**d**) nano-TCP substrate after 20 h immersion. (c1, d1) top view and (c2, d2) cross-sectional view. (c3) and (d3) are higher magnifications of (c2) and (d2)

28.3.2 Later Stage of Overgrowth

Figure 28.3a, b, respectively, show powder XRD and thin-film in-plane XRD profiles of the micro-TCP substrate after 20 h. Both XRD profiles of the nano-TCP substrate are almost the same. In the powder XRD profile, the (002) and (004) peaks are strong, while the other peaks are very weak. In the thin-film in-plane XRD profile, the peaks in the a-axis direction, (100), (200), and (010), are strong, while the peak in the c-axis direction, (002), is weak. This is due to the c-axial orientation of the OCP crystals on the substrate. The overgrown crystals are identified as OCP by combined analysis of both XRDs.

On both substrates, OCP crystals grew in the same manner. As the immersion period increased, the length of OCP crystals in the c-axis direction increased: 4–6 μm after 60 min, 10 μm after 3 h, 15–20 μm after 5 h, and 66–70 μm after 20 h. In the case of the nano-TCP substrate, plate-like OCP crystals (PL) grew on the layer of small flake-like crystals (F-layer), under which the layer of string-like precipitates (S-layer) had formed, and as a result, a three-layer structure was observed (Fig. 28.3d3). On the contrary, in the case of the micro-TCP substrate, OCP crystals grew directly on β-TCP particles, and no such structure was observed (Fig. 28.3c3).

Inside of the substrates, tiny OCP crystals (Fig. 28.3c3) and small amounts of HAp-nanofibers precipitated in the micro-TCP substrate (Fig. 28.4a, c), whereas

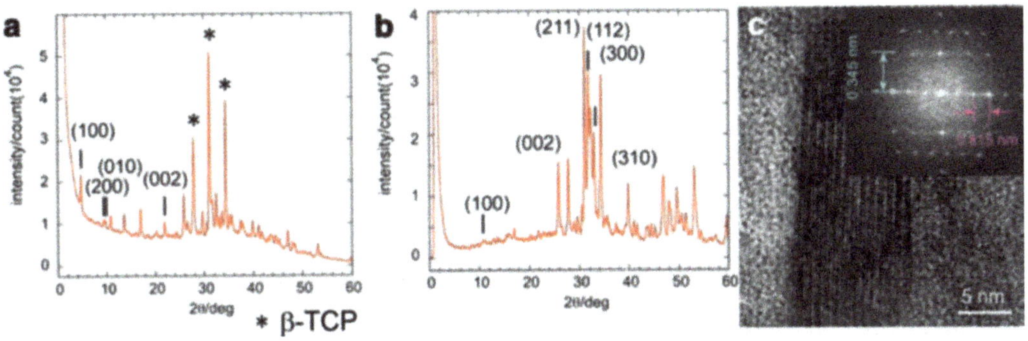

Fig. 28.4 2θ-intensity converted microbeam XRD profile of (**a**) micro-TCP substrate and (**b**) nano-TCP substrate after 20 h immersion. Characteristic XRD peaks of OCP (JCPDF 26-1056) and HAp (JCPDF 09-0432) are labeled, respectively, in (**a**, **b**). (**c**) HR-TEM image of a HAp-nanofiber formed inside of the micro-TCP substrate and its FFT

only HAp-nanofibers were formed in the nano-TCP substrate (Fig. 28.4b). HAp-nanofibers were formed much more in the nano-TCP substrate than in the micro-TCP substrate, and they were localized around particles less than 500 nm in the micro-TCP substrate (Iijima and Onuma 2017). Thus, it was concluded that nano-TCP particles induced the formation of HAp-nanofibers (Onuma and Iijima 2017).

Thus, varying the particle size of the β-TCP had great effect on the early stage of overgrowth and precipitates inside the substrates. Various types of OCP-coating layers were formed on β-TCP substrate. There is a general consensus that the physical properties of the coating layer, i.e., its thickness and topography, affect the in vivo performance of the coated material (Curtis and Wilkinson 1997; Anselme and Bigerelle 2011). These findings will facilitate the structural design of OCP-coating layers on a β-TCP scaffold.

Acknowledgments This study was supported by a Grant-in-Aid for Scientific Research from the Japan Society for the Promotion of Science (JSPS KAKENHI C; 16K04954).

References

Anselme K, Bigerelle M (2011) Role of materials surface topography on mammalian cell response. Int Mater Rev 56:243–266

Brown WE, Smith JP, Lehr JR, Fraier AW (1962) Crystallographic and chemical relation between octacalcium phosphate and hydroxyapatite. Nature 196:1050–1055

Curtis A, Wilkinson C (1997) Topographical control of cells. Biomaterials 18:1573–1583

Hench LL, Polak JM (2002) Third-generation biomedical materials. Science 295:1014–1017

Iijima M, Onuma K (2017) Particle-size-dependent octacalcium phosphate overgrowth on β-tricalcium phosphate substrate in calcium phosphate solution. Ceram Int. https://doi.org/10.1016/j.ceramint.2017.10.167

Karageogiou V, Kaplan D (2005) Porosity of 3D biomaterial scaffolds osteogenesis. Biomaterials 26:5474–5491

Kato A, Miyaji H, Ogawa K, Momose T, Nishida E, Murakami S, Yoshida T, Tanaka S, Sugaya T (2016) Bone-forming effects of collagen scaffold containing nanoparticles on extraction sockets in dogs. Jpn J Conserv Dent 59:351–358

Onuma K, Iijima M (2017) Nanoparticles in β-tricalcium phosphate substrate enhance modulation of structure and composition of an octacalcium phosphate grown layer. Cryst Eng Comm 19:6660–6672

Suzuki O, Nakamura M, Miyasaka Y, Kagayama M, Sakurai M (1991) Bone formation on synthetic precursors of hydroxyapatite. Tohoku J Exp Med 164:37–50

Suzuki O, Kamakura S, Katagiri T, Nakamura M, Zhao B, Honda Y, Kamijo R (2006) Bone formation enhanced by implanted octacalcium phosphate involving conversion into Ca-deficient hydroxyapatite. Biomaterials 27:2671–2681

Wang L, Hu YY, Wang Z, Li X, Li DC (2015) Flow perfusion culture human fetal bone cells in large beta-tricalcium phosphate scaffold with controlled architectures. Ceram Int 41:2654–2667

Zhang F, Chang C, Lin K, Lu J (2008) Preparation, mechanical properties and in vitro degradability of wollastonite/tricalcium phosphate macroporous scaffolds from nanocomposite powders. J Mater Sci Mater Med 19:167–173

Part VII
Biominerals for Environmental and Paleoenvironmental Sciences

Chapter 29
Coral-Based Approaches to Paleoclimate Studies, Future Ocean Environment Assessment, and Disaster Research

Atsushi Suzuki

Abstract Global warming causes serious harm to the Earth's environment. A more sophisticated and accurate climate model can be developed by reconstructing climatic change since the Industrial Revolution and for other past periods of global warming. Coral skeletons are an important archive of past climate changes, and advances in the ability to read sea surface temperature and salinity in the coral record have been made by applying state-of-the-art technology. Coral skeletal climatology has been successfully applied to characterize both the recent global warming trend in the Western Pacific and the mid-Pliocene warming that occurred 3.5 million years ago, and it has also been used to investigate biological and environmental issues such as ocean acidification and coral bleaching, which is caused by unusually high seawater temperatures. Coral skeletal climatology methods have also been used to study *Porites* boulders cast ashore by historical tsunamis; such studies have high social value from the perspective of regional disaster prevention. Nevertheless, aspects of coral skeletal climatology still need clarification, including the basic mechanism by which seawater temperature is recorded in coral skeletons, and further research on biomineralization will improve predictions of the future responses of marine calcifying organisms to ocean acidification.

Keywords Coral · Global warming · Ocean acidification · Coral bleaching · Tsunami

29.1 Introduction

Annual banding in the skeletons of modern corals was first described by Ma (1934), then a PhD student at Tohoku University, after a field trip to the northern Ryukyu Islands of Japan (Fig. 29.1). The annual bands of coral skeletons became the subject

A. Suzuki (✉)
Geological Survey of Japan, National Institute of Advanced Industrial Science and Technology (AIST), Tsukuba, Ibaraki, Japan
e-mail: a.suzuki@aist.go.jp

K. Endo et al. (eds.), *Biomineralization*,
https://doi.org/10.1007/978-981-13-1002-7_29

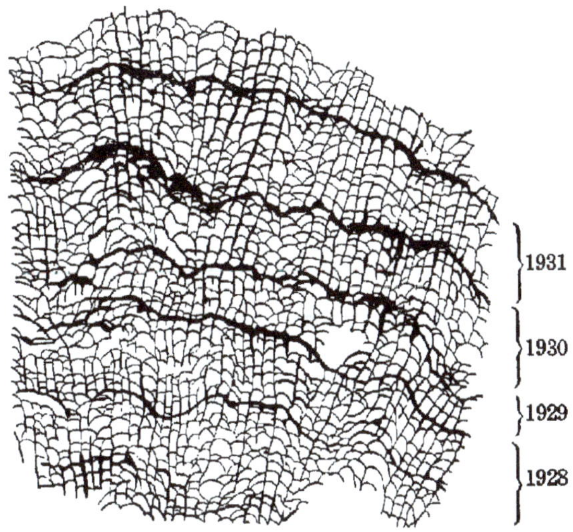

Fig. 29.1 First published illustration of annual banding in modern corals. (Reprinted from Ma 1934 with permission from the Institute of Geology and Paleontology Sendai, Tohoku University)

of active research in the 1990s, but only recently has the research developed into the field of coral skeletal climatology (see Suzuki 2012). Corals provide rich archives of past climatic variability in tropical regions, where instrumental records are relatively few. In this review, I explain why the coral skeleton is such an excellent archive of past global climate change and describe some of the major ways in which coral skeletal analyses have been successfully applied to biological and environmental issues, including coral bleaching events and ocean acidification, as well as to paleo-tsunami research.

29.2 Coral Skeletal Climatology

Geochemists have found useful climate proxies in the coral skeleton. For example, the strontium/calcium (Sr/Ca) ratio is a good, and pure, proxy for sea surface temperature; that is, the skeletal Sr/Ca ratio is controlled only by seawater temperature. In contrast, the oxygen isotope ratio ($\delta^{18}O$) is a mixed proxy for both seawater temperature and salinity, and the uranium/calcium (U/Ca) ratio is a mixed proxy for seawater temperature and pH. By a combined analysis of two proxies, Sr/Ca and $\delta^{18}O$ or Sr/Ca and U/Ca, referred to as a "dual proxy method," it is possible to extract past salinity variation (McCulloch et al. 1994) or past seawater pH from the coral skeletal record (Fig. 29.2).

Two examples of twentieth century coral oxygen isotope records from coral reefs in Japan are shown in Fig. 29.3. Fluctuations of $\delta^{18}O$ in corals from Ishigaki Island (124°E, 24°N), which is very close to Taiwan (Mishima et al. 2010), and Chichijima Island (142°E, 27°N) in the Ogasawara island chain, due south of Tokyo (Felis et al. 2009), record seasonal variations of seawater temperature. In addition, both curves show a shift toward more negative values with time, indicating a long-term seawater temperature increase. Moreover, by applying the dual proxy method, the Ogasawara

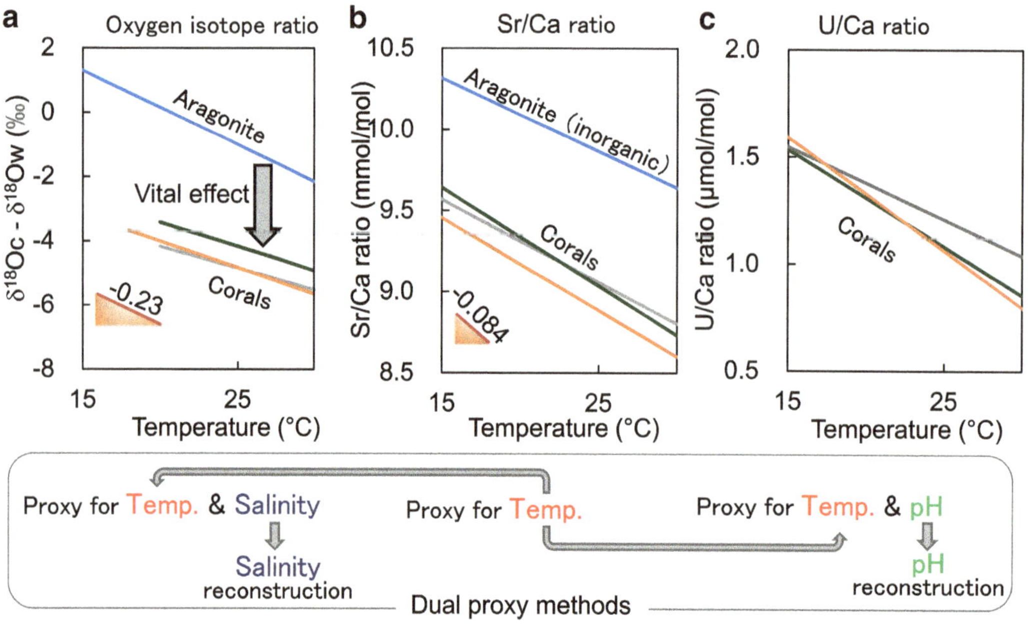

Fig. 29.2 Coral climate proxies that have been developed by geochemists: (**a**) oxygen isotope ratio ($\delta^{18}O$); (**b**) Sr/Ca ratio; and (**c**) U/Ca ratio. The $\delta^{18}Oc$ and $\delta^{18}Ow$ denote oxygen isotope ratio of coral skeleton and seawater, respectively. The skeletal Sr/Ca ratio is controlled only by seawater temperature, whereas $\delta^{18}O$ is a mixed proxy for seawater temperature and salinity and the U/Ca ratio is a mixed proxy for seawater temperature and pH. Through a combined analysis of Sr/Ca and $\delta^{18}O$ (U/Ca), the seawater salinity (pH) variation can be extracted. Ideal temperature dependency of $\delta^{18}O$ and Sr/Ca ratio proposed by Gagan et al. (2012) are shown in panels (**a**, **b**), respectively

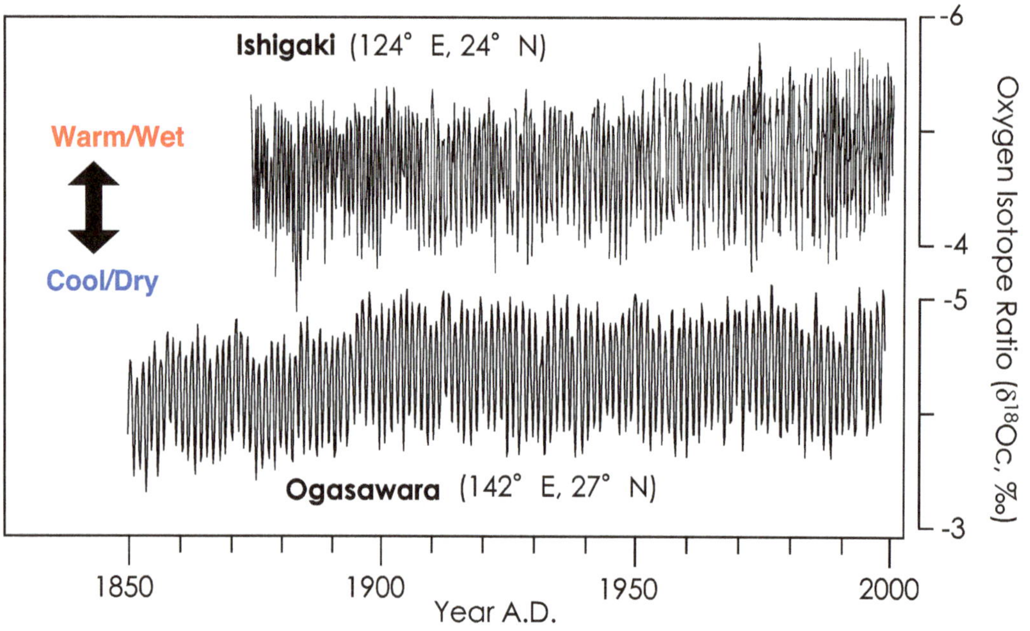

Fig. 29.3 Times series of coral $\delta^{18}O$ records from Ishigaki Island in the southern Ryukyus (Mishima et al. 2010) and Chichijima Island in the Ogasawara Islands (Felis et al. 2009) in the Western Pacific

corals were found to record a long-term freshening of seawater (decrease in salinity) in the region. The long-term warming trend revealed by Ishigaki coral can be attributed to anthropogenic climate change.

Conditions during the Pliocene warm period, about 4.6–3 million years ago, are thought to be similar to the climate conditions expected to result from global warming in the near future. Watanabe et al. (2011), who compared analysis results obtained by the same method between modern corals and well-preserved fossil corals from Luzon Island, the Philippines, showed that El Niño occurred on about the same cycle during the Pliocene warm period as at present. Their study is an example of the successful application of coral skeletal climatology to the distant past.

29.3 Application to Environmental Issues

Coral skeletal climatology can also be applied to the investigation of biological and environmental issues such as coral-bleaching events and ocean acidification.

Coral bleaching at a scale unseen before occurred in coral reefs around the Ryukyu Islands in August 1998, and another major coral bleaching event occurred in the southern Ryukyu Islands, especially around Ishigaki Island, in summer 2016. Suzuki et al. (2003) examined skeletal records of bleached corals and observed an abrupt rise, corresponding to the bleaching period, in the $\delta^{18}O$ profile analyzed at high resolution along the growth axis of the skeleton. They interpreted this jump to reflect a cessation of coral skeletal growth for a few months immediately after bleaching. As global warming progresses and high seawater temperatures occur more frequently, environmental conditions can be expected to further inhibit coral growth.

Another good proxy for the pH of seawater, or, more precisely, that of the calcifying fluid of the organism, is the boron isotope ratio of the coral skeleton. Kubota et al. (2017) conducted high-precision boron isotope measurements of two coral cores collected from Kikai Island (Ryukyu Islands) and Chichijima Island (Ogasawara Islands) and reported that the ratios from the two islands decreased over the long term, indicating decreasing pH. Interestingly, in both cases, the rate of decline increased in the latter half of the twentieth century. Although seawater pH changes have been observed by shipboard measurements since 1985, the coral record confirms the existence of an ocean acidification trend in the Western Pacific.

29.4 Application to Disaster Research

The 2011 Tohoku-oki earthquake (Great East Japan Earthquake) occurred on 11 March 2011, and the tsunami generated by the earthquake caused major damage to the Pacific coasts of the Tohoku and Kanto regions of Japan. To mitigate the effects of future tsunamis, it is urgent to reevaluate past tsunami damage throughout Japan.

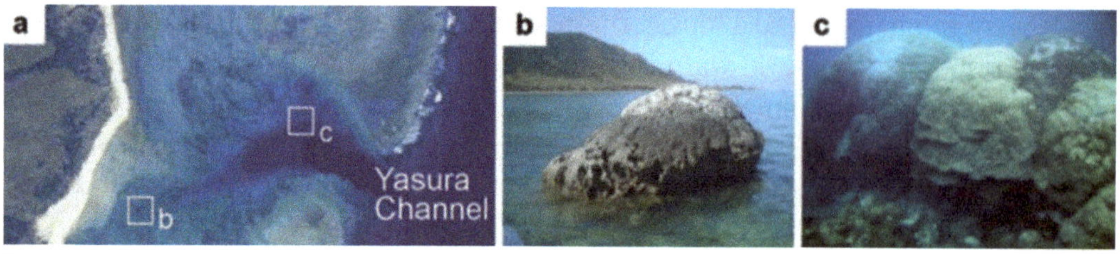

Fig. 29.4 (**a**) Aerial photograph of the fringing coral reef on the eastern shore of Ishigaki Island, Japan (from the Geospatial Information Authority of Japan). (**b**) A tsunami boulder composed of a massive *Porites* coral on the reef flat. This coral was dated to about AD 1771 (Araoka et al. 2010). (**c**) Massive *Porites* coral colonies in the reef channel

Coral skeletal climatology methods have been applied to the analysis of *Porites* boulders cast ashore by past tsunamis (Suzuki et al. 2008; Fig. 29.4). By applying radiocarbon dating and coral skeletal climatological techniques to *Porites* boulders scattered along the eastern coast of Ishigaki Island, southern Ryukyus, Araoka et al. (2010) demonstrated that some of the boulders, at least, were washed ashore by the Meiwa tsunami in 1771. Araoka et al. (2013) extended this approach to neighboring islands in the southern Ryukyus. They selected non-eroded *Porites* coral boulders along shorelines for radiocarbon dating, because they retain characteristics that make it possible to determine the probable timing of their deposition by tsunamis. Their results demonstrate that the southern Ryukyu Islands have repeatedly experienced tsunami events since at least 2400 years ago, with a recurrence interval of about 150–400 years. Their study demonstrates that by reliably dating large numbers of coral boulders, it is possible to ascertain the timing, recurrence interval, and magnitude of past tsunamis in a location where few survey sites exist that include sandy tsunami deposits.

29.5 Future Directions

Several points still need clarification, including the basic mechanisms by which climatological factors such as seawater temperature are recorded in the chemical and isotope compositions of coral skeletons. Further, the influence of the coral growth rate on coral climate proxies such as $\delta^{18}O$ is still problematic (Fig. 29.5). Special attention needs to be paid to diagenetic alteration of coral proxy signals. In addition to the geochemical methods, culture experiments should be conducted and molecular biological methods should be applied to clarify the biological mechanism of calcification. Recent papers have recognized that coral primary polyps are particularly suitable for biomineralization studies because of their small size and simple form (Iwasaki et al. 2016; Ohno et al. 2017). An integrated approach that brings various perspectives to bear on these problems is needed, because coral biomineralization reflects synergetic effects (Fig. 29.6).

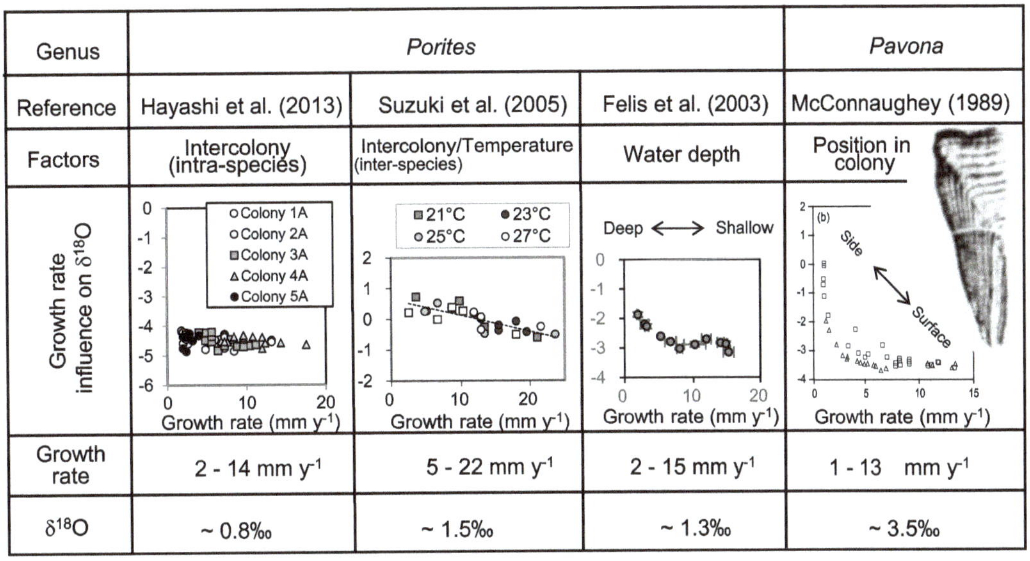

Fig. 29.5 Influence of the skeletal growth rate on the skeletal oxygen isotope ratio ($\delta^{18}O$) as reported in the literature (The image of the coral skeleton has been reprinted from McConnaughey 1989 with permission from Elsevier). Hayashi et al. (2013) reported a relatively small growth rate dependency of skeletal $\delta^{18}O$ values, but most previous studies have reported considerable dependence of climate proxies on the skeletal growth rate (Felis et al. 2003; Suzuki et al. 2005)

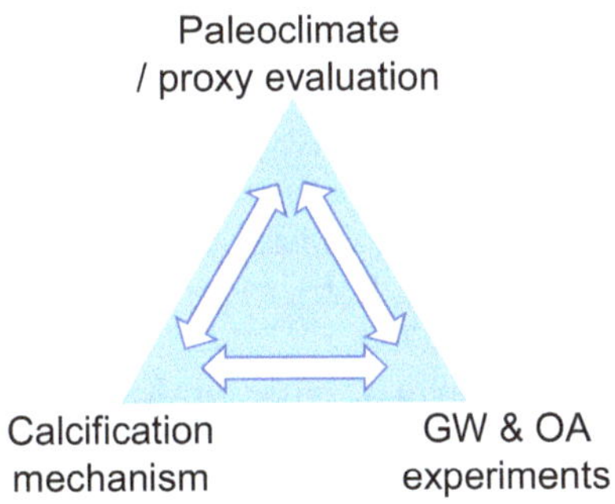

Fig. 29.6 Graphical summary of the integrated approach used by the author's research group. Research is conducted from various perspectives simultaneously because we expect synergetic effects for better understanding biomineralization of corals. *GW* global warming, *OA* ocean acidification

Acknowledgments This paper is based on joint research with H. Kawahata, A. Iguchi, Y. Ohno, M. Inoue, D. Araoka, T. Watanabe, and many other collaborators. To all of them, I express my sincere gratitude. This study was supported by KAKENHI grant 15H02813 and 18H03366 to AS.

References

Araoka D, Inoue M, Suzuki A, Yokoyama Y, Edwards RL, Cheng H, Matsuzaki H, Kan H, Shikazono N, Kawahata H (2010) Historic 1771 Meiwa tsunami confirmed by high-resolution U/Th dating of massive *Porites* coral boulders at Ishigaki Island in the Ryukyus, Japan. Geochem Geophys Geosyst 11:Q06014

Araoka D, Yokoyama Y, Suzuki A, Goto K, Miyagi K, Miyazawa K, Matsuzaki H, Kawahata H (2013) Tsunami recurrence revealed by *Porites* coral boulders in the southern Ryukyu Islands, Japan. Geology 41:919–922

Felis T, Pätzold J, Loya Y (2003) Mean oxygen-isotope signatures in *Porites* spp. corals: inter-colony variability and correction for extension-rate effects. Coral Reefs 22:328–336

Felis T, Suzuki A, Kuhnert H, Dima M, Lohmann G, Kawahata H (2009) Subtropical coral reveals abrupt early 20th century freshening in the western North Pacific Ocean. Geology 37:527–530

Gagan MK, Dunbar GB, Suzuki A (2012) The effect of skeletal mass accumulation in *Porites* on coral Sr/Ca and $\delta^{18}O$ paleothermometry. Paleoceanography 27:PA1203

Hayashi E, Suzuki A, Nakamura T, Iwase A, Ishimura T, Iguchi A, Sakai K, Okai T, Inoue M, Araoka D, Murayama S, Kawahata H (2013) Growth-rate influences on coral climate proxies tested by a multiple colony culture experiment. Earth Planet Sci Lett 362:198–206

Iwasaki S, Inoue M, Suzuki A, Sasaki O, Kano H, Iguchi A, Sakai K, Kawahata H (2016) The role of symbiotic algae in the formation of the coral polyp skeleton: 3-D morphological study based on X-ray microcomputed tomography. Geochem Geophys Geosyst 17:3629–3637. https://doi.org/10.1002/2016GC006536

Kubota K, Yokoyama Y, Ishikawa T, Suzuki A, Ishii M (2017) Rapid decline in pH of coral calcification fluid due to incorporation of anthropogenic CO_2. Sci Rep 7:7694

Ma TYH (1934) On the growth rate of reef corals and the sea water temperature in the Japanese Islands during the latest geological times. Science reports of the Tohoku Imperial University 2nd series. Geology 16(3):165–189

McConnaughey T (1989) ^{13}C and ^{18}O isotopic disequilibrium in biological carbonates: I. Patterns. Geochim Cosmochim Acta 53:151–162

McCulloch MT, Gagan MK, Mortimer GE, Chivas AR, Isdale PJ (1994) A high resolution Sr/Ca and ^{18}O coral record from the Great Barrier Reef, Australia, and the 1982–1983 El Niño. Geochim Cosmochim Acta 58:2747–2754

Mishima M, Suzuki A, Nagao N, Ishimura T, Inoue M, Kawahata H (2010) Abrupt shift toward cooler condition in the earliest 20th century detected in a 165 year coral record from Ishigaki Island, southwestern Japan. Geophys Res Lett 37:L15609

Ohno Y, Iguchi A, Shinzato C, Inoue M, Suzuki A, Sakai K, Nakamura T (2017) An aposymbiotic primary coral polyp counteracts acidification by active pH regulation. Sci Rep 7:40324

Suzuki A (2012) Paleoclimate reconstruction and future forecast based on coral skeletal climatology –understanding the oceanic history through precise chemical and isotope analyses of coral annual bands. Synthesiology 5:78–87

Suzuki A, Gagan MK, Fabricius K, Isdale PJ, Yukino I, Kawahata H (2003) Skeletal isotope microprofiles of growth perturbations in *Porites* corals during the 1997–1998 mass bleaching event. Coral Reefs 22:357–369

Suzuki A, Hibino K, Iwase A, Kawahata H (2005) Intercolony variability of skeletal oxygen and carbon isotope signatures of cultured *Porites* corals: temperature controlled experiments. Geochim Cosmochim Acta 69:4453–4462

Suzuki A, Yokoyama Y, Kan H, Minoshima K, Matsuzaki H, Hamanaka N, Kawahata H (2008) Identification of 1771 Meiwa Tsunami deposits using a combination of radiocarbon dating and oxygen isotope microprofiling of emerged massive *Porites* boulders. Quat Geochronol 3:226–234

Watanabe T, Suzuki A, Minobe S, Kawashima T, Kameo K, Minoshima K, Aguilar YM, Wani R, Kawahata H, Sowa K, Nagai T, Kase T (2011) Permanent El Niño during the Pliocene warm period not supported by coral evidence. Nature 471:209–211

Chapter 30
An Elemental Fractionation Mechanism Common to Biogenic Calcium Carbonate

Kotaro Shirai

Abstract Biological modulation of element incorporation presents a major hurdle in the interpretation of geochemical data as an environmental proxy, detailed understanding and quantitative evaluation of the mechanism of elemental fractionation both being essential for reliable reconstruction of an environment. Biogenic calcium carbonate has a specific skeletal microstructure, which is strongly controlled by biomineralization. Since primary processes are more likely reflected on a smaller spatial scale, elemental distribution patterns associated with skeletal microstructure should provide unique information on biological elemental fluctuations, which cannot be determined from large-scale analysis. To study elemental fractionation mechanisms, microscale elemental distribution patterns have been studied in coral skeletons and bivalve and foraminiferal shells and the skeletal microstructure, sulfur distribution, and organic features compared. The microanalytical studies revealed two characteristic patterns that were common to all studied biogenic calcium carbonates, even though the specimens examined represented different phyla: (1) significant compositional heterogeneities that could not be explained by changes in the ambient environment and (2) a strong correlation of "metal/Ca" ratios with all or some of sulfur distribution, skeletal microstructure, and organic character. Based on these common features, I propose a mechanism of elemental fractionation, commonly applicable to biogenic calcium carbonates and involving both composition and/or concentration of organics in the calcifying fluid, that facilitates preferential elemental incorporation into biogenic calcium carbonate.

Keywords Biogenic calcium carbonate · Proxy · Vital effect · Geochemistry · Trace element · Coral · Bivalve shell · Foraminifera · Sclerosponge

K. Shirai (✉)
Atmosphere and Ocean Research Institute, The University of Tokyo, Kashiwa, Chiba, Japan
e-mail: kshirai@aori.u-tokyo.ac.jp

K. Endo et al. (eds.), *Biomineralization*,
https://doi.org/10.1007/978-981-13-1002-7_30

30.1 Introduction

Mg/Ca and Sr/Ca ratios in biogenic calcium carbonate are widely used as proxies for estimating past seawater temperatures (e.g., Henderson 2002; Lea 2003). However, such ratios are also more or less affected by biological processes, so-called vital effects (Cohen and McConnaughey 2003). For example, the Sr/Ca ratio in a coral skeleton (aragonite) and Mg/Ca ratio in a foraminiferan test (calcite) reflect temperature relatively precisely (Lea 2003), whereas Mg/Ca in the former and Sr/Ca in the latter, and both ratios in bivalve shells (both aragonite and calcite), are susceptible to biological modulation (Schöne 2013). Although the vital effect is considered to be species-specific, it remains a major hurdle to interpreting geochemical data as an environmental proxy, as the ultimate mechanism governing elemental fractionation, a detailed understanding and quantitative evaluation of which is essential for reliable past environment reconstruction, is still unclear.

A fundamental question concerns the common existence or otherwise of an elemental fractionation mechanism in any biogenic calcium carbonate. Biomineralization can be interpreted as inorganic mineralization strongly controlled by soluble and insoluble organic materials, as well as physiological control, such as that exerted by pH, physical structure, space regulations, and ion transportation (e.g., Marin et al. 2008). Thus, the relationship between micrometer-scale elemental distribution and microstructure may provide a unique opportunity to investigate the mechanism of element fractionation by biological processes. The aim of the present study was to examine a common, cross-phylum fractionation mechanism based on microscale elemental distribution in coral skeletons and bivalve and foraminiferal shells, comparing elemental distribution, skeletal/shell microstructure, sulfur distribution, and organic features.

30.2 Materials and Methods

The examined samples included the reef building branching coral *Acropora nobilis* (Shirai et al. 2008a), deep sea solitary coral *Caryophyllia ambrosia ambrosia* (Shirai et al. 2005), ocean quahog *Arctica islandica* (Shirai et al. 2014), deep sea hydrothermal mussel *Bathymodiolus platifrons* (Shirai et al. 2008b), and planktonic foraminifera *Globorotalia menardii* (Kunioka et al. 2006). Samples were cleaned, embedded in epoxy resin, sectioned, polished, metal coated where necessary, and analyzed by electron probe microanalysis (EPMA) or high lateral resolution secondary ion mass spectrometry (NanoSIMS). The microstructure was observed by SEM or optical microscope following etching/staining by Mutvei's solution (Schöne et al. 2005). Specific details of sample origin and preparation and analytical methods are included in the above-cited references.

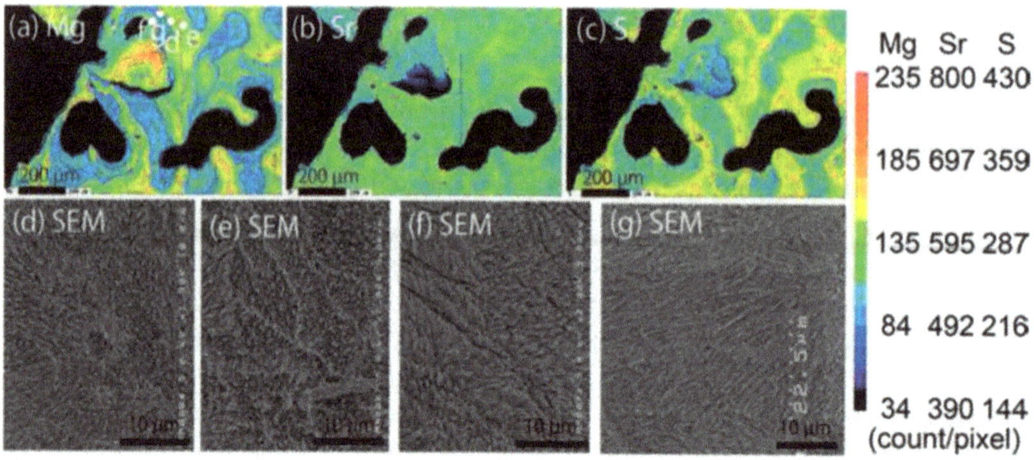

Fig. 30.1 Elemental distribution and skeletal microstructure of branching coral *Acropora nobilis*. (**a**) EPMA Mg map. (**b**) EPMA Sr map. (**c**) EPMA S map. (**d–g**) Skeletal microstructure of polished-etched surface by SEM. (Figures modified from Shirai et al. 2008a). Color scale bar on right indicates gross count per pixel

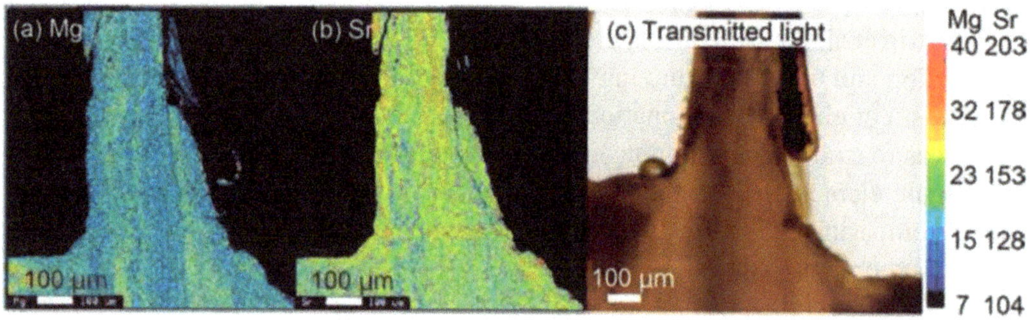

Fig. 30.2 Elemental distribution and skeletal microstructure of deep sea coral *Caryophyllia ambrosia ambrosia*. (**a**) EPMA Mg map. (**b**) EPMA Sr map. (**c**) Skeletal microstructure observed in thin section under transmitted light microscopy. (Figures modified from Shirai et al. 2005). Color scale bar on right indicates gross count per pixel

30.3 Results

Elemental distribution and skeletal/shell microstructure of the examined samples are shown in Figs. 30.1, 30.2, 30.3, 30.4, and 30.5. Regardless of mineralogy and phylum, the following were common at the microscale level in all of the examined biogenic carbonates: (1) large compositional heterogeneity and (2) element/Ca ratios, skeletal/shell microstructure, sulfur distribution, and insoluble skeletal organic characters all correlated (nonlinear) with one another.

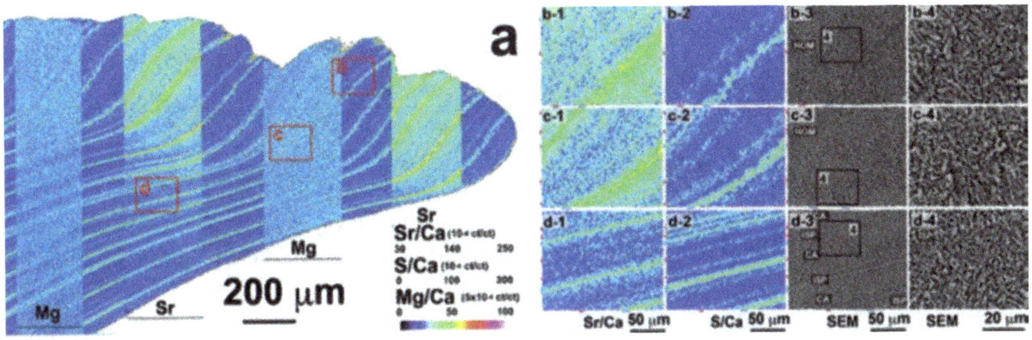

Fig. 30.3 Elemental distribution and shell microstructure of ocean quahog *Arctica islandica*. (**a**) Sr/Ca and Mg/Ca maps partly overlapped on S/Ca map. (**b–d**) High-magnification images of elemental maps and shell microstructure along sixth annual growth line from ventral margin (red rectangles in (**a**)). From left to right, (1) EPMA Sr/Ca map, (2) EPMA S/Ca map, (3) SEM microstructure image, and (4) inset of (3). *HOM* homogeneous structure, *ISP* irregular simple prismatic structure, *CA* crossed acicular structure, *N.C.* shell microstructure is not clear. (Figures modified from Shirai et al. 2014). Color scale bar on bottom right in panel (**a**) indicates gross count ratio (*ct/ct* count/count) per pixel

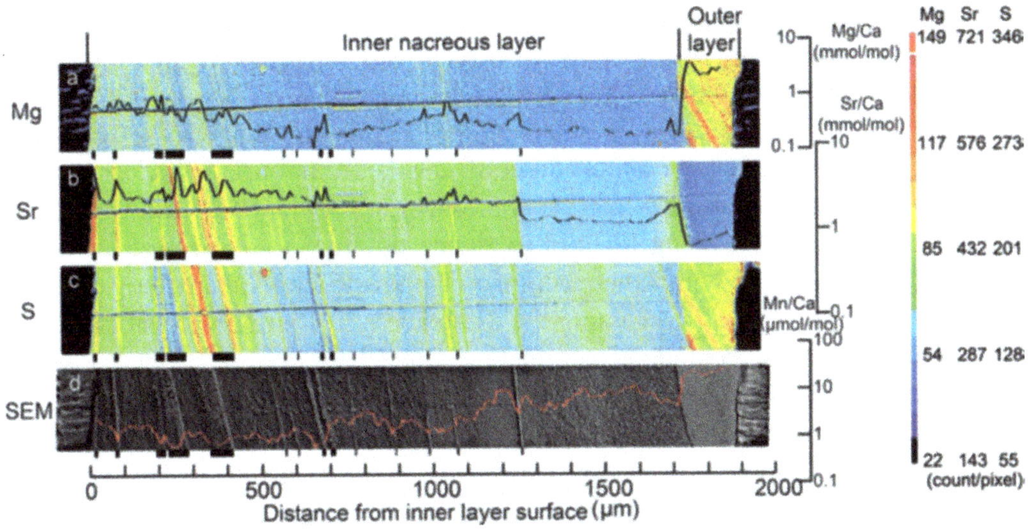

Fig. 30.4 Elemental distribution and shell microstructure of hydrothermal mussel *Bathymodiolus platifrons*. (**a**) EPMA Mg map with NanoSIMS Mg/Ca profile overlaid (right axis for scale). (**b**) EPMA Sr map with NanoSIMS Sr/Ca profile overlaid. (**c**) EPMA S map. (**d**) Shell microstructure of polished-etched surface by SEM with NanoSIMS Mn/Ca profile overlaid. (Figures modified from Shirai et al. 2008b)

30.4 Discussion

The correlation with microstructure suggests that microscale heterogeneity is likely induced by the biomineralization processes, the magnitude of variation being too great to be explained by ambient environmental changes. Similar correlations between chemical composition and microstructure have been documented in other coral skeleton studies (e.g., Meibom et al. 2004, 2008), bivalve shell

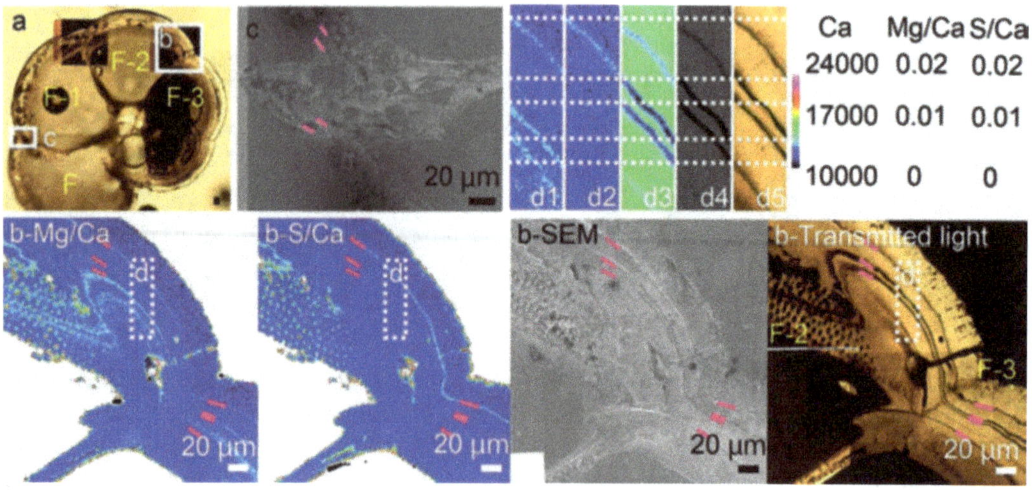

Fig. 30.5 Elemental distribution and shell microstructure of planktonic foraminifera *Globorotalia menardii*. (**a**) Shell microstructure under transmitted light microscopy after EPMA analysis (**b**) From left to right, EPMA Mg/Ca map, EPMA S/Ca map, shell microstructure of polished-etched surface by SEM and transmitted light microscope image. (**c**) SEM microstructure image, enlargements of inset of (**a**). (**d**) Enlargements of inset of (**b**). From left to right, (d1) EPMA Mg/Ca map, (d2) EPMA S/Ca map, (d3) EPMA Ca map, (d4) EPMA backscattered electron image, and (d5) transmitted light microscope image. Pink bars represent organic membrane. White dashed lines in (**d**) act as a guide for comparing each figure on the same position

(Dauphin et al. 2005, 2013; Füllenbach et al. 2017), foraminifera (Sadekov et al. 2005; Kunioka et al. 2006), brachiopod (Pérez-Huerta et al. 2011), and Ostracoda (Morishita et al. 2007), being lines of evidence pointing to an almost universal relationship between elemental distribution and microstructure in any biogenic calcium carbonate, as well as suggesting the existence of a common physiochemical mechanism governing elemental fractionation.

Recent studies have reported that organic molecules present in the calcifying solution enhance Mg incorporation in inorganically precipitated calcite (Stephenson et al. 2008) and amorphous calcium carbonate (Wang et al. 2009). In the latter model, aqueous carboxylated molecules, which have greater selectivity for binding to Ca than Mg, increase the relative activity of Mg against Ca in the solution, producing high Mg/Ca amorphous calcium carbonate, considered a precursor phase of crystalline carbonate (e.g., Pouget et al. 2009). Thus, organically mediated fractionation processes may occur in the early stages of crystallization (Wang et al. 2009), with the mechanism that determines the composition of amorphous calcium carbonate also likely controlling biogenic calcite composition. Since the organic membrane has a characteristic electrostatic structure regulating biomineralization (e.g., Marin et al. 2008; Ren et al. 2011), it is also possible that such a structure of insoluble organics influences elemental incorporation into carbonate. Since biomineralization occurs in calcifying fluid (or calcifying space), the organic (and inorganic) composition of which is highly regulated by the organism, I suggest that both soluble and insoluble organic composition and concentration in calcifying fluids control the microscale elemental distribution commonly found in biogenic calcium carbonate. Changes in the microstructure and sulfur distribution can be considered as signatures of change in the organic composition and sulfur-containing organic matrix in the calcifying medium, respectively. These processes are likely common in any biomineralization. Such an organically mediated fractionation hypothesis can also explain why elemental composition is not correlated with other elements in a quantitative manner, since the function of macromolecules in calcium carbonate precipitation depends not only on their structure and composition but also on their supramolecular assemblage (e.g., Marin et al. 2008). A detailed discussion of this elemental fractionation mechanism is reported in Shirai et al. (2014) and Füllenbach et al. (2017).

References

Cohen AL, McConnaughey TA (2003) Geochemical perspectives on coral mineralization. Rev Mineral Geochem 54:151–187

Dauphin Y, Cuif JP, Salome C, Susini J (2005) Speciation and distribution of sulfur in a mollusk shell as revealed by in situ maps using X-ray absorption near-edge structure (XANES) spectroscopy at the SK-edge. Am Mineral 90:1748–1758

Dauphin Y, Ball AD, Castillo-Michel H, Chevallard C, Cuif JP, Farre B, Pouvreau S, Salome M (2013) In situ distribution and characterization of the organic content of the oyster shell *Crassostrea gigas* (Mollusca, Bivalvia). Micron 44:373–383

Füllenbach CS, Schöne BR, Shirai K, Takahata N, Ishida A, Sano Y (2017) Minute co-variations of Sr/Ca ratios and microstructures in the aragonitic shell of *Cerastoderma edule* (Bivalvia)–are geochemical variations at the ultra-scale masking potential environmental signals? Geochim Cosmochim Acta 205:256–271

Henderson GM (2002) New oceanic proxies for paleoclimate. Earth Planet Sci Lett 203:1–13

Kunioka D, Shirai K, Takahata N, Sano Y, Toyofuku T, Ujiie Y (2006) Microdistribution of Mg/Ca, Sr/Ca, and Ba/Ca ratios in *Pulleniatina obliquiloculata* test by using a Nano-SIMS: implication for the vital effect mechanism. Geochem Geophys Geosyst 7:Q12P20

Lea DW (2003) Elemental and isotopic proxies of past ocean temperatures. Treat Geochem 6:365–390

Marin F, Luquet G, Marie B, Medakovic D (2008) Molluscan shell proteins: primary structure, origin, and evolution. Curr Top Dev Biol 80:209–276

Meibom A, Cuif JP, Hillion FO, Constantz BR, Juillet-Leclerc A, Dauphin Y, Watanabe T, Dunbar RB (2004) Distribution of magnesium in coral skeleton. Geophys Res Lett 31:L23306

Meibom A, Cuif JP, Houlbreque F, Mostefaoui S, Dauphin Y, Meibom KL, Dunbar R (2008) Compositional variations at ultra-structure length scales in coral skeleton. Geochim Cosmochim Acta 72:1555–1569

Morishita T, Tsurumi A, Kamiya T (2007) Magnesium and strontium distributions within valves of a recent marine ostracode, *Neonesidea oligodentata*: implications for paleoenvironmental reconstructions. Geochem Geophys Geosyst 8:GC001585

Pérez-Huerta A, Cusack M, Dalbeck P (2011) Crystallographic contribution to the vital effect in biogenic carbonates Mg/Ca thermometry. Earth Env Sci Trans Roy Soc Edinbur 102:35–41

Pouget EM, Bomans PHH, Goos JACM, Frederik PM, de With G, Sommerdijk NAJM (2009) The initial stages of template-controlled CaCO3 formation revealed by Cryo-TEM. Science 323:1455–1458

Ren D, Feng Q, Bourrat X (2011) Effects of additives and templates on calcium carbonate mineralization in vitro. Micron 2:228–245

Sadekov AY, Eggins SM, De Deckker P (2005) Characterization of Mg/Ca distributions in planktonic foraminifera species by electron microprobe mapping. Geochem Geophys Geosyst 6:GC000973

Schöne BR (2013) *Arctica islandica* (Bivalvia): a unique paleoenvironmental archive of the northern North Atlantic Ocean. Glob Planet Chang 111:199–225

Schöne BR, Dunca E, Fiebig J, Pfeiffer M (2005) Mutvei's solution: an ideal agent for resolving microgrowth structures of biogenic carbonates. Palaeogeogr Palaeoclimatol Palaeoecol 228:149–166

Shirai K, Kusakabe M, Nakai S, Ishii T, Watanabe T, Hiyagon H, Sano Y (2005) Deep-sea coral geochemistry: implication for the vital effect. Chem Geol 224:212–222

Shirai K, Kawashima T, Sowa K, Watanabe T, Nakaniori T, Takahata N, Arnakawa H, Sano Y (2008a) Minor and trace element incorporation into branching coral *Acropora nobilis* skeleton. Geochim Cosmochim Acta 72:5386–5400

Shirai K, Takahata N, Yamamoto H, Omata T, Sasaki T, Sano Y (2008b) Novel analytical approach to bivalve shell biogeochemistry: a case study of hydrothermal mussel shell. Geochem J 42:413–420

Shirai K, Schöne BR, Miyaji T, Radermacher P, Krause RA Jr, Tanabe K (2014) Assessment of the mechanism of elemental incorporation into bivalve shells (*Arctica islandica*) based on elemental distribution at the microstructural scale. Geochim Cosmochim Acta 126:307–320

Stephenson AE, DeYoreo JJ, Wu L, Wu KJ, Hoyer J, Dove PM (2008) Peptides enhance magnesium signature in calcite: insights into origins of vital effects. Science 322:724–727

Wang DB, Wallace AF, De Yoreo JJ, Dove PM (2009) Carboxylated molecules regulate magnesium content of amorphous calcium carbonates during calcification. Proc Natl Acad Sci U S A 106:21511–21516

Chapter 31
Biomineralization of Metallic Tellurium by Bacteria Isolated From Marine Sediment Off Niigata Japan

Madison Pascual Munar, Tadaaki Matsuo, Hiromi Kimura, Hirokazu Takahashi, and Yoshiko Okamura

Abstract Three facultative anaerobe mesophilic bacteria were isolated from marine sediment collected off Niigata, Japan. Sequencing of complete 16S ribosomal DNA revealed 99% homology with *Shewanella algae*, *Pseudomonas pseudoalcaligenes*, and *P. stutzeri*. Phylogenetic analyses suggest novel strain status thus new strains were designated as *S. algae* strain Hiro-1, *P. pseudoalcaligenes* strain Hiro-2, and *P. stutzeri* strain Hiro-3. Minimum inhibitory concentration assays using increasing concentrations of Na_2TeO_3 revealed resistance of *S. algae* strain Hiro-1 at 15 mM, and *P. pseudoalcaligenes* strain Hiro-2 and *P. stutzeri* strain Hiro-3 both showed resistance at 4 mM. Transmission electron microscopy revealed intracellular aggregation of metallic tellurium nanorods with a minimum unit size of 60-nm nanoparticle.

Keywords Marine sediment · *Pseudomonas pseudoalcaligenes* · *Pseudomonas stutzeri* · *Shewanella algae* · Tellurite reduction · Tellurium nanorods

31.1 Introduction

Tellurite is a strong oxidizing agent that is highly toxic to most microorganisms (Fleming 1932; Taylor 1999; Chasteen et al. 2009; Arenas-Salinas et al. 2016). The compound's toxicity was reported to induce oxidative stress, which eventually leads to cell death. Some microorganisms can resist this toxicity, either by enzymatic reduction with the aid of nitrate reductase or by overexpression of glutathione (GSH) to maintain homeostasis inside the cell (Avazeri et al. 1997; Sabaty et al. 2001; Turner 2001; Turner et al. 2012; Pugin et al. 2014). Tellurate (TeO_4^{2-}) and tellurite (TeO_3^{2-}) oxyanions can also serve as electron acceptors in anaerobic

M. P. Munar · T. Matsuo · H. Kimura · H. Takahashi · Y. Okamura (✉)
Department of Molecular Biotechnology, Graduate School of Advanced Sciences of Matter, Hiroshima University, Higashihiroshima, Japan
e-mail: ziphiro@hiroshima-u.ac.jp; okamuray@hiroshima-u.ac.jp

K. Endo et al. (eds.), *Biomineralization*,
https://doi.org/10.1007/978-981-13-1002-7_31

respiration by purple sulfur bacteria (Csotonyi et al. 2006; Baesman et al. 2007). Reduction of tellurite into pure metallic elemental tellurium (Te^0) can be observed as formation of black tellurium precipitate (Tucker et al. 1962).

Production and recovery of this scarce metalloid is required for the sustainability of green technologies such as solar cells in the future. However, the exact mechanism of tellurium reduction is still unknown. Most studies conducted on tellurite reduction (TR) employed bacterial species with very low resistance to the element, and the poor survival of cells in the presence of tellurite is a major impediment to fully elucidating the enigmatic reduction mechanism (Arenas-Salinas et al. 2016). Biomineralization of tellurium nanoparticles (TeNPs) has been documented in several bacterial genera including *Rhodobacter*, *Escherichia*, *Shewanella*, *Geobacter*, *Sulfurospirillum*, *Bacillus*, *Pseudomonas*, *Erwinia*, *Agrobacter*, *Staphylococcus*, and *Selenihalanaerobacter* (Moore and Kaplan 1994; Avazeri et al. 1997; Trutko et al. 2000; Sabaty et al. 2001; Di Tomaso et al. 2002; Borsetti et al. 2003; Oremland et al. 2004; Csotonyi et al. 2006; Baesman et al. 2007, 2009; Turner et al. 2012; Borghese et al. 2014). Some species within these bacterial genera possess innate resistance to the toxic metalloid and are thereby potential candidates for microbiological reduction and recovery of the valued rare Earth element. Here, we report the isolation and identification of tellurite-resistant and tellurite-reducing bacterial strains that can be used for the development of efficient metal recovery strategies. Further analyses of these strains may add additional insights into factors prerequisite for efficient bioremediation.

31.2 Materials and Methods

31.2.1 Isolation and Cultivation

A marine sediment sample collected at a depth of 100 m off Niigata, Japan (38°05′N, 139°04′E) was generously provided by Dr. Takeshi Terahara of the Tokyo University of Marine Science and Technology. The sediment was inoculated and incubated at a final volume of 50 mL with RCVBN medium (Burgess et al. 1991) in completely filled 50-mL centrifuge tubes (Falcon) under continuous illumination for 1 month. The culture showed prominent growth of a biofilm-forming purple bacteria as observed by the deep purple pigment production in the media. A 1-mL sample of the resulting culture was transferred into 7-mL fresh RCVBN medium supplemented with 1-mM sodium tellurite and cultured in completely filled 8-mL screw-capped tubes at 24 °C under continuous illumination (38 $\mu mol/m^2/s$). TR activity was visually recorded by the formation of black tellurium precipitate. The successive pour plate method and streak plate method were used to isolate tellurite-resistant and tellurite-reducing bacteria on RCVBN agar media (pH 7.6, 37 °C). Purified colonies were re-streaked in RCVBN agar plates with 1 mM Na_2TeO_3 to observe TR activity. Colony characteristics were observed after 72 h of growth. To determine the TR activity and minimum inhibitory concentration (MIC), the cultures were incubated with varying concentrations of Na_2TeO_3 (1, 2, 4, 6, 8, 10, 12, and 15 mM). Inoculum was standardized by using culture with similar OD values for each strain. Bacterial growth in pH and temperature optimum experiments was measured using spectrometer at OD_{550} nm (WPA CO-7500 Colorimeter, Biochrom Ltd., UK).

31.2.2 16S rDNA Amplification, Cloning, and Sequencing

The 16S rDNA was amplified using PCR mix including 10X KOD Plus-Neo Buffer, 2 mM dNTPs, 25 mM $MgSO_4$ (TOYOBO Co., Ltd., Osaka, Japan), 10 μM each forward and reverse primer 16S 27F (F-5′-AGAGTTTGATCNTGGCTCAG-3′) and 16S ipRSR2 (R-5′-AAGGAGGTGATCCANCCGC-3′) (Eurofins Genomics, Tokyo, Japan), 0.05 U/μL KOD Neo POL (TOYOBO Co., Ltd., Osaka, Japan), and 2 μL genomic DNA. Thermal cycling conditions were as follows: pre-denaturation 2 mins at 94 °C for 1 cycle, followed by 35 cycles of denaturation at 95 °C for 10 s, annealing at 60 °C for 10 s, and extension at 68 °C for 60 s, and final extension at 68 °C for 60 s (T100™ Thermal Cycler, Bio-Rad, CA, USA).

After PCR, amplified fragments were excised from the gel. Purified 16S rDNA fragments were cloned into the ZERO-Blunt TOPO vector following the kit protocol (Invitrogen, USA). Clones able to grow on LB/Kanamycin plates were used for colony PCR to verify insertion using M13 primers (F-5′-TGTAAAACGACGGCCAGT-3′; R-5′-CAGGAAACAGCTATGACC-3′) (Eurofins Genomics, Tokyo Japan). Thermal cycling conditions were as follows: pre-denaturation 5 mins at 94 °C for 1 cycle, followed by 28 cycles of denaturation at 94 °C for 10 s, annealing at 70 °C for 20 s, and extension at 72 °C for 45 s. Positive clones with verified inserts were sub-cultured and plasmids were extracted using a Fastgene plasmid mini kit (Nippon Genetics Co., Ltd., Tokyo, Japan) following the manufacturer's protocol. The sequences of the resulting clones were analyzed by Eurofins Genomics Co., Ltd. (Tokyo, Japan). SnapGene (SnapGene Software, www.snapgene.com) was used to check chromatogram quality and to guide quality trimming. High quality reads were assembled using CodonCode Aligner (CodonCode Corporation, www.codoncode.com) and assembled sequences were used for BLAST analysis (NCBI).

31.2.3 Phylogenetic Analysis

With MEGA6 software, Neighbor-Joining, Maximum-Likelihood, Minimum Evolution and Maximum Parsimony with Kimura-2-parameter distance correction and 1000 bootstrap value were used to identify the three pure cultures (Kimura 1980; Felsenstein 1985; Saitou and Nei 1987; Rzhetsky and Nei 1992; Nei and Kumar 2000; Tamura et al. 2013). NCBI GenBank database was surveyed for closely related strains with partial and complete 16S ribosomal DNA sequences included in the phylogenetic analyses. The 16S rDNA sequences of all species identified were aligned with the muscle DNA alignment method in MEGA 6 software.

Aligned sequences were visually evaluated to ensure that the subsequent cladogram would result from polymorphisms rather than sequence errors, gaps, and branch pulling due to differences in sequence directions or sizes. A total of 26 *Shewanella* and 24 *Pseudomonas* species and strains were included in the phylogenetic analyses with equal length of final quality trimmed sequences of 1360 bp and 1391 bp, respectively.

31.2.4 Benchmarking of New Isolates with Type Strains

Type strains *Shewanella algae* (NBRC 103173^T), *Pseudomonas pseudoalcaligenes* (NBRC 14167^T), and *Pseudomonas stutzeri* (NBRC 14165^T) were obtained from the National Institute of Technology and Evaluation Biological Resource Center (NBRC) in Japan. The type cultures were initially revived using the prescribed growth medium for each culture, then were grown in RCVBN media to compare colony morphology with our new isolates. Cultures were streaked onto plates to observe single pure colonies of the type strains and new isolates. RCVBN agar spread with 200 μL 1 mM Na_2TeO_3 was used to evaluate the TR activity of the type strains. Plates were incubated at 37 °C for 6 days were used for observation of morphology and TR activity under stereomicroscope (TW-360, WRAYMER, Japan).

31.2.5 Electron Microscopy of New Isolates

Transmission electron microscopy (TEM) was performed on the three new isolates to observe their crystal morphologies and localizations. Enrichment cultures of each strain exposed at 1 mM Na_2TeO_3 incubated for 101 days were used for TEM. The long incubation period would allow for the observation of all possible crystal morphologies. A 1-mL culture of each strain was washed twice with milliQ water by centrifugation at 10,000 × g for 5 min. The harvested cells were resuspended in milliQ water and mounted on 150-mesh copper grids coated with collodion (Nisshin EM Co., Ltd., Tokyo, Japan).

31.3 Results

31.3.1 Three Marine Mesophiles with Tellurite Resistance and Reduction Activity

The mesophiles isolated into pure culture included two *Pseudomonas* species and one *Shewanella* species. BLAST search using the full-length 16S rDNA sequences of the three isolates revealed 99% homology to *P. pseudoalcaligenes* (Query length: 1529 bp),

P. stutzeri (Query length: 1529 bp), and *S. algae* (Query length: 1538 bp) with E-value of 0.00. Based on phylogenetic analyses using four different building methods, the three isolates were found to be unique strains. Representative trees are shown in Fig. 31.1. Thus, we designate new strains on *S. algae*, *P. pseudoalcaligenes*, and *P. stutzeri* with strain Hiro-1 (DDBJ Accession no.: LC339942), Hiro-2 (DDBJ Accession no.: LC339940), and Hiro-3 (DDBJ Accession no.: LC339941), respectively. The two *Pseudomonas* isolates showed TR activity up to 4 mM tellurite with a MIC of 6 mM tellurite.

The *S. algae* isolate showed TR activity up to 10 mM tellurite with a MIC of 15 mM tellurite (Fig. 31.2). Negative control samples containing only RCVBN (Fig. 31.2, tube C1) or RCVBN spiked with 1 mM Na_2TeO_3 (data not shown) showed no visible TR or bacterial growth indicating no spontaneous reduction or contamination, respectively.

31.3.2 Colony Characteristics of New Isolates

S. algae strain Hiro-1 formed colonies with round form, entire margin, convex elevation, mucoid consistency, and orange-brown color. *P. pseudoalcaligenes* strain Hiro-2 formed colonies with irregular form, undulate margin, raised elevation, viscid consistency, and translucent color. *P. stutzeri* strain Hiro-3 formed colonies with wrinkled form, undulate margin, raised elevation, rugose consistency, and yellow color. The morphology and TR activity were also compared to the type strains, and the new isolates showed similar colony morphology and TR activity to the type cultures (Fig. 31.3). All three new strains grew optimally at pH 7.0. Growth at pH 7.0 was significantly higher than growth at all other pH levels tested based on unpaired *t*-test with 95% confidence level (p-value <0.05). Optimum growth temperature coincided with mesophilic cardinal temperatures. For all three strains, there was no significant difference between the growth at 25 °C, 37 °C, and 45 °C based on unpaired *t*-test with 95% confidence level (p-value >0.05). Little to no growth was observed at 4 °C.

31.3.3 Intracellularly Deposited Tellurium Particles

TEM revealed that tellurium particles were deposited within the cell for all three strains (Fig. 31.4). In *S. algae* strain Hiro-1, 60-nm minimum units of nanorod particles were conjugated along the crystallographic axis, forming long rod crystals that finally assembled into a bundle within the cell (Fig. 31.4a). However, this culture was too old, and the cells were easily lysed. External, inorganically growing crystals were also found (data not shown). Strain Hiro-2, interestingly, formed needle-shaped particles 60 nm in size (Fig. 31.4b), whereas strain Hiro-3 formed rod-shaped crystals resembling the nanorods from the strain Hiro-1 (Fig. 31.4c).

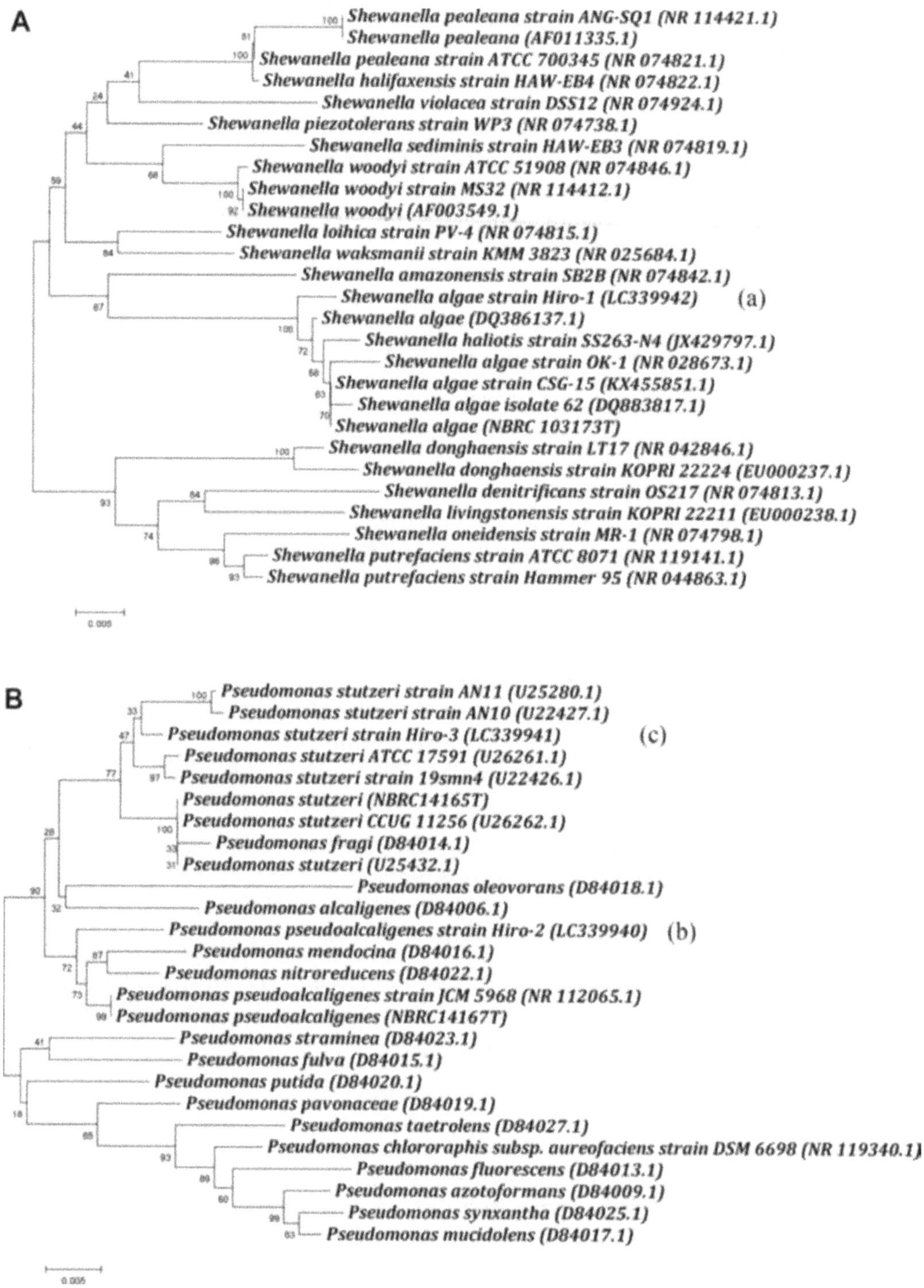

Fig 31.1 Unrooted neighbor-joining tree. (**a**) *S. algae* strain Hiro-1 (a). (**b**) *P. pseudoalcaligenes* strain Hiro-2 (b). P. stutzeri strain Hiro-3 (c). Accession numbers are in parentheses. Numbers at nodes represent bootstrap values from 1000 resampled datasets. Scale bar indicates 0.5% sequence divergence. Kimura-2-parameter was used for distance correction

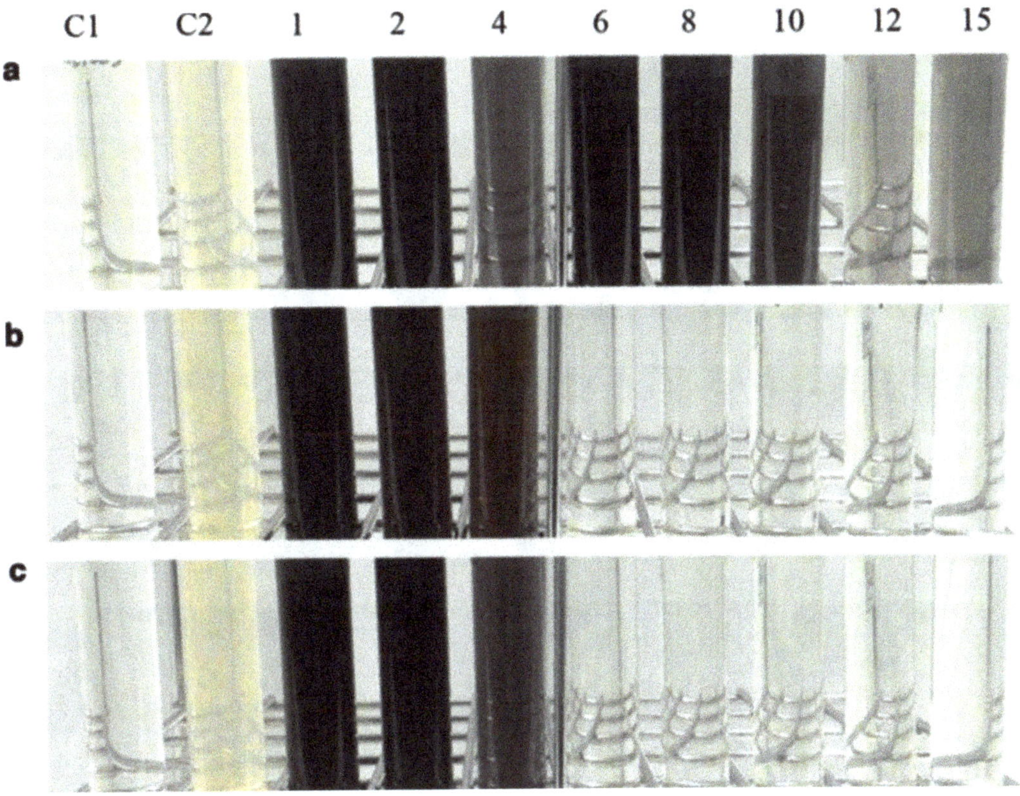

Fig. 31.2 Tellurite reduction activity (TR activity) and minimum inhibitory concentration (MIC) of tellurite. Control tube C1 is RCVBN media alone and control tube C2 is RCVBN with culture inoculum. The other tubes are labeled with the concentration (mM) of Na_2TeO_3 added to the RCVBN media inoculated with the culture. Image shown is representative of two replicate reactions taken after 3 weeks of incubation. (**a**) *S. algae*, (**b**) *P. pseudoalcaligenes*, and (**c**) *P. stutzeri*

Both *Pseudomonas* spp. maintained cell integrity, and both showed smaller and scattered nanoparticles within the cell. Long crystals were observed in ripped cells, suggesting that the length of tellurium crystal must be regulated within the cellular environment.

31.4 Discussion

Deep marine sediments support the growth of anaerobic microorganisms that may use various metals as final electron acceptors in the respiratory chain, such as purple sulfur bacteria. *S. algae* has bioremediation potential against uranium, plutonium, tellurite ions, nitrite, and halogenated organic compounds (Almagro et al. 2005; Klonowska et al. 2005). Mucoid, round colonies are common colony morphologies for *Shewanella* species (Simidu et al. 1990; Nozue et al. 1992; Venkateswaran et al. 1998; Holt et al. 2005; Gao et al. 2006; Kim et al. 2007) which is also evident in our isolate. *P. pseudoalcaligenes* and *P. stutzeri* have bioremediation potential against cyanide and tellurite (Romero et al. 1998). *P. pseudoalcaligenes* subsp. *citrulli*,

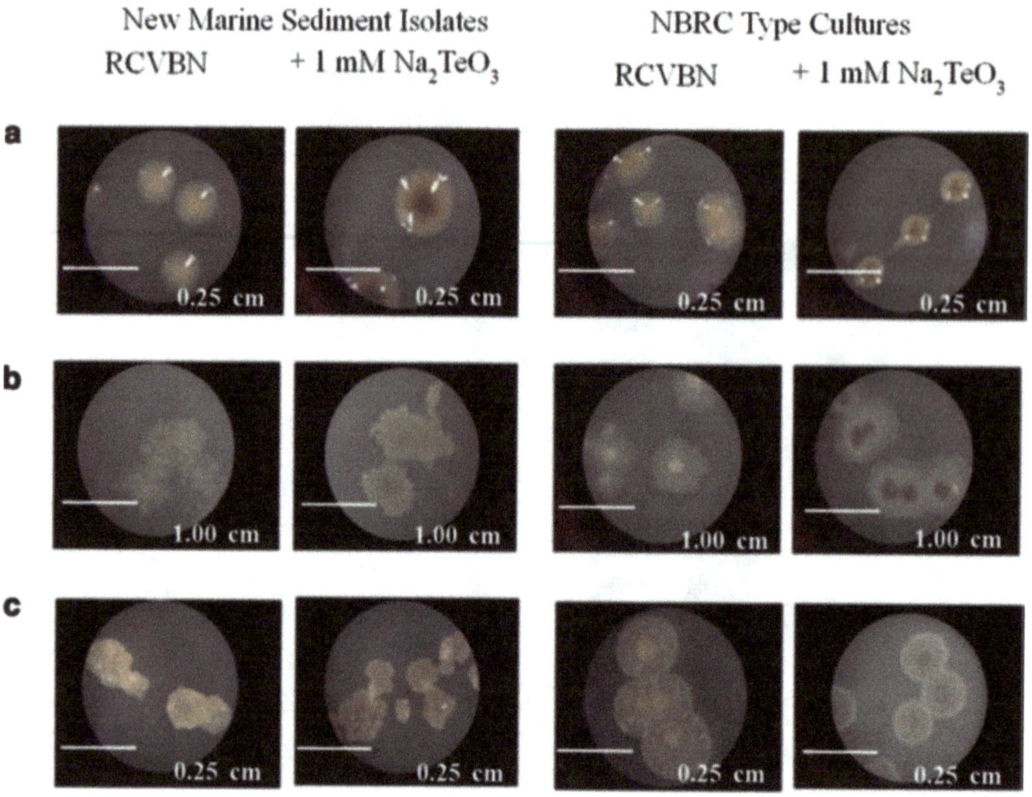

Fig. 31.3 Colony morphology and TR activity of the three new isolates and their corresponding type cultures, *S. algae* (**a**), *P. pseudoalcaligenes* (**b**), and *P. stutzeri* (**c**)

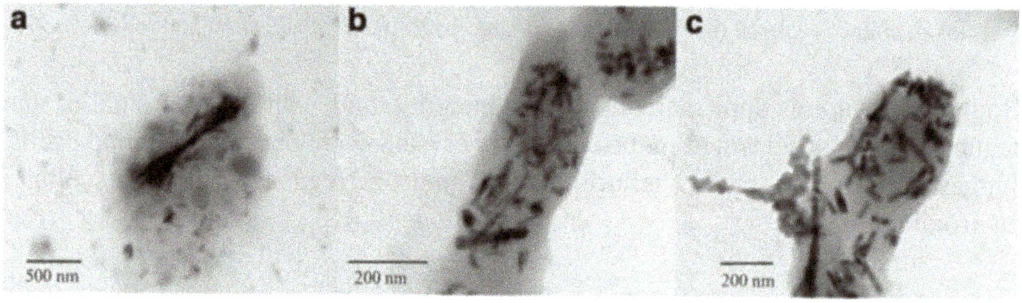

Fig. 31.4 TEM observation of intracellular tellurium particles in *S. algae* strain Hiro-1 (**a**), *P. pseudoalcaligenes* strain Hiro-2 (**b**), and *P. stutzeri* strain Hiro-3 (**c**)

isolated from diseased watermelon, and *P. alcaligenes*, a human opportunistic pathogen, are both reported to have translucent consistency (Monias 1928; Ralston-Barrett et al. 1976; Schaad et al. 1978) which is consistent with our isolate. *P. stutzeri* isolated as an opportunistic human pathogen has wrinkled and hard/dry characteristics (Lalucat et al. 2006) which is also observed in our isolate.

Our new isolates from deep marine sediment have also shown extreme resistance and reduction activity in very high concentrations (above 1 mM) of tellurite ions. This extreme resistance could be attributed to the species-specific reduction mechanisms, differential cell physiology, or genetic adaptation mechanisms in extremely toxic environments.

Species-specific biomineralization has been observed in several bacterial strains. Common tellurium morphologies vary from spheres to nanospheres and from rods to nanorods (Turner et al. 2012). Spatial distribution of nanoparticles also shows species-specific variation. The most common localization of metal biodeposition is at the cell surface or in the cytoplasm (Turner et al. 2012). The new isolates showed intracellular mineralization of metallic tellurium nanorods. This was also evident from the blackening of bacterial colonies, while surrounding tellurite ions present in the agar media were unaffected. Intracellular crystal formation denotes influx of metal ions into the cell cytoplasm, and thus unknown ion transporters or channels might be involved in this phenomenon. Once inside the cell, enzyme-catalyzed reduction of tellurite ions into elemental tellurium precedes crystal nucleation and growth. Tellurium crystals showed minimum unit size of 60 nm which falls under the category of nanoparticles (<100 nm) and therefore has a potential use for nanotechnology applications (Arenas-Salinas et al. 2016).

Together, these results show that the three new isolates identified in this study effectively reduce tellurite even at high concentrations. This reduction occurs within the cell, but determining the exact mechanisms will require further study. These strains may be useful for bioremediation, as well as for recovery of this valuable metalloid for use in manufacturing.

References

Almagro VM, Blasco R, Huertas MJ, Luque MM, Vivian CM, Castillo F, Roldan MD (2005) Alkaline cyanide biodegradation by *Pseudomonas pseudoalcaligenes* CECT5344. Biochem Soc Trans 33:168–169

Arenas-Salinas M, Perez JI, Morales W, Pinto C, Diaz P, Cornejo FA, Pugin B, Sandoval JM, Vasquez WA, Villagran C, Rojas FR, Morales EH, Vasquez CC, Arenas FA (2016) Flavoprotein-mediated tellurite reduction: structural basis and applications to the synthesis of tellurium-containing nanostructures. Front Microbiol 7:1–14

Avazeri C, Turner RJ, Pommier J, Weiner JH, Giordano G, Vermeglio A (1997) Tellurite and selenite reductase activity of nitrate reductases from *Escherichia coli*: correlation with tellurite resistance. Microbiology 143:1181–1189

Baesman SM, Bullen TD, Dewald J, Zhang DH, Curran S, Islam FS, Beveridge TJ, Oremland RS (2007) Formation of tellurium nanocrystals during anaerobic growth of bacteria that use Te oxyanions as respiratory electron acceptors. Appl Environ Microbiol 73:2135–2143

Baesman SM, Stolz JF, Kulp TR, Oremland RS (2009) Enrichment and isolation of *Bacillus beveridgei* sp. nov., a facultative anaerobic haloalkaliphile from Mono Lake, California, that respires oxyanions of tellurium, selenium, and arsenic. Extremophiles 13:695–705

Borghese R, Baccolini C, Francia F, Sabatino P, Turner RJ, Zannoni D (2014) Reduction of chalcogen oxyanions and generation of nanoprecipitates by the photosynthetic bacterium *Rhodobacter capsulatus*. J Hazard Mater 269:24–30

Borsetti F, Borghese R, Francia F, Randi MR, Fedi S, Zannoni D (2003) Reduction of potassium tellurite to elemental tellurium and its effect on the plasma membrane redox components of the facultative phototroph *Rhodobacter capsulatus*. Protoplasma 221:152–161

Burgess JG, Miyashita H, Sudo H, Matsunaga T (1991) Antibiotic production by the marine photosynthetic bacterium *Chromatium purpuratum* NKPB 031704: localization of activity to the chromatophores. FEMS Microbiol Lett 68:301–305

Chasteen TG, Fuentes DE, Tantalean JC, Vasquez CC (2009) Tellurite: history, oxidative stress, and molecular mechanisms of resistance. FEMS Microbiol Rev 33:820–832

Csotonyi JT, Stackebrandt E, Yurkov V (2006) Anaerobic respiration on tellurate and other metalloids in bacteria from hydrothermal vent fields in the eastern Pacific Ocean. Appl Environ Microbiol 72:4950–4956

Di Tomaso G, Fedi S, Carnevali M, Manegatti M, Taddei C, Zannoni D (2002) The membrane-bound respiratory chain of *Pseudomonas pseudoalcaligenes* KF707 cells grown in the presence or absence of potassium tellurite. Microbiology 148(Pt 6):1699–16708

Felsenstein J (1985) Confidence limits on phylogenies: an approach using the bootstrap. Evolution 39:783–791

Fleming A (1932) On the specific antibacterial properties of penicillin and potassium tellurite. Incorporating a method of demonstrating some bacterial antagonisms. J Pathol Bacteriol 35:831–842

Gao H, Obraztova A, Stewart N, Popa R, Fredrickson JK, Tiedje JM, Nealson KH, Zhou J (2006) *Shewanella loihica* sp. nov., isolated from iron-rich microbial mats in the Pacific Ocean. Int J Syst Evol Microbiol 56:1911–1916

Holt HM, Gahrn-Hansen B, Bruun B (2005) *Shewanella algae* and *Shewanella putrefaciens*: clinical and microbiological characteristics. Clin Microbiol Infect 11:347–352

Kim D, Baik KS, Kim MS, Jung BM, Shin TS, Chung GH, Rhee MS, Seong CH (2007) *Shewanella haliotis* sp. nov., isolated from the gut microflora of abalone, *Haliotis discus hannai*. Int J Syst Evol Microbiol 57:2926–2931

Kimura M (1980) A simple method for estimating evolutionary rate of base substitutions throughcomparative studies of nucleotide sequences. J Mol Evol 16:111–120

Klonowska A, Heulin T, Vermeglio A (2005) Selenite and tellurite reduction by *Shewanella oneidensis*. Appl Environ Microbiol 71:5607–5609

Lalucat J, Bennasar A, Bosch R, García-Valdés E, Palleroni NJ (2006) Biology of *Pseudomonas stutzeri*. Microbiol Mol Biol Rev 70:510–547

Monias B (1928) Classification of *Bacterium alcaligenes pyocyaneum* and *fluorescens*. J Infect Dis 43(4):330–334

Moore MD, Kaplan S (1994) Members of the family Rhodospirillaceae reduce heavy metal oxyanions to maintain redox poise during photosynthetic growth. ASM News 60:17–24

Nei M, Kumar S (2000) Molecular evolution and phylogenetics. Oxford University Press, New York

Nozue H, Hayashi T, Hashimoto Y, Ezaki T, Hamasaki K, Ohwada K, Terawaki Y (1992) Isolation and characterization of *Shewanella alga* from human clinical specimens and emendation of the description of *S. alga* Simidu et al., 1990, 335. Int J Syst Bacteriol 42:628–634

Oremland RS, Herbel MJ, Blum JS, Langley S, Beveridge TJ, Ajayan PM, Sutto T, Ellis AV, Curran S (2004) Structural and spectral features of selenium nanospheres produced by Se-respiring bacteria. Appl Environ Microbiol 70:52–60

Pugin B, Cornejo FA, Muñoz-Diaz P, Muñoz-Villagrán CM, Vargas-Pérez JI, Arenas FA, Vásquez CC (2014) Glutathione reductase-mediated synthesis of tellurium-containing nanostructures exhibiting antibacterial properties. Appl Environ Microbiol 80:7061–7070

Ralston-Barrett E, Palleroni NJ, Duodoroff M (1976) Phenotypic characterization and deoxyribonucleic acid homologies of the "*Pseudomonas alcaligenes*" group. Int J Syst Bacteriol 26:421–426

Romero JM, Orejas RD, Lorenzo VD (1998) Resistance to tellurite as a selection marker for genetic manipulations of *Pseudomonas* strains. Appl Environ Microbiol 64:4040–4046

Rzhetsky A, Nei M (1992) A simple method for estimating and testing minimum evolution trees. Mol Biol Evol 9:945–967

Sabaty M, Avazeri C, Pignol D, Vermeglio A (2001) Characterization of the reduction of selenate and tellurite by nitrate reductases. Appl Environ Microbiol 67:5122–5126

Saitou N, Nei M (1987) The neighbor-joining method: A new method for reconstructing phylogenetic trees. Mol Biol Evol 4:406–425

Schaad NW, Sowell G, Goth RW, Colwell RR, Webb RE (1978) *Pseudomonas pseudoalcaligenes* subsp. *citrulli* subsp. nov. Int J Syst Bacteriol 28:117–125
Simidu U, Kita-Tsukamoto K, Yasumoto T, Yotsu M (1990) Taxonomy of four marine bacterial strains that produce tetrodotoxin. Int J Syst Bacteriol 40:331–336
Tamura K, Stecher G, Peterson D, Filipski A, Kumar S (2013) MEGA6: molecular evolutionary genetics analysis version 6.0. Mol Biol Evol 30:2725–2729
Taylor DE (1999) Bacterial tellurite resistance. Trends Microbiol 7:111–115
Trutko SM, Akimenko VK, Suzina NE, Anisimova LA, Shlyapnikov MG, Baskunov BP, Duda VI, Boronin AM (2000) Involvement of the respiratory chain of gram-negative bacteria in the reduction of tellurite. Arch Microbiol 173:178–186
Tucker FL, Walper JF, Appleman MD, Donohue J (1962) Complete reduction of tellurite to pure tellurium metal by microorganisms. J Bacteriol 83:1313–1314
Turner RJ (2001) Tellurite toxicity and resistance in gram-negative bacteria. Recent Res Dev Microbiol 5:69–77
Turner RJ, Borghese R, Zannoni D (2012) Microbial processing of tellurium as a tool in biotechnology. Biotechnol Adv 30:954–963
Venkateswaran K, Dollhopf ME, Aller R, Stackebrandt E, Nealson KH (1998) *Shewanella amazonensis* sp. nov., a novel metal-reducing facultative anaerobe from Amazonian shelf muds. Int J Syst Bacteriol 48:965–972

Chapter 32
Calcium Oxalate Crystals in Plant Communities of the Southeast of the Pampean Plain, Argentina

Stella Maris Altamirano, Natalia Borrelli, María Laura Benvenuto, Mariana Fernández Honaine, and Margarita Osterrieth

Abstract Calcium oxalate crystals (COC) are one of the most prevalent and widely distributed biomineralizations in plants. The aim of this work is to analyze and compare the data previously reported about the presence and production of COC in leaves of plant species from forests, wetlands, and agroecosystems of the southeast of the Pampean Plain. Diaphanization, clearing of tissues with 50% sodium hypochlorite, and cross sectioning of the leaves were realized. The material was mounted with gelatin–glycerin, and COC were identified and described with optical, polarization, and scanning electron microscopes. Crystal size and density were calculated. Calcification mainly occurred in leaf mesophyll. In terrestrial species, crystals were closely associated with vascular bundles, while in aquatic species, they were associated with aerenchyma. Druses, prisms, and raphides were observed in the leaves of all species analyzed. Average crystal size was smaller in terrestrial species than aquatic ones (12 and 80 μm, respectively), but average crystal density was higher (246 and 23 crystals/mm^2, respectively). These different patterns in COC production and distribution may be related to taxonomical characteristics, the types of cells where crystals precipitate, their function, and the differential transpiration rates, among other factors.

Keywords Biomineralizations · Phytoliths · Calcium oxalate crystals · Terrestrial and aquatic ecosystems · Forest · Agroecosystem · Pampean plain

---

S. M. Altamirano · N. Borrelli (✉) · M. L. Benvenuto · M. F. Honaine · M. Osterrieth
Instituto de Geología de Costas y del Cuaternario (IGCyC), FCEyN, UNMdP – CIC, Mar del Plata, Argentina

Instituto de Investigaciones Marinas y Costeras (IIMyC), CONICET – UNMdP, Mar del Plata, Argentina
e-mail: nlborrel@mdp.edu.ar; fhonaine@mdp.edu.ar; mosterri@mdp.edu.ar

K. Endo et al. (eds.), *Biomineralization*,
https://doi.org/10.1007/978-981-13-1002-7_32

32.1 Introduction

Biomineralizations in plants are called phytoliths (Coe et al. 2014), and calcium oxalate crystals (COC) are one of the most common (Metcalfe 1985). The calcium absorbed from the environment through the roots is combined with oxalate (one of the products of plant metabolism) to produce crystals of different morphologies such as prisms, styloids, raphides, druses, and crystal sand that precipitate within the vacuole of specific cells called idioblasts (Franceschi and Horner 1980; Franceschi and Nakata 2005; Bauer et al. 2011).

COCs play essential structural and physiological functions (Franceschi and Horner 1980; Franceschi and Nakata 2005). COCs serve as a Ca^{+2} sink and source, preventing Ca accumulation and ensuring the normal cells functions, protect against herbivory and chewing insects, and play structural functions (Ilarslan et al. 1997; Prychid and Rudall 1999; Molano-Flores 2001; Braissant et al. 2004; Franceschi and Nakata 2005; Korth et al. 2006; Bauer et al. 2011). They also have taxonomic importance since their morphology and distribution in plant tissues and organs are characteristic of taxa (Franceschi and Horner 1980; Franceschi and Nakata 2005; Lersten and Horner 2008). Moreover, once in the soil, oxalotrophic bacteria promote COC oxidation because they function as a carbon, energy, and electron source, influencing the carbon and calcium cycle in soils (Braissant et al. 2004; Verrecchia et al. 2006).

In spite of the biological, ecological and biogeochemical importance of COC in plants, there are few researches about the COC description and quantification in relation to the type of community and/or environment, especially in our country. The aim of this work is to analyze and compare the data previously reported about the presence and production of COC in leaves of plant species from forests, wetlands, and agroecosystems of the southeast of the Pampean Plain, Argentina.

32.2 Materials and Methods

32.2.1 *Study Sites*

The southeast of Buenos Aires province (38°12′ S, 57°48′ W) belongs to the geomorphological unit known as "Perinange aeolian hills," which comprises a relief of morphologically complex hills, with relative heights of up to 30 m and concave–convex profiles with intermediate straight patches and slopes between 6% and 8% (Osterrieth et al. 1998) (Fig. 32.1). The hills originated from processes of primary aeolian accumulation, modified later by superficial wash (Osterrieth and Martínez 1993). In this region, the climate is mesothermic and subhumid, with little or no water deficiency, including an annual precipitation of 809 mm (Burgos and Vidal 1951). Los Padres Basin (37° 55′ 14.47″ and 38° 1′ 50.56″ S, 57° 52′ 21.96″ and

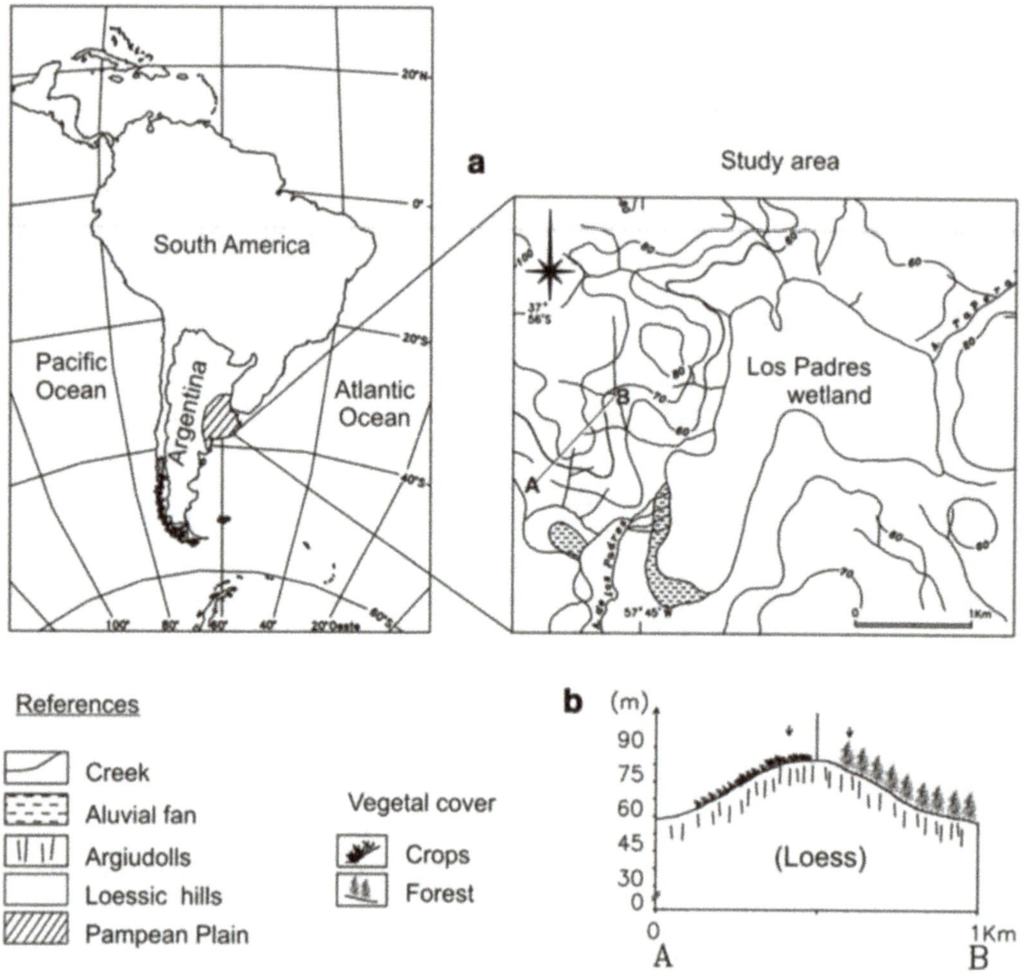

Fig. 32.1 (**a**) Location of the study area. (**b**) Topographic profile of the study sites (Line A–B in **a**)

57° 43′ 0.95″ W) is also located in the southeast of the Pampean region. Los Padres wetland is a shallow permanent lake (maximum depth 2.4 m) with an area of 216 ha bounded by the Tandilia Range, a block mountain system (Cionchi et al. 1982). The main processes that produced the wetland were tectonic events and wind erosion (Cionchi et al. 1982). The waterbody receives input from rainwater and groundwater and constitutes open systems recharge–discharge (Cionchi et al. 1982).

Grasslands were the pristine vegetation predominant in the study area across the Quaternary (Cabrera 1976). Approximately 150 years ago, because of the intense agricultural and horticultural activity in the Pampean Plain, these native plant communities had been replaced by crops, where the soybean is one of the most representative (Aizen et al. 2009). Also, at about 50 years ago, a process of artificial forestation with the aim of creating recreation areas generated the introduction of forest species like *Eucalyptus* sp., *Pinus* sp., *Cupressus* sp., and *Acacia* sp., among others.

32.2.2 Sample Units

Terrestrial and aquatic vegetation was collected from these environments:

(a) Forest mainly composed of *Acacia melanoxylon* R. Brown (Fabaceae: Mimosoideae) and *Eucalyptus globulus* Labill (Myrtaceae), both associated with *Celtis ehrenbergiana* (Klotzsch) Liebm. (Celtidaceae), a native species.
(b) Agroecosystem with soybean (*Glycine max* L., Fabaceae: Faboideae) crop.
(c) Los Padres wetland with these dominant aquatic species: *Alternanthera philoxeroides* (Mart.) Griseb. (Amaranthaceae), *Ludwigia peploides* (Kunth) P.H. Raven (Onagraceae), *Polygonum hydropiperoides* Michx. (Polygonaceae), *Rumex crispus* L. (Polygonaceae), *Hydrocotyle bonariensis* Lam. (Apiaceae), *Typha latifolia* L. (Typhaceae).

32.2.3 Description and Quantification of Calcium Oxalate Crystals

For each species, leaves from at least two plants at flowering or fruiting stage were sampled, washed with distilled water, and cleaned with an ultrasound bath (Test-Lab, TBC 10 model) in order to remove any adhered material. Afterward, tissue clarification (Dizeo de Strittmater 1973) and cross-sectioning were applied. The material was mounted with gelatine–glycerine, and calcium oxalate crystals were identified and described with a petrographic (Olimpus BX 51P) and optical microscope (Leitz Wetzlar D35780) at 400× magnification. Photographs were taken with a Kodak EasyShare CX7530 digital camera.

Average crystals size was calculated from the measuring of about 10–90 crystals per species, depending on the COC production of the species. Crystal density (n° crystals/mm^2) was determined within an area of 0.196 mm^2 in the clarified leaf samples. Between five and ten areas per leaf were analyzed according to the size of the leaves.

32.3 Results and Discussion

COC were mainly located in parenchyma tissue and randomly distributed in the mesophyll (Fig. 32.2a, f–j). Moreover, in terrestrial species (*A. melanoxylon*, *E. globulus*, *C. ehrenbergiana*, *G. max*, *H. bonariensis*), COC were associated to vascular bundles (Fig. 32.2a–e), whereas in some aquatic species (*T. latifolia*, *R. crispus*) COC were also distributed in the cells around the air spaces of aerenchyma tissue (Fig. 32.2k) (Graciotto Silva-Brambilla and Moscheta 2001; Jáuregui-Zúñiga et al. 2003; Cervantes-Martínez et al. 2005; Torres Boeger et al. 2007; Borrelli et al. 2009, 2011, 2016). These COC distribution patterns could be related with their

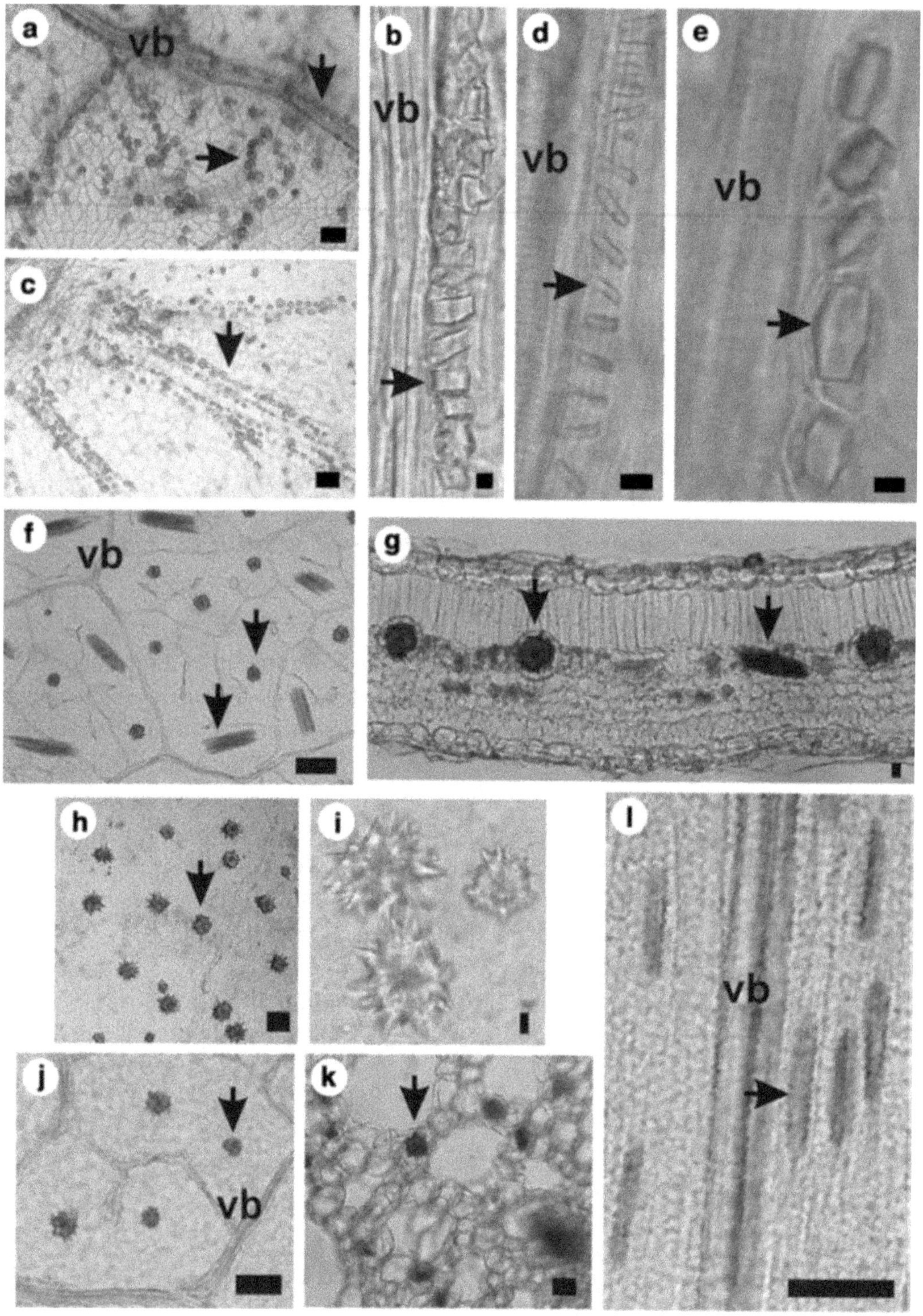

Fig. 32.2 Calcium oxalate crystals in leaves of the terrestrial and aquatic species analyzed. Druses in the mesophyll and prisms associated to vascular bundles in *E. globulus* (**a**). Prisms associated with vascular bundles in *E. globulus* (**b**), *A. melanoxylon* (**c**), and *G. max* (**d–e**). Druses and raphides in the mesophyll of *L. peploides* (**f–g**). Druses in the mesophyll of *P. hydropiperoides* (**h–i**) and *R. crispus* (**j**). Druses in the aerenchyma of *R. crispus* (**k**). Raphides in *T. latifolia* (**l**). vb: vascular bundles. Arrows: COC. Scale bars: 10 μm (**a–e**, **g**, **i**), 100 μm (**f**, **h**, **j–k**)

Table 32.1 Size and density of COC in the analyzed species

Plant species		Average COC size (μm)			Average COC density (N° crystals/mm^2)		
		Druses	Prisms	Raphides	Druses	Prisms	Raphides
Terrestrial vegetation	*Acacia melanoxylon*		12			283	
	Eucalyptus globulus	15			120		
	Celtis ehrenbergiana	9			243		
	Glycine max		14			340	
	Hydrocotyle bonariensis	9			247		
Aquatic vegetation	*Ludwigia peploides*	45		210	32		7
	Polygonum hydropiperoides	58			38		
	Rumex crispus	37			14		
	Typha latifolia			76			20

different functions. The sequestration of Ca^{+2} in the COCs lets the normal functioning of chlorenchyma cells and could be also involved in the diffraction of light improving the photosynthesis process (Franceschi and Nakata 2005; Horner 2012). Moreover, the presence of COCs closely associated with vascular bundles in terrestrial species could be explained by their higher transpiration rate. As Ca^{+2} is distributed along the entire plant via xylem, it is possible that the precipitation of biomineralizations in these areas prevents the mobilization of calcium excess through cells (Prychid and Rudall 1999; Franceschi and Nakata 2005; Lersten and Horner 2008; Gilliham et al. 2011). On the other hand, the differential COC distribution in leaf tissues between terrestrial and aquatic species could be explained by the reduced xylem system and the important aerenchyma tissue characteristic of aquatic plants (Fahn 1990). In addition to the structural function of COCs in the aerenchyma (Kuo-Huang et al. 1994; Prychid and Rudall 1999), the presence of calcium could increase cell wall plasticity around air spaces (Kausch and Horner 1983).

As it was previously reported, there are differences about COC morphologies between species (Franceschi and Horner 1980; Franceschi and Nakata 2005; Lersten and Horner 2008). Terrestrial species produced druses (*E. globulus*, *C. ehrenbergiana*, *H. bonariensis*) and prisms (*E. globulus*, *A. melanoxylon*, *G. max*) (Fig. 32.2a–e, Table 32.1) (O'Connell et al. 1983; Ilarslan et al. 1997; Borrelli et al. 2009, 2016; He et al. 2012, 2013), while aquatic plants produced druses (*R. crispus*, *P. hydropiperoides*, *L. peploides*, *A. philoxeroides*) and raphides (*T. latifolia*, *L. peploides*) (Fig. 32.2f–l, Table 32.1) (Kausch and Horner 1983; Kuo-Huang et al. 1994; Prychid and Rudall 1999; Graciotto Silva-Brambilla and Moscheta 2001; Lytle 2003; Duarte and Debur 2004; Borrelli et al. 2011). This differential production of morphologies is related to taxonomical characteristics, the types of cells where crystals precipitate and their function (Franceschi and Nakata 2005; Borchert 1984).

Differences were also observed in relation with crystals size and density (Table 32.1). Generally, in terrestrial species, average crystal size was smaller than aquatic species (12 and 80 μm, respectively), but average crystal density was higher (246 and 23 crystals/mm^2, respectively) (Table 32.1). This trend could be related with the differential transpiration rates between aquatic and terrestrial species, among others.

In summary, calcium is an important macronutrient necessary for the normal development of plants. COC production let the different species to regulate Ca^{+2} concentration in cells along with many other physiological and structural functions that enhance the normal cell functioning. Differences in terrestrial and aquatic environments influence the COC production and distribution among leaf tissues.

Acknowledgments This work was supported by the Agencia Nacional de Promoción Científica y Tecnológica (PICT 1583/2013), the Universidad Nacional de Mar del Plata (EXA 741/15), and CONICET PIP (11220130100145CO).

References

Aizen MA, Garibaldi LA, Dondo M (2009) Expansión de la soja y diversidad de la agricultura Argentina. Ecol Austral 19:45–54

Bauer P, Elbaumb R, Weissc IM (2011) Calcium and silicon mineralization in land plants: transport, structure and function. Plant Sci 180:746–756

Borchert R (1984) Functional anatomy of the calcium excreting system of *Gleditsia triacanthos* L. Bot Gaz 145:474–482

Borrelli N, Osterrieth M, Marcovecchio J (2009) Calcium biominerals in typical Argiudolls from the Pampean Plain, Argentina: an approach to the understanding of their role within the calcium biogeochemical cycle. Quat Int 193:61–69

Borrelli N, Fernández Honaine M, Altamirano SM, Osterrieth M (2011) Calcium and silica biomineralization in leaves of eleven aquatic species of the Pampean Plain, Argentina. Aquat Bot 94:29–36

Borrelli N, Benvenuto ML, Osterrieth M (2016) Calcium oxalate crystal production and density at different phenological stages of soybean plants (*Glycine max* L.) from the southeast of the Pampean Plain, Argentina. Plant Biol 18(6):1016–1024

Braissant O, Cailleau G, Aragno M, Verrecchia EP (2004) Biologically induced mineralization in the iroko *Milicia excelsa* (*Moraceae*): its causes and consequences to the environment. Geobiology 2:59–66

Burgos JJ, Vidal A (1951) Los climas de la República Argentina según la nueva clasificación de Thornthwaite. Meteor-Forschung 1:3–32

Cabrera AL (1976) Regiones fitogeográficas argentinas. Editorial ACME SACI, Buenos Aires, 85 pp

Cervantes-Martinez T, Horner H, Palmer R, Hymonwitz T, Brown A (2005) Calcium oxalate crystal macropatterns in leaves of species from groups *Glycine* and *Shuteria* (Glycininae; Phaseoleae; Papilionoideae; Fabaceae). Can J Bot 83:1410–1421

Cionchi J, Schnack E, Alvarez J, Bocanegra E, Bogliano J, del Río JL (1982) Caracterización hidrogeológica y físico-ambiental preliminar de la Laguna de Los Padres, Partido de General Pueyrredón, provincia de Buenos Aires. Centro de Geología de Costas y del Cuaternario (CGCyC) – Municipalidad de General Pueyrredón (MGP), 100 pp

Coe HH, Osterrieth M, Fernández Honaine M (2014) Phytoliths and their applications. In: Gomes Coe H, Osterrieth M (eds) Synthesis of some phytolith studies in South America. Nova Publishers, New York, pp 1–26

Dizeo de Strittmater CG (1973) Nueva técnica de diafanización. Bol Soc Arg Bot 15:126–129

Duarte MR, Debur MC (2004) Characters of the leaf and stem morpho-anatomy of *Alternanthera brasiliana* (L.) O. Kuntze, Amaranthaceae. Braz J Pharm Sci 40:85–92

Fahn A (1990) Plant anatomy, 4th edn. Pergamon Press, Oxford

Franceschi VR, Horner HT (1980) Calcium oxalate crystals in plants. Bot Rev 46:361–427

Franceschi V, Nakata P (2005) Calcium oxalate in plants: formation and function. Annu Rev Plant Biol 56:41–71

Gilliham M, Dayod M, Hocking BJ, Xu B, Conn SJ, Kaiser BN, Leigh RA, Tyerman SD (2011) Calcium delivery and storage in plant leaves: exploring the link with water flow. J Exp Bot 62:2233–2250

Graciotto Silva-Brambilla M, Moscheta IS (2001) Anatomia foliar de Polygonaceae (Angiospermae) da planície de inundac¸ ão do alto rio Paraná. Maringá 23:571–585

He H, Bleby TM, Veneklaas EJ, Lambers H, Kuo J (2012) Morphologies and elemental compositions of calcium crystals in phyllodes and branchlets of *Acacia robeorum* (Leguminosae: Mimosoideae). Ann Bot 109:887–896

He H, Bleby TM, Veneklaas EJ, Lambers H, Kuo J (2013) Precipitation of calcium, magnesium, strontium and barium in tissues of four *Acacia* species (Leguminosae: Mimosoideae). PLoS One 7:e41563

Horner HT (2012) *Peperomia* leaf cell wall interface between the multiple hypodermis and crystal-containing photosynthetic layer displays unusual pit fields. Ann Bot 109:1307–1315

Ilarslan H, Palmer RG, Imsande J, Horner HT (1997) Quantitative determination of calcium oxalate and oxalate in developing seeds of soybean (Leguminosae). Am J Bot 84:1042–1046

Jáuregui-Zúñiga D, Reyes-Grajeda JP, Sepulveda-Sanchez JD, Whitaker JR, Moreno A (2003) Crystallochemical characterization of calcium oxalate crystals isolated from seed coats of *Phaseolus vulgaris* and leaves of *Vitis vinifera*. Plant Physiol 160:239–245

Kausch AP, Horner HT (1983) The development of mucilaginous raphide crystal idioblasts in young leaves of *Typha angustifolia* L. (Typhaceae). Am J Bot 70:691–705

Korth K, Doege SJ, Park S-H, Goggin FL, Wang Q, Gomez SK, Liu G, Jia L, Nakata PA (2006) *Medicago truncatula* mutants demonstrate the role of plant calcium oxalate crystals as an effective defense against chewing insects. Plant Physiol 141:188–195

Kuo-Huang LL, Chiou-Rong S, Yuen-Po Y, Shu-Hwa TC (1994) Calcium oxalate crystals in some aquatic angiosperms of Taiwan. Bot Bull Acad Sin 34:179–188

Lersten NR, Horner HT (2008) Crystal macropatterns in leaves of Fagaceae and Nothofagaceae: a comparative study. Plant Syst Evol 271:239–253

Lytle ST (2003) Adaptation and acclimation of populations of *Ludwigia repens* to growth in high- and lower-CO2 springs. Dissertation, University of Florida, 157pp

Metcalfe CR (1985) Secreted mineral substances. Crystals. In: Metcalfe CR, Chalk L (eds) Anatomy of the Dicotyledons II. Word structure and conclusion of the general introduction. Clarendon Press, Oxford, pp 82–97

Molano-Flores B (2001) Herbivory and calcium concentrations affect calcium oxalate crystal formation in leaves of *Sida* (Malvaceae). Ann Bot 88:387–391

O'Connell AM, Malajczuk N, Gailitis V (1983) Occurrence of calcium oxalate in Karri (*Eucalyptus diversicolor* F, Muell.), Forest ecosystems of South Western Australia. Oecología (Berlin) 56:239–244

Osterrieth M, Martínez G (1993) Paleosols on late Cainozoic sequences in the northeastern side of tandilia range, Buenos Aires, Argentina. Quat Int 17:57–65

Osterrieth M, Fernández C, Bilat Y, Martínez P, Martínez G, Trassens M (1998) Geoecología de Argiudoles típicos afectados por prácticas hortícolas en la Llanura Pampeana, Buenos Aires, Argentina. Abstracts XVI Congreso Mundial de la Ciencia del Suelo, pp 1–8

Prychid CJ, Rudall PJ (1999) Calcium oxalate crystals in monocotyledons: a review of their structure and systematics. Ann Bot 84:725–739

Torres Boeger MR, Barbosa de Oliveira Pil MW, Filho NB (2007) Arquitetura foliar comparativa de *Hedychium coronarium* J. Koenig (Zingiberaceae) ede *Typha domingensis* Pers (Typhaceae). Iheringia, Sér Bot Porto Alegre 62:113–120

Verrecchia EP, Braissant O, Cailleau G (2006) The oxalate-carbonate pathway in soil carbon storage: the role of fungi and oxalotrophic bacteria. In: Gadd M (ed) Fungi in biogeochemical cycles. Cambridge Univ. Press, Cambridge, pp 289–310

Chapter 33
Iron and Calcium Biomineralizations in the Pampean Coastal Plains, Argentina: Their Role in the Environmental Reconstruction of the Holocene

Margarita Osterrieth, Celia Frayssinet, and Lucrecia Frayssinet

Abstract Biomineralizations are biogenic composites, crystalline or amorphous, produced by the metabolic activity of organisms distributed all over the world. The aim of this work was to evaluate the presence of iron and calcium biomineralizations and their influence in the physicochemical and mineralochemical variations in paleo and actual pedosedimentary sequences of the coastal plains in Mar Chiquita. The complex interaction of calcium with iron biomineralizations, as framboidal and poliframboidal pyrites associated with gypsum, barite, calcite, halite, and iron oxy-hydroxides, have demonstrated the active and complex biogeochemistry that occurs in the temperate–wet paleoesturaries and estuaries of the coastal Pampean Plains. Particularly the consequences that different human activities could have, such as the possible acidification processes as result of the iron sulfide oxidation.

Keywords Framboidal pyrite · Poliframboidal pyrite · Calcium oxalate · Calcite · Biogeochemistry · Soil acidification

33.1 Introduction

Biominerals are deposited in intra- or extracellular spaces as the consequence of metabolic activity. Biomineralizations processes are genetically controlled and are also a widespread phenomenon in nature that can take place on both marine and terrestrial systems, acting as a global source and sink of soluble ions (Lowenstam 1981; Osterrieth 2004). Among the most common biomineralizations can be mentioned those ones composed by calcium, iron, and amorphous silica (Mann 2001),

M. Osterrieth (✉) · C. Frayssinet · L. Frayssinet
Instituto de Geología de Costas y del Cuaternario (IGCyC), FCEyN, UNMdP – CIC, Mar del Plata, Argentina

Instituto de Investigaciones Marinas y Costeras (IIMyC), CONICET – UNMdP, Mar del Plata, Argentina

K. Endo et al. (eds.), *Biomineralization*,
https://doi.org/10.1007/978-981-13-1002-7_33

particularly in coastal environments, where the interaction between marine and terrestrial processes is very intense, as well as the biotic and anthropic activity.

The geomorphological and biotic factors in concordance with the pedological processes have created a complex soil system, where the active iron and calcium biogeochemistry might allow the acidification processes, as result of the iron sulfide oxidation, when biogenic calcium is available (Osterrieth et al. 2017).

In Argentina, the first record about framboidal pyrites biomineralizations associated with paleo-salt marshes environments dates from 1992 (Osterrieth 1992), without further information, while in other regions, there is a large number of reports about the pyrites formation and its biogeochemical implications (Stribling 1997; Wilkin et al. 1996; Roychoudhury et al. 2003).

The research of calcium biomineralizations at pedesodimentary sequences associated to bioclastic levels and bioerosion processes is very scarce in Argentina (Osterrieth et al. 2000, 2016, 2017).

In the Pampean plains, coastal morphodynamics throughout the Holocene (10,000 BP until now) have been very active and have produced variations linked to the installation of coastal barriers, conditioning the evolution of dunes, marshes, and the unique coastal lagoon of Argentina: Mar Chiquita lagoon (Osterrieth 2005).

The aim of this work was to evaluate the presence of iron and calcium biomineralizations and their influence in the physicochemical and mineralochemical variations in paleo and actual pedosedimentary sequences of the coastal plains in Mar Chiquita, Argentina.

33.2 Materials and Methods

33.2.1 Study Site

Study site is located in the coastal area of Mar Chiquita, Buenos Aires province (Fig. 33.1).

The regional weather is mesothermic and subhumid. The vegetation is characterized by communities of psammophytic, halophytic, and freshwater plants, as well as by woodlands. The main soils at the study area are Udolls and Aquents (Osterrieth 2005).

33.2.2 Methods

The soils and exhumed soils were analyzed across a coastal section of 10 km length (Fig. 33.1); description of the modal profiles was reported according Soil Survey Staff (1996). Different pedosedimentary sequences of the Holocene present in geomorphological units (UG): paleoestuarine (UG1) and estuarine-salt marsh (UG2) were analyzed (Fig. 33.1a, b).

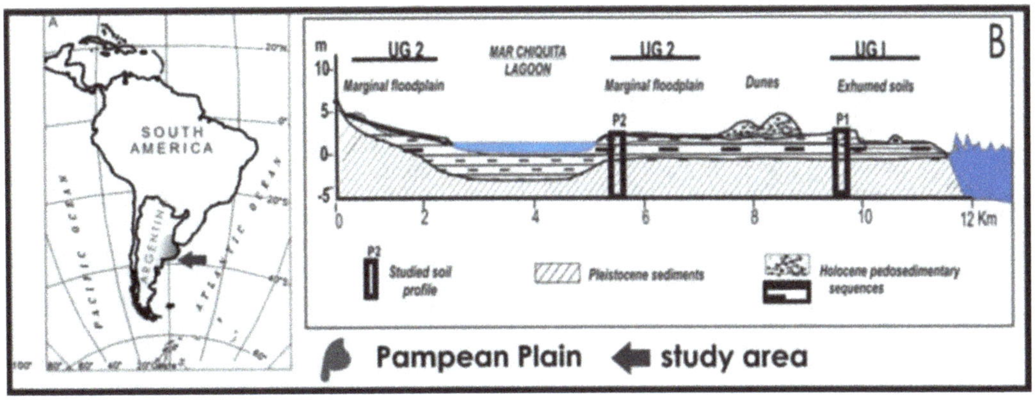

Fig. 33.1 Study area. Toposequence, geopedological units (UG1, UG2), and profiles studies (P1–P2)

Dating by ^{14}C acceleration mass spectrometry (AMS) was performed (Beta Analytic, USA; LATIR-UNLP) on soil organic matter and bioclastic material.

Organic matter content, pH, calcium carbonate, and particle size distribution were done by routine methods (Walkley and Black 1965; Dawis 1970; Galehouse 1971, respectively).

Disturbed and undisturbed samples at different scales of resolution were analyzed using polarization microscope (Olympus BX 51P) and scanning electron microscope (SEM: JEOL JSM6460LV). Mineralochemical studies were performed using an energy dispersive X-ray spectrometer (EDXS, between 15 and 25 kV).

33.3 Results and Discussion

Mar Chiquita region is mostly included in the Biosphere Reserve (Man and Biosphere Reserve Program, UNESCO) called "Parque Atlántico Mar Chiquita" (UNESCO 2016). This reserve is a coastal ecosystem with specific organism diversity and, affected by complex biogeochemical processes, is a shallow body of brackish water affected by low amplitude tides and constitutes an estuarine environment with a very particular behavior (Marcovecchio et al. 2006). The morphodynamics of this area is unique as marine, estuarine, and eolian deposits interdigitate and intercalate between them (Osterrieth 2005).

33.3.1 Paleoestuarine: Exhumed Soils (UG1)

33.3.1.1 Morphological and Physicochemical Characteristics

The exhumed soils were affected by an active erosion and showed diagenetic and biogeochemical specific characteristics associated with ancient coastal deposits, linked to the last Holocene transgressive–regressive cycle (Fig. 33.2a, b, d-1). Soils

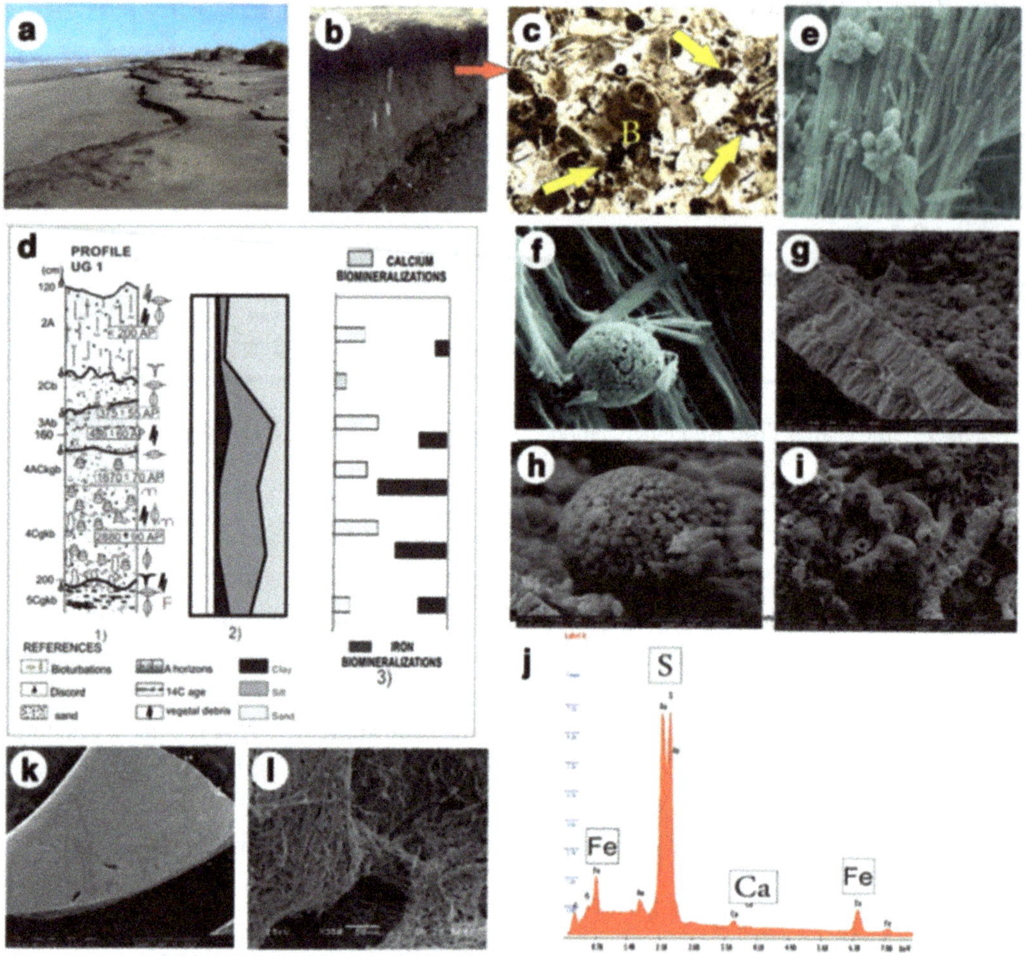

Fig. 33.2 (**a**) Panoramic view of the exhumed soils (UG 1). (**b**) Photo of del modal profile. (**c**) Micromorphological photo (3Ab). (**d**) Geological profile, grain size analysis, and biomineralizations present in the profile. (**e**) Framboidal pyrites and gypsum in the soil matrix. (**f**) Framboidal pyrites, gypsum, and barite on vegetal debris, (**g**) associated with bioclast. (**h**) Detailed view of framboidal pyrites. (**i**) Tubes calcium biomineralizations (CB) in matrix soil. (**j**) EDXS result of soil matrix, in the profile, (**k**) bioclast bioeroded. (**l**) CB on clast and matrix exhumed soil. BC: bioclasts. Yellow arrow: framboidal pyrites (FP). **e**–**l**: SEM photos

were characterized as Hapludolls (2A-2Cb horizons), Sulfaquents (3Ab and 4ACkgb-4Cgkb horizons), and Fluvaquents (5Cgkb horizons), all of them with low to moderated pedological development (Fig. 33.2d-1).

At the subsuperficial horizons, pH values were alkaline (8–9), as consequence of the saline and/or brackish water influence, with high exchangeable sodium contents and with abundant bioclastic materials that were affected by processes of bioerosion and calcium carbonates and oxalates reprecipitation (Fig. 33.2k) (Osterrieth 2005). The superficial horizon was slightly alkaline to neutral (7–8) due to the high organic matter content. The grain size distribution showed a sandy texture in 2A level, changing to silt loam towards the bottom of the profile. In all the exhumed soils, the clay content was very scarce (Fig. 33.2d).

The organic matter content was medium (between 6% and 10%) and has decreased with depth.

Carbonates were present in all the profile, as whole or fragmented shells, scattered in the soil mass. The calcium carbonate content was variable and increased toward the lower horizons, with an average between 6% in 2A and 15% in 2Cb, 3Ab horizons, but rising to more than 35% in paleosols (level 4 and 5), associated with bioclastic materials.

33.3.1.2 Iron and Calcium Biomineralizations

Previous research on exhumed paleo marshes have determined that the iron content was between 56 and 95 μmol Fe/g and have reflected that the largest iron proportion was in the form of crystalline iron oxides (28–76%) and lepidocrocite (6–16%), while the proportion associated with ferrihydrite and pyrite was lower (0–9% and 1–17%, respectively), especially at the upper levels of the exhumed soils (2A and 3Ab in Fig. 33.2d-1). According with the chemical fractionation data on these horizons, well defined framboidal pyrites were found associated with the plant debris cover (Fig. 33.2d-3, j). These pyrites increased in quantity and morphological variety toward the bottom of the profile, where the anoxic conditions were more resistant (Osterrieth et al. 2016).

The presence of framboidal and poliframboidal pyrites associated with gypsum, barite, calcite, halite (Fig. 33.2c, e–h), and iron oxyhydroxides was frequent all along the profile. The sequences of pyrite formation (sulfidation) as well as their metastable forms (mackinawite and greigite) were observed. Framboidal pyrites showed diverse morphologies: combined microcrystals, octahedral–dodecahedral subedrals, and cubic and irregular octahedral microcrystals subedrals to anedrals with sizes between 0.2 and 5 μm, closely associated with plant debris, bioclasts, and pores and channels of the soil matrix (Fig. 33.2g, h). Degradation processes (sulfurization) were inferred by geochemical and EDXS results, as presence of crystalline iron oxides, lepidocrocite, and ferrihydrite were observed immersed in the matrix of the peds. This sulfurization was related to the complex redox processes of these environments, such as the aeration that is generated in the rhizosphere and also by the intense bioturbation of invertebrates (Osterrieth et al. 2016). Once the sequence was exposed to oxic conditions and eroded by storm episodes, the oxidation of sulfides and the intense dissolution and transformation of framboidal pyrite into iron crystalline phases could have been the responsible for the acidic conditions, mainly in the surface horizons (Roychoudhury et al. 2003)

The association of framboidal pyrites have originated elongated and subspherical poliframboidal pyrites, with sizes of 50–80 μm wide and 190–140 μm length. They were immersed and cemented by thin films of amorphous silica and iron (Fig. 33.2c). These secondary framboidal pyrites were authigenic, generated "in situ" under anoxic conditions (Osterrieth 1992). The framboidal pyrite genesis in these coastal soils of the Pampean Plain was bacterial, through biogeochemical reduction processes that have produced a certain type of microcrystals, very different from those generated by purely chemical action (Osterrieth et al. 2016; Wilkin et al. 1996).

A lot of isolated octahedral and dodecahedral pyrite's crystals associated with framboids and with different types of biofilms, mainly composed by silica were observed. These biofilms might be related to the high amounts of diatoms and silicophytoliths found that could have been altered by the extreme pH values consequence of the framboidal pyrites generation and degradation cycle.

These paleoestuarine deposits, with abundant wholly and partially fragmented bioclasts, included mollusk shells such as *Heleobia* sp., dated 1,670 ± 70 year BP by ^{14}C, and *Tagelus plebeius* dated between 1,710 ± 60 and 2,880 ± 90 year BP (Osterrieth, 2005). Also, soil organic carbon was dated, ranging from < 200 year BP to 486 ± 60 year BP.

This bioclastic material constituted by calcite/aragonite biomineralizations was affected by dissolution, bioerosion (Fig. 33.2k), and reprecipitation of biogenic calcium carbonates and oxalates (bacteria, fungi, and algae). The reprecipitation processes were relevant on the bioclasts (Fig. 33.2i, l) and in the matrix between grains and bioclasts (Fig. 33.2l). The matrix of the peds had dense calcified filaments, raphides, styloids, tubes, rods, and short and long needles with sharp or straight ends, composed by whewellite (monohydrate calcium oxalate) or weddellite (polyhydrated calcium oxalate) (Fig. 33.2i, l) (Verrecchia and Verrecchia 1994, Verecchia et al. 1995; Osterrieth et al. 2000, 2017). In general, all the morphologies found here could be associated with microbial activity at the matrix, coating peds, pores, and the bioclastic-matrix interface (Fig. 33.2i, l). Moreover, it was common to see framboidal pyrite associated to bioclasts, being part of a complex biofilm composition dominated by calcium (41%), chlorine (29%), silica (13%), carbon (5%), iron (5%), sodium (4%), and aluminum (3%) (Fig. 33.2j).

33.3.2 Estuarine Actual Soils (UG2)

33.3.2.1 Morphological and Physicochemical Characteristics

The soils (Profile 2) were located within the marginal plain and the tidal channels of the Mar Chiquita lagoon (Fig. 33.1b) affected by the lagoon's level variation and also by the episodic sea advances that had increased the presence of iron sulfides in the surface. These soils classified as oxyaquic Udifluvents (Fig. 33.3b) were affected by the presence of mollusk shells and intensely bioturbated by *Uca uruguayensis and Neohelice granulate* (Fig. 33.3).

The vegetation community was composed of *Cortaderia selloana*, *Panicum racemosum*, *Sacocornia* sp., *Juncus* sp., etc. (Fig. 33.3a, b).

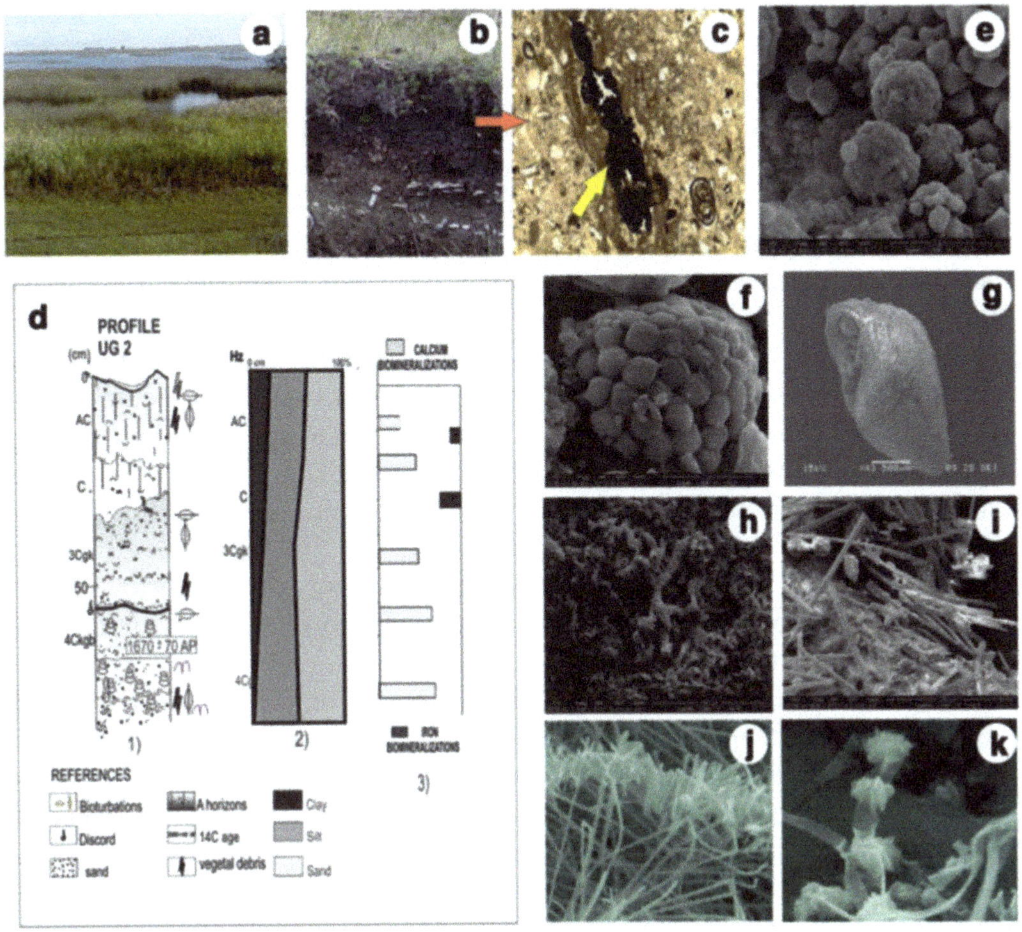

Fig. 33.3 (**a**) Panoramic view of the UG2. (**b**) Photo of del modal profile (P2). (**c**) Micromorphological slide (AC). (**d**) Geological profile, grain size analysis, and biomineralizations in the profile. (**e**) Framboidal pyrites in and isolates pyrite crystals in the marsh soil matrix. (**f**) Detailed view of framboidal pyrites. (**g**) *Heleobia* sp. bioeroded; (**h**) SEM, soil matrix with CB; (**i**) matrix with filaments, rods CB; (**j**) detailed view of CB: rods, raphides, and styloids associated with the bacterium; (**k**) detailed view of *rosettes* CB associated with fungi. Yellow arrow: framboidal pyrites (FP). (**e**–**k**): SEM photos

Soil reaction ranged from moderately alkaline in the surface to alkaline at the base of the sequence (pH:7.5–9). The organic matter content was moderate in the AC horizon (6.5%) and has descended sharply toward the bottom of the profile (1.3%). The calcium carbonate content was scarce (6%) in the superficial horizon (AC) and increased at the lower horizons (3Cgk and 4Cgkb horizon) associated with the presence of bioclastic materials (33%).

The sequence was texturally homogeneous with fine and very fine sand fractions being dominant, while the AC horizon showed a slight increase in clays and silts (Fig. 33.3d-2).

33.3.2.2 Iron and Calcium Biomineralizations

In these soils the presence of iron and calcium biomineralizations was common too, but the framboidal and poliframboidal pyrites were less abundant when compared to the paleoesturine soils. The quantity and morphologies of the calcium biomineralizations observed in this profile were similar to those registered in UG1.

The low degree of pyritization registered here, which is below the typical values reported for modern estuarine sediments of tropical environments (Wilkin et al. 1996), could be explained by the lower proportion of iron obtained here (36–75 μmol Fe/g.) (Osterrieth et al. 2016). The sequences of pyrite formation (*sulfidation*) were observed with diverse morphologies, for example, octahedral–dodecahedral microcrystals and irregular octahedral microcrystals subedrals to anedrals (Fig. 33.3c, f). The presence of gypsum or barite associated to framboidal pyrites was very scarce, although the oxic conditions were more common in this soils than in the paleomarisms.

In these soils, the aeration generated by the high density of crab burrows and *S. densiflora* has promoted the oxic conditions that leaded to a lower pyrite framboidal production (Osterrieth et al. 2016).

Bioclasts were affected by bioerosion through the action of microorganisms with a subsequently calcium reprecipitation as secondary oxalates and carbonates biomineralizations (Fig. 33.3g–k). These biomineralizations were also added or weakly bound to the skeletal components, which allowed them to be incorporated into the matrix of soils and sediments. Mineralochemical studies confirmed the presence of calcium and variable carbon contents, subject to the crystal's development stage. Thus, it was possible to define the genetic sequence of calcite via calcium oxalate (weddellite and whewellite) associated with hyphae, algae, soil bacteria, and actinomycetes. A remarkable variety of dichotomous tubes was found as clear evidence of fungal genesis, added to elongated tubes of multiple sizes and diameters, and complex interdigitated crystalline textures of oxalate and calcium carbonates, that also indicated biological production (Fig. 33.3g–k). Type and diversity of calcium biomineralizations increased directly in relation with the bioclastic parental material and biogeochemical conditions (Fig. 33.3d-3).

33.4 Final Remarks

The important role of the iron and calcium biomineralizations lies on the possibility to further understand the biogeochemical processes and to deepen the knowledge about the complex interaction of the pedological processes on the paleo and recent coastal environments. They also allow us to deduce that many environmental processes do not correlate with chronological evolution, while biogeochemical aspects related to biomineralizations do.

The presence of iron biominerals allowed us to define the redoxymorphic conditions in paleoestuarine and estuarine pedosedimentary sequences.

Calcium biomineralizations were found and associated with processes of dissolution and reprecipitation of calcium carbonates and oxalates associated to fungus, algae, and bacteria in actual and exhumed soils.

Calcium and iron biomineralizations with other cations and organic components allowed the formation of organomineral complex which plays an important role in the availability of macro- and micronutrients for the biota development and in the persistence of the aggregates and the resistance to erosion processes in these coastal soils.

Iron and calcium biomineralizations found in paleo marshes allow us to make inferences related to the management of actual salt marshes, warning us about the possible acidification processes generated by the iron sulfide oxidation associated to different human activities in the temperate–wet coastal environments of the Pampean Plains.

Acknowledgments This work was supported by the AGENCIA-PICT 1583/2013, UNMDP-EXA 741/15, and CONICET- PIP-11220130100145CO.

References

Dawis JF (1970) Physiological and chemical methods of soil and water analysis. Soil Bull 10:39–51

Galehouse JS (1971) Sedimentation analysis. In: Carver (ed) Procedures in sedimentary petrology. Wiley Interscience, Hoboken, pp 69–94

Key facts and figures on Argentina – UNESCO cooperation (2016) Available in; https://es.unesco.org/system/files/countries/Home/arg_facts_figures.pdf?language

Lowenstam HA (1981) Minerals formed by organisms. Science 211:1126–1131

Mann S (2001) Biomineralization: principles and concepts in bioinorganic materials chemistry. Oxford University Press, New York

Marcovecchio J et al (2006) Seasonality of hydrographic variables in a coastal lagoon: Mar Chiquita, Argentina. Aquat Conserv Mar Freshwat Ecosyst 16:335–347

Osterrieth M (1992) Pirita framboidal en secuencias sedimentarias del Holoceno tardío en Mar Chiquita, Buenos Aires, Argentina. IV R Arg de Sedimentol 2:73–80

Osterrieth M (2004) Biominerales y Biomineralizaciones. In: Sociedad Mejicana de Cristalografía (eds) Cristalografía de Suelos, pp 206–218

Osterrieth M (2005) Biomineralizaciones de hierro y calcio, su rol en procesos biogeoquímicos de secuencias sedimentarias del sudeste bonaerense. XVI Congreso Geol Argent III:255–262

Osterrieth M et al (2000) Biominerales de oxalato de calcio en suelos de Laguna de los Padres, Buenos Aires. Rev Argent Cienc del Suelo 18(1):50–58

Osterrieth M et al (2016) Iron biogeochemistry in Holocene palaeo and actual salt marshes in coastal areas of the Pampean plain, Argentina. Environ Earth Sci 75:671–672

Osterrieth M, et al. (2017) Calcium Biomineralizations associated with bioclastic deposits in coastal pedostratigraphic sequences of the Southeastern Pampean Plain, Argentina. In: Rabassa J (ed) Advances in geomorphology and quaternary studies in Argentina, vol 11. Springer, Cham, pp 261–287

Roychoudhury A et al (2003) Pyritization: a palaeoenvironmental and redox proxy reevaluated. Estuar Coast Shelf Sci 57:1183–1193

Soil Survey Staff (1996) Keys to soil taxonomy, 7th edn. United States Department of Agriculture, Washington, DC

Stribling J (1997) The relative importance of sulfate availability in the growth of *Spartina alterniflora* and *Spartina cynosuroides*. Aquat Bot 56:131–143

Verrecchia E, Verrecchia K (1994) Needle-fiber calcite: review and classification. J Sediment Res 64(3):650–664

Verrecchia E et al (1995) Role of calcium oxalate biomineralization by fungi in the formation of calcretes: a case study from Nazareth, Israel. J Sediment Petrol 65:1060–1066

Walkley A, Black A (1965) In: Black C (ed) Methods of soil analysis. American Society of Agronomy, Madison, pp 1372–1375

Wilkin RT et al (1996) The size distribution of framboidal pyrite in modern sediments: an indicator of redox conditions. Geochim Cosmochim Acta 60(20):3897–3912

Part VIII
Mollusk Shell Formation

Chapter 34
Skeletal Organic Matrices in Molluscs: Origin, Evolution, Diagenesis

Frédéric Marin, Aurélien Chmiel, Takeshi Takeuchi, Irina Bundeleva, Christophe Durlet, Elias Samankassou, and Davorin Medakovic

Abstract The mollusc shell comprises a small amount of organic macromolecules, mostly proteins and polysaccharides, which, all together, constitute the skeletal organic matrix (SOM). In the recent years, the study of the SOM of about two dozens of mollusc species via transcriptomics and/or proteomics has led to the identification of hundreds of shell-associated proteins. This rapidly growing set of data allows several comparisons, shedding light on similarities and differences at the primary structure level and on some peculiar evolutionary mechanisms that may have affected SOM proteins. In addition, it constitutes a prerequisite for investigating the SOM repertoires of sub-fossils or fossil specimens, closely related to known extant species, in order to revisit diagenetic processes, i.e. how SOM proteins degrade during fossilization. These two aspects are briefly exemplified here: on the one hand, *Aplysia californica*, the sea hare, exhibits a vestigial internal shell that has kept a proteomic signature similar to that found in fully functional external shells. On the other hand, subfossil specimens of the giant clam *Tridacna*, collected in French Polynesia, precisely dated and analysed by proteomics for their SOM content, comprise several preserved proteins that can still be identified by their peptide signature, in spite of information losses likely due to diagenetic transformations.

F. Marin (✉) · A. Chmiel · I. Bundeleva · C. Durlet
UMR CNRS 6282 Biogéosciences, Bâtiment des Sciences Gabriel,
Université de Bourgogne Franche-Comté, Dijon, France
e-mail: frederic.marin@u-bourgogne.fr; irina.bundeleva@u-bourgogne.fr; christophe.durlet@u-bourgogne.fr

T. Takeuchi
Marine Genomics Unit, Okinawa Institute of Science and Technology Graduate University, Okinawa, Japan

E. Samankassou
Department of Earth Sciences, University of Geneva, Geneva, Switzerland
e-mail: Elias.Samankassou@unige.ch

D. Medakovic
Center for Marine Research Rovinj, Rudjer Boskovic Institute, Rovinj, Croatia
e-mail: medakovic@cim.irb.hr

K. Endo et al. (eds.), *Biomineralization*,
https://doi.org/10.1007/978-981-13-1002-7_34

Keywords Mollusc · Shell · Proteomics · Protein · Sequences · Functional domains · Diagenesis

34.1 Introduction

The mollusc shell is a remarkable composite material made of calcium carbonate at 99% and of a minor organic fraction, the skeletal organic matrix (SOM). During the mineral deposition process, the SOM is secreted by the shell-forming organ, the mantle, and remains occluded. It is considered to be the main regulator of crystallization. In addition, it exhibits an interesting potential for preservation in fossil or subfossil samples (Hare et al. 1980). Classical biochemical characterizations indicate that the SOM consists in a mixture of proteins and polysaccharides (Marin et al. 2012). For decades, the SOM was considered as a 'black box' and analysed biochemically in bulk. Nowadays, high-throughput screening of SOMs, via the combined use of proteomics and transcriptomics, has allowed the identification of hundreds of shell proteins that are putatively involved in shell biosynthesis, in about two dozens of model mollusc genera comprising mostly bivalves, gastropods, and, in a lesser extent, cephalopods (Marin et al. 2016). This wealth of molecular data has considerably blurred the outlines of the SOM. However, taken individually, each of these 'shell repertoires' represents a key component of the calcifying machinery for making a shell, and shell repertoires can be compared to each other, shedding light on the macroevolution of calcifying matrices (Kocot et al. 2016; Marie et al. 2017). In addition to giving information on the calcification process and its macroevolution, molecular data collected from shells of extant molluscs is a prerequisite for obtaining – whenever possible – similar proteins in archaeological or fossil shell samples, an emerging field defined as paleoproteomics (Demarchi et al. 2016; Wallace and Schiffbauer 2016).

In the present paper, we briefly describe two unpublished examples on the use of proteomics to identify shell proteins: the first example relates to the Californian sea hare, *Aplysia californica*, a heterobranch gastropod that belong to a family, the Aplysiidae, characterized by an internal atrophied shell which is weakly calcified. The second example relates to subfossil specimens of the giant clam, *Tridacna* sp., collected in French Polynesia and precisely dated. In both cases, proteomics was performed from their extracted SOM.

34.2 Materials and Methods

34.2.1 Materials

Fresh shells of the Californian sea hare *Aplysia californica* were obtained from RSMAS at the University of Miami (Ph. Gillette) after sacrifice of the living animals according to ethical rules. Six shells of the giant clam *Tridacna* sp., including fresh, recent and subfossil specimens, were collected by one of us (E. S) on two sites of French Polynesia: Motu Piti Aau, Motu Mute, Bora Bora (Society Islands) and Motu Tepapuri, Mangareva (Gambier archipelago). The fresh *Tridacna* specimens were used as reference material.

34.2.2 Structural and Geochemical Characterizations

Series of structural characterizations of the shells were performed by SEM observations on polished sections or on freshly broken shell pieces that were slightly etched (EDTA 1% wt/vol, 3–5 min.). Minute fragments were sampled and powdered and the powder analysed by FT-IR spectroscopy, in order to check the mineralogy (aragonite). For *Tridacna* samples, thick sections were made for cathodoluminescence, epifluorescence and XRD analyses. In addition, the subfossil samples were dated via ^{14}C measurements (Beta Analytic, Miami, FL, USA).

34.2.3 Extraction of the Aplysia *and* Tridacna *SOMs*

All *Tridacna* shells were scrupulously abraded and cleaned (two or three extended bleaching treatments with sodium hypochlorite) in order to remove putative contaminants. The clean powders were decalcified overnight with acetic acid, and the soluble and insoluble fractions were fractionated by centrifugation. All the subsequent steps leading to freeze-dried matrices were performed as previously described (Ramos-Silva et al. 2014). For *Aplysia californica*, the thinness of shells required adapting the cleaning/extraction protocol, which consisted first in protein desorption in successive bathes of TBS buffer containing Tween 20 (0.1%), NaN_3 (0.001%), pH 9.2 for 1 week. After drying and reduction into powder, the samples were decalcified and centrifuged, leading to the fractionation of the soluble and insoluble matrices. The soluble fraction was desalted by several centrifugations/resuspension in water, in Vivaspin 20 cells (3 kDa cutoff), while the insoluble was rinsed with water. Both fractions were freeze-dried.

34.2.4 Proteomics on SOMs

All lyophilized samples were submitted to proteomic analysis (3P5 platform, Institut Cochin, Université Paris Descartes, Paris), after trypsic digestion, as previously described (Immel et al. 2016). For *Aplysia californica*, assigning identified peptides to known proteins was performed by using Mascot program (version 2.5, MatrixScience, London, UK) against the nonredundant NCBInr database. The search was restricted to 'Other Metazoa' dataset, which comprises a large collection of transcriptomic and genomic sequences from *Aplysia californica*, publicly accessible at NCBI (www.ncbi.nlm.nih.gov/). For *Tridacna* sp., an unpublished EST database provided by one of us (Dr. T. Takeuchi) from mantle tissues of the coral reef-associated crocus giant clam *Tridacna crocea* was used for protein identification.

34.3 Results

34.3.1 *Proteomics on* Aplysia californica *Shell Matrices*

The internal shell of *Aplysia californica* is lightly calcified, chitinous, made of aragonite of the crossed-lamellar type (see Fig. 34.1a, b). It was submitted to a complete structural, chemical, biochemical and proteomic characterization that will be the subject of an extended publication in preparation. In the present paper, we simply summarize few of the outcomes obtained by proteomics. Our investigations generated several hits with proteins – known or unknown – from *Aplysia californica*. In total, we obtained 40 hits with proteins identified by more than two peptides and several additional hits with proteins identified with one peptide. We classified the protein hits according to the similarity of each of their primary structure to known functional domains or domains with a peculiar signature in terms of amino acid composition. As shown in Fig. 34.1c, we obtained six categories: enzymes, protease inhibitors, ECM/ECM-like (extracellular matrix), cation-interacting proteins, proteins containing LCDs/RLCDs (repetitive low complexity domains). The last category (others) comprises proteins that cannot be included in the five others. It is to note that the heterogeneous class of proteins containing LCDs/RLCDs represents the biggest group of shell proteins. It contains hydrophobic proteins in addition to P-rich, D-rich and S-rich proteins.

34.3.2 *Proteomics on Subfossil* Tridacna *Samples from French Polynesia*

The subfossil samples of the giant clam *Tridacna* sp. were carefully checked for their preservation state, taking the fresh shells as reference. In particular, microsamplings made across the thickness of the shell to identify the mineralogy via FT-IR spectroscopy showed that all shells were fully aragonitic and not recrystallized (data not shown). All of them exhibited the classical crossed-lamellar microstructure. In the subfossil shells, we however saw important alterations and perforations in their outermost and innermost layers (which were subsequently discarded) while the core layer was intact.

Proteomic investigations performed on the fresh shells generated up to 134 protein hits, 46 of which corresponding to proteins identified by at least two peptides.

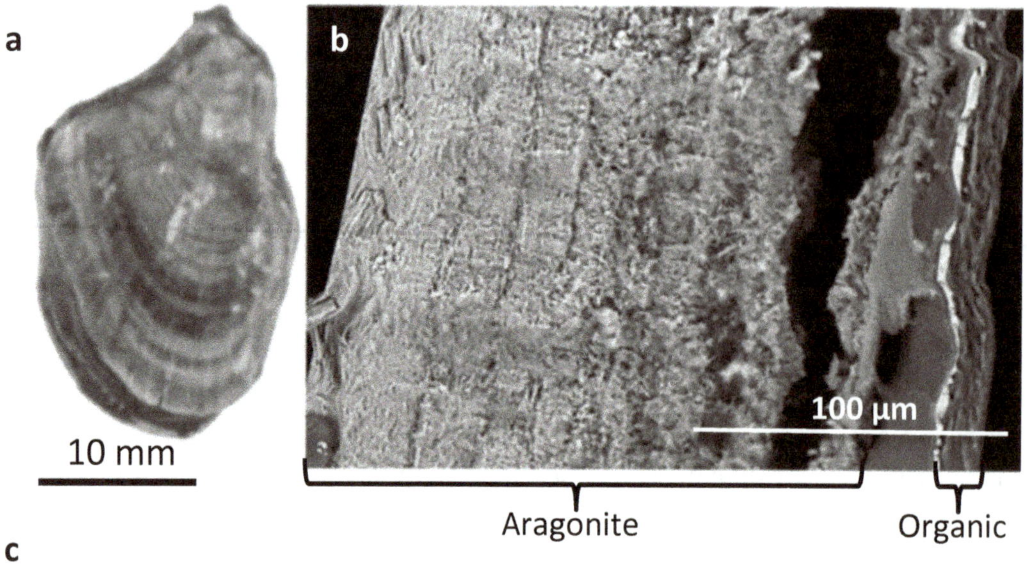

c

FUNCTIONAL DOMAINS	Protein name	MW (kDa)	pI	SP
ENZYMES	Tyrosinase-3-like	47.9	5.5	N
	Hybrid signal transduction histidine kinase A-like	40.4	9.7	N
PROTEASE INHIBITORS	CD109 antigen-like	134.7	7.9	Y
	BPTI/Kunitz-domain containing protein 4-like	25.0	8.9	Y
ECM / ECM-like	Collagen alpha-VI / BMPS *M. edulis* (partial)	158.2	6.4	N
CATION-INTERACTING	Seductin (ependymin-related): Ca	20.2	5.1	N
	Hephaestin-like: Fe/Cu	78.7	5.2	N
LCDs / RLCDs containing proteins	Proline-rich protein HaeIII subfamily 1-like	19.4	12.3	N
	Ser/Arg repetitive matrix protein 1-like	88.1	9.8	N
	Fibroin heavy chain-like	71.0	10.9	N
	Basic proline-rich protein-like	53.7	4.8	N
	Several uncharacterized proteins (>10) (hydrophobic, D-rich, S-rich)			
OTHERS	Microtubule-associated futsch-like	198.6	4.3	N
	Cytoplasmic intermediate filament protein A	65.1	5.5	N
	Vacuolar protein-sorting associated protein 36-like	35.6	9.6	Y

Fig. 34.1 (**a**) The internal shell of *Aplysia californica*; the shell is lightly calcified. Top, apex (posterior); bottom, anterior part, which corresponds to the non-calcified growing shell margin. (**b**) Microstructure of the shell, observed in cross section; the dorsal side is on the right, the ventral, on the left. (**c**) Abridged list of proteins identified in the SOM of *A. californica* by proteomics. LCDs/RLCDs stands for low complexity domains/repetitive low complexity domains, ECM for extracellular matrix. The columns on the right indicate their theoretical molecular weight (MW) in kDaltons, their calculated isoelectric point (pI) and the presence (Y) or absence (N) of signal peptides. Signal peptides were identified by SignalP 4.1, while molecular weights and isoelectric points were calculated by ProtParam (after removal of the signal peptides when present). Both tools are accessible at http://www.expasy.ch/tools/. The fact that several secreted proteins do not exhibit a signal peptide could indicate that some of the sequences are not complete

For subfossil shells, these numbers decreased drastically. For example, the GAM-14 sample, the age of which was precisely determined at 2880 ± 30 BP (before present), exhibited a total of 40 hits, but only 4 of them correspond to proteins identified by at least 2 peptides. Figure 34.2 shows an example of a new LCD-containing protein (P-rich), unambiguously identified in the fresh *Tridacna* sample, owing to

TRINITY_DN253411_c2_g2_i3|m.459507

A

*ETMNKVILIVFSGLLAVQLVSAQ*SHTTWAAAQVPGLGRMTPPTTDYPEYMLHMAVG
EIMRAPTENKAAYAAAKVYNPVMDMSDKVQQALEDRVLQLRHPPGTPYYRRKLDFD
VMQLVIGAYYKTLNISAPQQLGSFYGPPPANHWAGASQPVGPPARQPGPLPPAGPP
AGPAMGPPTSIRRGFRPRAQGIYSPFEPTPWELDRAVQDIHMARTEKQAVKAAAGVH
RIGLDLADIVVNALEEKIARLRRPNWTGFRPPPIPRGLNVHGLVRHAFYEIQRIAQAKAA
ADAAAAAAAAAKAKKTPPPPTPRAGSKIPTTLPPTPPPKPYKKPRQPSKPNPPPSPKKT
KPPKRDFMTDFIQNRRKQRQPPPAPKLFKQAQITRPPFVQPVRRQTLNPFPTQPSVPP
YFEPTKITRPPYVQPQRRDPVDPFFSQPSYRPKPQVEPFRPPPNVPRPPKINWKKKAAA
KPVPTSVSLTEKGPTSISAASSNSNKSPVSYETIPSQNSAKPAFMKIPKPNVPPAPFRSEP
PKPKSLFPKGNSGRPSDIPKAVLSSNKGKGKRPSSKTVEPLFQSTETTPSPEEQQLFNRY
PGLFENKARMRVANLAQHRLETVGPSAEISKPPLKGPNPQPPKVSNKKMPVSKPPQQ
AAVKVAPKIIKPSKVWSPLGNLGSNINEILKFSIDGPSESVPIPTAAPLTTKAPTTTTKKPT
TTTPRKQEKVKPIRKTKVKRRRKVVSKAKSKSFAIKLAKKKPEKPKKPQGADKLTQLHKLL
EGISPSQLQTLVDLIKAKANEGKPKPLPKPEPLPKPKPIFAPPPPPGSEHKGPPREFRSQ
MQSSRSGPYRPNSDYGPPPDNRGPPPDWARGPGGRPRGPPGPPGPGGPGGPGMR
GGPDLSNPQIARLIRVMKQGGHPKNNFLSGRTPGSSAAAAGGEAPEAGEGPTGLLGN
PLMMSMLMNRGGQGGGGGIASLLGGGAAGGANPLAALMPGGAGGAGGGEGGM
NPAMLAAIMGGGQGGGGGGMGALGGGYGGMLAGLGL

Protein sequence coverage: 38%

B

*ETMNKVILIVFSGLLAVQLVSAQ*SHTTWAAAQVPGLGRMTPPTTDYPEYMLHMAVG
EIMRAPTENKAAYAAAKVYNPVMDMSDKVQQALEDRVLQLRHPPGTPYYRRKLDFD
VMQLVIGAYYKTLNISAPQQLGSFYGPPPANHWAGASQPVGPPARQPGPLPPAGPP
AGPAMGPPTSIRRGFRPRAQGIYSPFEPTPWELDRAVQDIHMARTEKQAVKAAAGVH
RIGLDLADIVVNALEEKIARLRRPNWTGFRPPPIPRGLNVHGLVRHAFYEIQRIAQAKAA
ADAAAAAAAAAKAKKTPPPPTPRAGSKIPTTLPPTPPPKPYKKPRQPSKPNPPPSPKKT
KPPKRDFMTDFIQNRRKQRQPPPAPKLFKQAQITRPPFVQPVRRQTLNPFPTQPSVPP
YFEPTKITRPPYVQPQRRDPVDPFFSQPSYRPKPQVEPFRPPPNVPRPPKINWKKKAAA
KPVPTSVSLTEKGPTSISAASSNSNKSPVSYETIPSQNSAKPAFMKIPKPNVPPAPFRSEP
PKPKSLFPKGNSGRPSDIPKAVLSSNKGKGKRPSSKTVEPLFQSTETTPSPEEQQLFNRY
PGLFENKARMRVANLAQHRLETVGPSAEISKPPLKGPNPQPPKVSNKKMPVSKPPQQ
AAVKVAPKIIKPSKVWSPLGNLGSNINEILKFSIDGPSESVPIPTAAPLTTKAPTTTTKKPT
TTTPRKQEKVKPIRKTKVKRRRKVVSKAKSKSFAIKLAKKKPEKPKKPQGADKLTQLHKLL
EGISPSQLQTLVDLIKAKANEGKPKPLPKPEPLPKPKPIFAPPPPPGSEHKGPPREFRSQ
MQSSRSGPYRPNSDYGPPPDNRGPPPDWARGPGGRPRGPPGPPGPGGPGGPGMR
GGPDLSNPQIARLIRVMKQGGHPKNNFLSGRTPGSSAAAAGGEAPEAGEGPTGLLGN
PLMMSMLMNRGGQGGGGGIASLLGGGAAGGANPLAALMPGGAGGAGGGEGGM
NPAMLAAIMGGGQGGGGGGMGALGGGYGGMLAGLGL

Protein sequence coverage: 4%

Fig. 34.2 Example of a novel protein identified in the fresh (**a**) and in the subfossil (**b**) *Tridacna* sample. This protein is the translation of the sequenced transcript TRINITY_DN253411_c2_g2_i3|m.459507. This protein is rich in proline (17.2%), glycine (10.1) and alanine (9.6%) residues and its theoretical calculated pI is basic (10.63). Its function in biomineralization is unknown. In grey italic, signal peptide. The peptides identified by proteomics are underlined. Note that the full protein sequence is well covered (38%) in the case of the fresh *Tridacna* shell while the coverage is poor (4%) for the subfossil shell. This drop may be explained by information losses at the peptide level due to diagenetic transformations (hydrolysis, modification of chemical groups on amino acids) good protein sequence coverage by peptides (38%, 17 peptides) all along the sequence. In the subfossil sample, the percentage of coverage of this protein sequence by peptides drops to 4% only (5 peptides), which suggests that the other non-covered parts of the sequence may be submitted to diagenetic transformation and/or hydrolysis. A complete view of all the results will be resumed in a publication in preparation.

34.4 Discussion

This paper illustrates how proteomics contributes to answer questions related to the functions, evolution and diagenesis of SOMs in mollusc shell. In the first case, we explored the protein composition of the internal shell of the Californian sea hare, *Aplysia californica.* Aplysiidae are usually considered as a very derived gastropod family that has emerged only 25 million years ago (Klussmann-Kolb 2004) during the Oligocene epoch. This family is characterized by the presence of an atrophied and weakly calcified internal shell, which has completely lost its primary function, the protection of the soft tissues. In spite of this regressive evolution, it is remarkable to observe that the shell of *A. californica* has conserved a protein repertoire that exhibits a similar signature as the ones from fully functional external shells, in terms of diversity of protein families present in the matrix.

The second example deals with the diagenetic processes that affect organic matrices associated to calcium carbonate biominerals. In a previous paper, we showed that artificial diagenesis experiments performed on fresh nacre powder samples resulted in two phenomena recorded by proteomic analyses: a decrease of the number of identified proteins correlated to harsh diagenetic conditions and, in parallel, a decrease of the number of peptides identified per protein (Parker et al. 2015). Our analyses performed on the SOMs of subfossil *Tridacna* tend to correlate this finding. This example gives interesting perspectives for the coming time, i.e. the possibility to track the diagenetic pathway of each shell protein, taken individually, in sub-fossil/fossil of increasing age.

Acknowledgements This work was supported by NEWFELPRO programme (Dr. D. Medakovic), by funds from OIST (T. Takeuchi), by EC2CO project (I. Bundeleva, F. Marin) and by annual funds from UMR Biogeosciences (F. Marin).

References

Demarchi B, Hall S, Roncal-Herrero T, Freeman C et al (2016) Protein sequences bound to mineral surfaces persist into deep time. eLife 5:e17092

Hare PE, Hoering TC, King K (eds) (1980) Biogeochemistry of amino acids. Wiley, New York

Immel F, Broussard C, Catherinet B, Plasseraud L, Alcaraz G, Bundeleva I, Marin F (2016) The shell of the invasive bivalve species *Dreissena polymorpha*: biochemical, elemental and textural investigations. PlosOne 11:e0154264

Klussmann-Kolb A (2004) Phylogeny of the Aplysiidae (Gastropoda, Opisthobranchia) with new aspects of the evolution of seahares. Zool Scr 33:439–462

Kocot KM, Aguilera F, McDougall C, Jackson DJ, Degnan BM (2016) Sea shell diversity and rapidly evolving secretomes: insights into the evolution of biomineralization. Front Zool 13:23

Marie B, Arivalagan J, Mathéron L, Bolbach G, Berland S, Marie A, Marin F (2017) Deep conservation of bivalve nacre proteins highlighted by shell matrix proteomics of the Unionoida *Elliptio complanata* and *Villosa lienosa*. J R Soc Interface 14:pii20160846

Marin F, Le Roy N, Marie B (2012) The formation and mineralization of mollusk shell. Front Biosci S4:1099–1125

Marin F., Bundeleva I, Takeuchi T, Immel F, Medakovic D (2016) Organic matrices in metazoan calcium carbonate skeletons: composition, functions, evolution

Parker A, Immel F, Guichard N, Broussard C, Marin F (2015) Thermal stability of nacre proteins of the Polynesian pearl oyster: a proteomic study. Key Eng Mater 672:222–233

Ramos-Silva P, Kaandorp J, Herbst F, Plasseraud L, Alcaraz G, Stern C, Corneillat M, Guichard N, Durlet C, Luquet G, Marin F (2014) The skeleton of the staghorn coral *Acropora millepora*: molecular and structural characterization. Plos One 9:e97454

Wallace AF, Schiffbauer JD (2016) Paleoproteomics: proteins from the past. elife 5:e20877

Chapter 35
Functional Analysis on Shelk2 of Pacific Oyster

Jun Takahashi, Chieko Yamashita, Kenji Kanasaki, and Haruhiko Toyohara

Abstract Shelk2, a novel shell matrix protein from the Pacific oyster, *Crassostrea gigas*, is reported to be involved in shell biosynthesis of the prismatic layer. Results of RNAi experiment on *shelk2* showed that Shelk2 has a key role in shell regeneration. When dsRNA of *shelk2* was injected into the adductor muscle of Pacific oyster, the prismatic layer did not grow normally during shell regeneration. Observation of regenerated shell using scanning electron microscopy (SEM) revealed that the size of each column in the prismatic layer was reduced, and the edge of the column top looked rounder. From these results, it was deduced that the columns were less tightly bound with each other than in normally regenerated shells. Furthermore, the surface of the column appeared to be rough. Unexpectedly, the expression level of *shelk2* mRNA was not reduced but remarkably enhanced by the knockdown experiment. Further experiments including gene and protein expression will be necessary for a better understanding of its function and role in oyster shell regeneration.

Keywords Biomineralization · Knockdown · Mollusk · Pacific oyster · Shelk2 · Shell · Silk-like protein

35.1 Introduction

Mollusk is the second largest metazoan taxon with many members possessing mineralized hard tissues formed as a result of biomineralization. The molluscan shell is synthesized and maintained by the epithelial cells of the mantle, which is a specific tissue present only in mollusks. Generally, the molluscan shell is composed of >90% inorganic materials that mainly consist of $CaCO_3$ and <10% organic matrices, including polysaccharides and proteins. Various organic matrices play an important

J. Takahashi · H. Toyohara (✉)
Graduate School of Agriculture, Kyoto University, Kyoto, Japan
e-mail: juntaka@kais.kyoto-u.ac.jp; toyohara@kais.kyoto-u.ac.jp

C. Yamashita · K. Kanasaki
Progress Co., Ltd, Osaka, Japan
e-mail: c-yamashita@progress-water.com; k-kanasaki@progress-water.com

K. Endo et al. (eds.), *Biomineralization*,
https://doi.org/10.1007/978-981-13-1002-7_35

role in the crystallization and/or framework formation of the shell, while most of them reported so far do not share identity in their amino acid sequences among species, with the exception of acidic proteins (Takahashi et al. 2013).

The identification of most organic matrix substances, including proteins, so far has been accomplished by the decalcification of shells and subsequent extraction with specific solutions (Marin et al. 2000). This conventional method is suitable for the identification of relatively abundant proteins, but certain vital proteins cannot be obtained because of their low solubility and/or instability in solution.

Instead of the shell itself, we focused on the mantle where the genes involved in shell regeneration are expressed to identify essential proteins involved in shell biosynthesis. We have successfully cloned mantle edge-specific genes from Pacific oyster, *Crassostrea gigas*, by means of a subtractive hybridization method, then found two novel genes, *shelk1* and *shelk2* (Takahashi et al. 2012). The mRNA of *shelk2* was specifically expressed in the outer fold of the mantle edge, suggesting that it is possibly involved in the synthesis of the prismatic structure. *In situ* hybridization revealed gradual increase in *shelk2* mRNA expression during shell regeneration, suggesting the possible involvement of Shelk2 in shell formation (Takahashi et al. 2012).

Deduced amino acid sequences of both proteins were highly homologous to those of arthropod silk fibroins (Hayashi and Lewis 1998; Hinman and Lewis 1992). Interestingly, tandem repeats of poly-alanine (poly-Ala) motifs were identified in the amino acid sequence of Shelk2 of *C. gigas*. Poly-Ala motifs have also been reported in silk fibroins of arthropods (Guerette et al. 1996) and two shell matrix proteins of mollusks, including the MSI60 of Japanese pearl oyster (Sudo et al. 1997) and Shelk2 of *Crassostrea nippona* (Takahashi et al. 2012). However, the function of Shelk2 still remains unknown. Therefore, in this study, we made an attempt to elucidate their function *via* knockdown experiment.

35.2 Materials and Methods

Adult Pacific oysters (shell length, 5–7 cm; shell height, 7–11 cm) were purchased from the market and maintained in artificial seawater for a day before using them for the RNAi experiments.

For the synthesis of *shelk2* dsRNA, we used T7 RiboMAX Express RNAi System (Promega, Madison, WI, USA) following the manufacturer's instructions. The dsDNA templates of *shelk2* and *EF-1α* for both RNA syntheses were cloned into pTAC-2 plasmid (BioDynamics Laboratory, Tokyo, Japan), prepared using TaKaRa Ex Taq DNA polymerase (TaKaRa, Shiga, Japan) or PrimeSTAR GXL DNA polymerase (TaKaRa) with PCR primers shown in Table 35.1. These primers were designed on the basis of *C. gigas shelk2* sequence (GenBank ID: AB474183) and *EGFP* sequence. Thermal cycler T-Gradient Thermoblock (Biometra, Goettingen, Germany) was used for the amplification according to the conventional reaction program.

Table 35.1 Primers for dsRNA syntheses and qPCR analyses

Name	Sequence (5' -> 3')
dsRNA synthesis	
S2-101 Fw	ATGCTGAAGCTTGTCTCCATCGTTTGCCTT
S2-102 Rv	TTAATAGGTCTTTTTATGTCTGATGCCACC
T7 S2-117 Fw	GGATCCTAATACGACTCACTATAGGATGCTGAAGCTTGTCTCC
T7 S2-121 Rv	GGATCCTAATACGACTCACTATAGGTTAATAGGTCTTTTTATGTCTGATGCC
EGFP-903 Fw	ATGGTGAGCAAGGGCGAGGAGCTG
EGFP-904 Rv	TTACTTGTACAGCTCGTCCATGCC
T7 EGFP-901 Fw	GGATCCTAATACGACTCACTATAGGATGGTGAGCAAGGGCGAG
T7 EGFP-902 Rv	GGATCCTAATACGACTCACTATAGGTTACTTGTACAGCTCGTC
qPCR analysis	
Cg_EF1a-802 Fw	AAGTCTTGGAAGAGGCACCA
Cg_EF1a-803 Rv	CAGCCTTCTCAACCTCCTTG
S2-126 Fw	CTCCATCGTTTGCCTTTTTG
S2-127 Rv	AGTCCTCCAATGACACCACC

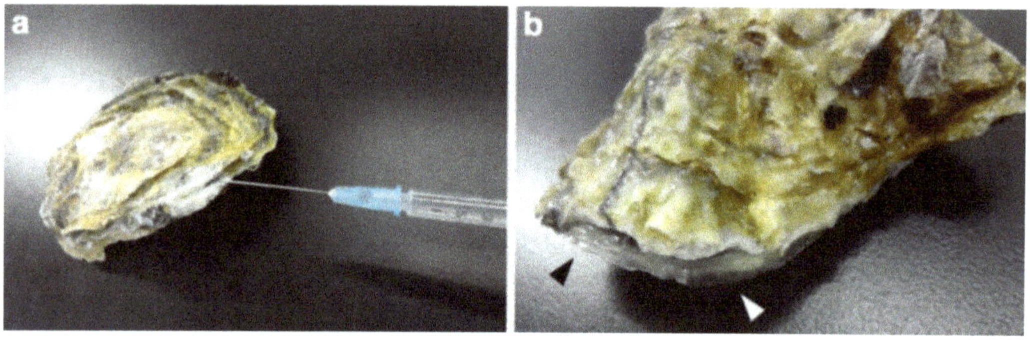

Fig. 35.1 Knockdown experiment and shell regeneration. (**a**) Shell surrounding the adductor muscle was excised by a pair of nippers within 3 cm, and dsRNA was injected into the adductor muscle. A constant volume (200 μl) of PBS solution containing 30 μg of *EGFP* dsRNA and 10 μg or 30 μg of *shelk2* dsRNA was injected into each group (n = 5). (**b**) Plastic-like structure of new shell was regenerated after a day of injection, and it was more clearly observed after the next 2 days (arrowheads). We collected the structure and the mantle edges after 7 days of injection

The Pacific oyster shells were cut on the ventral side near the adductor muscle into approximately 3-cm wide portions using a pair of nippers. To knock down the *shelk2*, the designed *shelk2* dsRNA (10 μg or 30 μg in 200 μL PBS) or *EGFP* dsRNA (30 μg in 200 μL PBS, for control) was injected into the adductor muscle of each oyster (Suzuki et al. 2009; Funabara et al. 2014; see Fig. 35.1a). The oysters were then kept in artificial seawater for 7 days without feeding. Then their mantles and the newly regenerated prismatic layers (Fig. 35.1b) were collected for qPCR experiments and SEM observation, respectively.

For SEM observation of the regenerated shell, Miniscope TM3000 (Hitachi High-Technologies, Tokyo, Japan) was used at two magnifications (×500 and ×2000).

For qPCR analyses, total RNA was extracted from the collected mantles using Sepasol-RNA I Super G (Nacalai tesque, Kyoto, Japan), while using Handy Sonic UR-20P (Tomy Seiko, Tokyo, Japan) for mantle homogenization. We used

PrimeScript RT Reagent Kit with gDNA Eraser (TaKaRa) for RT-PCR and first strand cDNA synthesis. Primers for qPCR were also designed on the basis of *C. gigas shelk2* sequence and *C. gigas EF-1α* sequence (GenBank ID: AB122066). For the qPCR reaction, KOD SYBR qPCR Mix (TOYOBO, Osaka, Japan) was used in StepOnePlus Real-Time PCR System (Life Technologies Japan, Tokyo, Japan) employing the comparative C_T ($\Delta\Delta C_T$) method.

35.3 Results and Discussion

35.3.1 Regeneration of Shell Prismatic Layer Observed by SEM

Figure 35.2 shows the SEM results (top view) of the newly generated plastic-like structure in the prismatic layer. In general, the prismatic layer gradually grew from the lower left to the upper right direction during the natural regeneration of a cracked shell, as shown in Fig. 35.2a. During this process, it is assumed that gap among the columns is filled densely. When dsRNA of *EGFP* was injected as the control experiment, the prismatic layer grew in a similar manner (Fig. 35.2c, d).

In contrast, when dsRNA of *shelk2* was injected, the prismatic layer did not grow normally (Figs. 35.2e–h). In particular, the size of each column was reduced, and the reduction was more remarkable by the 30-μg injection than by the 10-μg injection (Fig. 35.2g, h). In addition, the edge of the column top looked rounder; resultantly the columns were not tightly bound to each other compared with the control experiment as well as the natural regeneration. Furthermore, the surface of the column top looked rough, whereas those of the control experiment and the natural regeneration were smooth.

35.3.2 Real-Time PCR

To determine the effect of *shelk2* knockdown by RNAi, the expression of *shelk2* mRNA was evaluated (Fig. 35.3). Unexpectedly, the expression level of *shelk2* mRNA was considerably higher than that in the control experiment, in which *EGFP* dsRNA (Fig. 35.3) or PBS (data not shown) was injected. Generally, target gene expression is reduced in the knockdown experiments. Actually in the experiments of shells, the expression of *Pinctada fucata* genes including Pif and Nacrein were reduced by the previous knockdown experiment (Suzuki et al. 2009; Funabara et al. 2014), although their expressions were examined 7 or 8 days after injection similar to our experiments. In fact, reduction was observed in the knockdown experiment of another oyster silk-like gene, *shelk1*, in our experiment (data not shown).

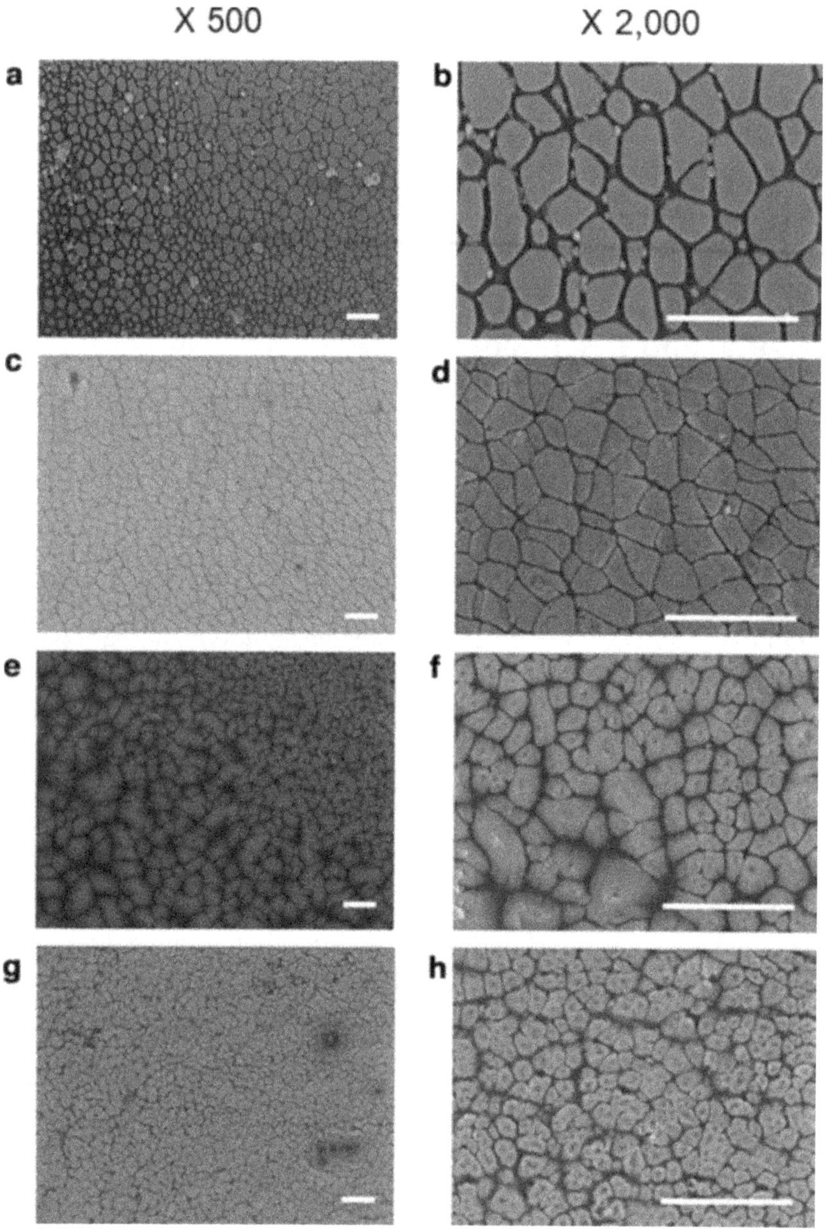

Fig. 35.2 SEM observation of the regenerated prismatic layers at two magnifications (×500 and ×2000). The bar indicates 30 μm. (**a**, **b**) Shell was excised, but no operation was performed. (**c**, **d**) dsRNA of *EGFP* was injected (control). (**e**, **f**) *Shelk2* dsRNA (10 μg) was injected. (**g**, **h**) *Shelk2* dsRNA (30 μg) was injected

As a result of *shelk2* knockdown, *shelk2* mRNA was expressed remarkably during shell regeneration, suggesting that Shelk2 would increase. Then the increase in the amount of the protein would induce the reduction in the column size of the prismatic layer. However, detailed studies on the change in expression levels of *shelk2* mRNA after injection are required for the full understanding of its remarkable expression.

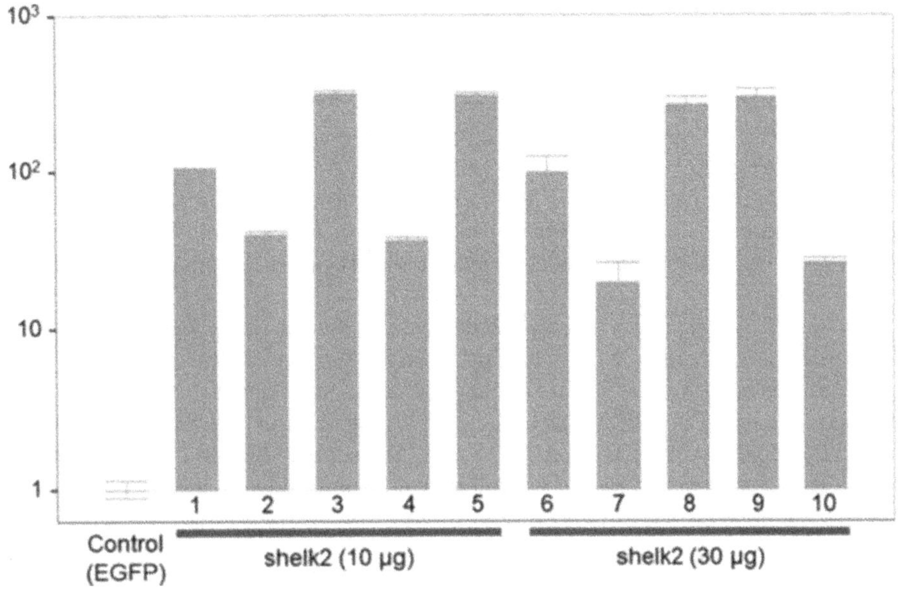

Fig. 35.3 Knockdown of *shelk2* by means of RNAi. The expression levels of *shelk2* mRNA in the mantle, which are normalized to those of *EF-1α*, were determined with real-time quantitative PCR. Five oysters were used in each experiment group. The graph bar shows the *shelk2* mRNA expression level of 7 days after injection with dsRNAs against 10 μg (bar number: 1–5) or 30 μg (6–10) of *shelk2*, and those of the *EGFP* group (average of 5 oysters) is attributed a relative value of 1.0. Unexpectedly, the *shelk2* expression levels increased more than ten times

35.3.3 Plan for Subsequent Studies

We have unexpectedly detected the remarkable expression of *shelk2* mRNA by real-time PCR analysis, but no information was available on the expression level of Shelk2. We are now trying to raise an antibody against Shelk2 for the detection of its expression and subsequent observation using SEM and western blotting during regeneration following knockdown experiments.

Since *shelk2* has multiple copies (Takahashi et al. 2012), the reactionary excess expression of the genes at multiple sites would be due to the temporal *shelk2* mRNA suppression caused by the RNAi. To validate the speculation, we attempt to identify the overexpressed gene after RNAi experiment. Further studies on the molecular mechanism of oyster shell synthesis, especially on the remarkably rapid regenerating process, would lead to the application in medical and cosmetic fields.

References

Funabara D, Ohmori F, Kinoshita S, Koyama H, Mizutani S, Ota A, Osakabe Y, Nagai K, Maeyama K, Okamoto K, Kanoh S, Asakawa S, Watabe S (2014) Novel genes participating in the formation of prismatic and nacreous layers in the pearl oyster as revealed by their tissue distribution and RNA interference knockdown. PLoS One 9:e84706

Guerette PA, Ginzinger DG, Weber BHF, Gosline JM (1996) Silk properties determined by gland-specific expression of a spider fibroin gene family. Science 272:112–115

Hayashi CY, Lewis RV (1998) Evidence from flagelliform silk cDNA for the structural basis of elasticity and modular nature of spider silks. J Mol Biol 275:773–784

Hinman MB, Lewis RV (1992) Isolation of a clone encoding a second dragline silk fibroin. J Biol Chem 267:19320–19324

Marin F, Corstjens P, Gaulejac B, Jong EVD, Westbroek P (2000) Mucins and molluscan calcification: molecular characterization of mucoperlin, a novel mucin-like protein from the nacreous shell layer of the fan mussel *Pinna nobilis* (Bivalvia, Pteriomorphia). J Biol Chem 275:20667–20675

Sudo S, Fujikawa T, Nagakura T, Ohkubo T, Sakaguchi K, Tanaka M, Nakashima K, Takahashi T (1997) Structures of mollusk shell framework proteins. Nature 387:563–564

Suzuki M, Saruwatari K, Kogure T, Yamamoto Y, Nishimura Y, Kato Y, Nagasawa H (2009) An acidic matrix protein, Pif, is a key macromolecule for nacre formation. Science 325:1388–1390

Takahashi J, Takagi M, Okihana Y, Takeo K, Ueda T, Touhata K, Maegawa S, Toyohara H (2012) A novel silk-like shell matrix gene is expressed in the mantle edge of the Pacific oyster prior to shell regeneration. Gene 499:130–134

Takahashi J, Kishida T, Toyohara H (2013) Poly-alanine protein Shelk2 from Crassostrea species of oysters. In: Watabe S, Meyama K, Nagasawa H (eds) Recent advances in pearl research. Terrapub, Tokyo, pp 167–181

Chapter 36
Mollusk Shells: Does the Nacro-prismatic "Model" Exist?

Yannicke Dauphin and Jean-Pierre Cuif

Abstract The "nacro-prismatic" shells are the most studied mollusks, and they are often said to be "the" model to unravel the biomineralization mechanisms. Nevertheless, the nacro-prismatic structure is not unique, despite most data are provided by only three genera. The aragonitic nacre is taxon dependent: in cephalopods and gastropods, nacre is columnar, whereas bivalves have a spiral or sheet nacre. The inner structure of gastropod and cephalopod columnar nacre differs. The shape of the tablets is specific of the taxa. Calcitic and aragonitic prisms exist. The composition of the organic matrices extracted from calcitic prisms with a similar shape and mineralogy strongly differs. The inner structure of aragonite prisms is complex, with a central zone and divergent elongated crystallites at the periphery. Additionally, the relationships between nacre and prisms are also taxonomically related. From these data, whatever the scale at which they are studied, every component of the "nacro-prismatic" model – nacre, prisms, and prism–nacre topographic relations – is highly variable, so that this "model" does not exist; it is a structure.

Keywords Mollusks · Nacre · Prismatic layer · Model

36.1 Introduction

The most common structure in mollusk shells is the aragonite crossed-lamellar layer, but the most studied is the "nacro-prismatic" arrangement. Almost all data about mollusks are from three bivalve genera with flat large shells: *Atrina*, *Pinna*, and *Pinctada*. These genera are taxonomically related (Pteriomorphia), with

Y. Dauphin (✉)
Institut de systématique, Evolution, Biodiversité, ISYEB – UMR 7205, Muséum national d'Histoire naturelle, Paris, France
e-mail: yannicke.dauphin@sorbonne-universite.fr

J.-P. Cuif
Centre de recherche sur la paléodiversité et les paléoenvironnements, CR2P – UMR 7207, Muséum national d'Histoire naturelle, Paris, France

K. Endo et al. (eds.), *Biomineralization*,
https://doi.org/10.1007/978-981-13-1002-7_36

large polygonal prismatic units and an inner nacreous layer, so that separating the two layers for detailed analyses is not difficult. They are often used as "the" model to understand the biomineralization processes. Sometimes, *Unio* and *Mytilus*, both with a nacro-prismatic structure, are also used as a model. The concept of model to describe this structure suggests that all these nacro-prismatic shells are identical in terms of structure and composition. The examination of the structure and composition of the layers and of the prismatic and nacreous units, as well as their relationships, demonstrates that the nacro-prismatic arrangement is not unique. It is impossible to enter into the detailed description of all mollusk shells. So, the present article will concentrate largely on the differences between the nacro-prismatic shells.

36.2 Materials and Methods

Details about the origin of the samples and preparative process and setup of the diverse used techniques are given in the relevant publications listed in the References.

36.2.1 Materials

Bivalves (*Pinctada, Pinna, Nucula, Neotrigonia, Unio*), gastropods (*Haliotis, Trochus, Turbo*), and cephalopods (*Nautilus, Sepia, Spirula*) were used. Depending on the genera, several species were studied (*Pinna, Sepia, Haliotis*, among others).

36.2.2 Methods

Micro- and nanostructures were studied using thin sections, fractures, and polished etched surfaces for the scanning electron microscope (secondary and backscattered electron modes, Philips SEM XL30, FEI Phenom) and atomic force microscope (Veeco Nanoscope Dimension 3100). Electron microprobes (energy- and wavelength-dispersive spectrometry) (Link AN10000, CAMECA SX50, SX100) were used for quantitative elemental chemical composition and distribution maps. Chemical distribution maps were also performed using NanoSIMS (CAMECA N50), TOF-SIMS (TOF-SIMS IV Ion-Tof GmbH), and XANES (ID21, ESRF). Thermogravimetric analyses allow to quantify the organic matrix content. Infrared and Raman spectrometry were used on both bulk samples and extracted organic matrices. Liquid chromatography and electrophoresis were used for molecular weights and acidity of the soluble matrices. Lipid content was known using thin-layer chromatography. Amino acid analyses were done on both soluble and insoluble matrices.

36.3 Results

36.3.1 Microstructures

Prisms are aragonite (*Neotrigonia*, Unionidae, Cephalopoda) or calcite (Pteriomorphia) (Fig. 36.1a–c) (Boggild 1930; Taylor et al. 1969, 1973; Ben Mlih 1983; Checa et al. 2014; Cuif et al. 2011). In some species, calcitic and aragonitic prisms coexist (Dauphin et al. 1989). The inner structure of the prisms is also variable, but the morphological and microstructural diversity is not related to the mineralogy (*Sepia*, Fig. 36.1b; *Haliotis*, Fig. 36.1c) but to the taxa. The inner structure of aragonite prisms is complex, with a central zone and divergent elongated crystallites at the periphery. Calcitic prisms are mono- or polycrystalline. The nacre is aragonite, but the tablets are deposited in vertical columns in gastropods and cephalopods, whereas they are in lenses in bivalves (Wise 1970). The inner structure of gastropod and cephalopod columnar nacre differs. Moreover, the shape and the inner structure of the tablets are species dependent (*Nautilus*, Fig. 36.1d; *Pinna*, Fig. 36.1e; *Sepia*, Fig. 36.1f) (Mutvei 1978, 1979). In coleoid cephalopods, the nacreous layer has no tablets (Mutvei 1963) (Fig. 36.1f).

Not only the shape, mineralogy, and inner structure of the prisms or tablets differ, but the transition between the two layers is also taxonomically dependent. When the prisms are calcite, there is no direct contact between the calcite and the nacre (Cuif et al. 2011). Both layers are separated by a thick organic membrane and an irregular layer of fibrous aragonite (*Pinctada*, Fig. 36.1g). In shells with aragonitic prisms, the transition is smooth, without an organic membrane (*Neotrigonia*, Fig. 36.1h) (Dauphin et al. 2014). Chemical differences also exist in the transition zone. Backscattered electron image of the calcitic–aragonitic transition demonstrates that the first aragonitic deposits are not nacre (*Pinctada*, Fig. 36.1i) (Dauphin et al. 2008). XANES map shows that the chemical composition of the end of the calcitic prisms is modified (*Pinctada*, Fig. 36.1j) (Dauphin et al. 2003), so that it cannot be said that the termination of prisms is "abrupt" (Hovden et al. 2015). No organic membrane exists between aragonitic prisms and nacre (*Neotrigonia*, Fig. 36.1k) (Checa and Rodriguez-Navarro 2001; Dauphin ct al. 2008, 2014). The amino acid content of the fibrous aragonite differs from that of the nacreous layer, as shown by TOF-SIMS maps (*Pinctada*, Fig. 36.1l, m) (Farre et al. 2011), and the N map confirms the difference between the nacre and the fibrous aragonite in calcitic–aragonitic shells (*Pinctada*, Fig. 36.1n) (Dauphin et al. 2008).

It must be added that the elemental chemical composition of a given structure (nacre, calcitic or aragonitic prisms) is species dependent (Fig. 36.1o) (Dauphin et al. 1989).

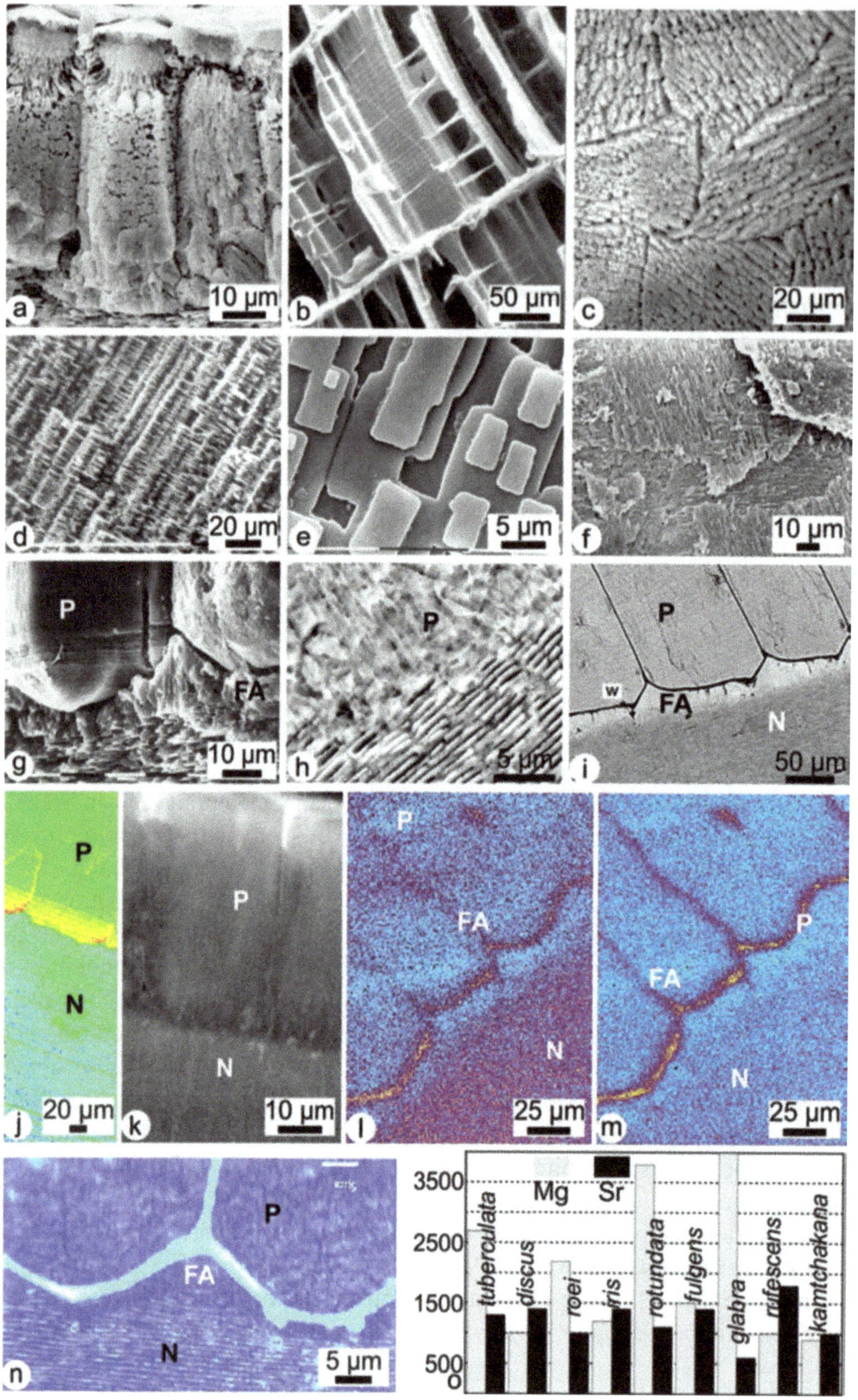

Fig. 36.1 (**a**) Unetched fracture showing the complex aragonitic prisms of *Neotrigonia*. (**b**) Aragonitic prismatic layer of the dorsal shield of *Sepia* – unetched fracture. (**c**) Calcitic prisms of *Haliotis rufescens,* polished and etched fracture. Formic acid 5%, 7 s, 20 °C. (**d**) Columnar nacreous layer of *Nautilus* – unetched fracture. (**e**) Rectangular nacreous tablets of *Pinna* – unetched sample. (**f**) Type 2 nacre: layered structure without tablets in a lamella of the ventral part of *Sepia* – unetched sample. (**g**) Unetched fracture showing the calcitic prismatic – aragonitic nacreous

36.3.2 Organic Components

It is now well-known that mollusk shells are organo-mineral biocomposites. For a given structure, the quantity and nature of the organic matrices differ and depend on the taxa as shown by TGA data of the nacre in *Nautilus* (Cephalopoda), *Trochus* (Gastropoda), and *Pinctada* (Bivalvia) (Fig. 36.2a, b). Insoluble matrices comprise proteins and lipids. It must be noted that the results differ following the sample preparation (decalcification or lipid extraction using organic solvents, Farre and Dauphin 2009). Using the same preparative process, the lipidic composition of the calcitic prisms of *Pinna* and *Pinctada* differs (Fig. 36.2c). The molecular weights of the soluble matrices of these prisms also differ (Fig. 36.1d) (Dauphin 2003). As for the insoluble matrices, most analyses are dedicated to the protein contents, mainly amino acid analyses (*Pinctada*, *Nautilus*, Fig. 36.2e). Nevertheless, infrared spectrometry of the insoluble matrices shows the presence of lipids and sugars in the insoluble matrices of nacreous layers (*Nautilus*, *Pinctada*, Fig. 36.2f). Despite the similarity of shape and mineralogy of the prisms of *Pinna* and *Pinctada*, the acidity (pI) and aliphatic index (indicative of the thermal stability for globular proteins) of the insoluble matrices differ (Fig. 36.2g).

36.4 Discussion and Conclusion

There is a strong contrast between the small number of studied taxa with a nacro-prismatic structure and the diversity of their shells. The examination of the shape, inner structure, mineralogy, and composition of both mineral and organic components of these shells show the large diversity of these characteristics (Samata 1990), despite some superficial similarities. The relationships between the two layers are also variable and controlled by the organism. However, the diversity is not hazardous: every characteristic is taxonomically dependent, usually at a specific level. Most often, the presence and role of acidic proteins in the biomineralization process is emphasized, but the role of sugars and lipids is neglected (Kocot et al. 2016). Up to now, proteomics and genomics data have not permitted to select the possible mechanisms of the secretion (Suzuki and Nagasawa 2013; Simkiss 2016).

Thus, not only the structure and composition of the nacre and prisms are heterogeneous, they are also dependent on the species, so that this heterogeneity does not

Fig. 36.1 (continued) transition in *Pinctada*, with a thick organic membrane and an irregular layer of fibrous aragonite. (**h**) Aragonitic prism – nacre transition in *Neotrigonia* – BSE image of a polished and etched section (HCl 1%10 s). (**i**) BSE map showing the organic membrane and the fibrous aragonite between the calcitic prisms and the nacre in *Pinctada*. (**j**) XANES map of S in amino acids in the shell of *Pinctada*. (**k**) XANES map of sulfate in *Neotrigonia*. (**l**) TOF-SIMS map of alanine in the shell of *Pinctada*. (**m**) TOF-SIMS map of glycine of the same section. (**n**) NanoSIMS map of N in *Pinctada*. (**o**): Mg and Sr contents of the prismatic calcitic layers in some species of *Haliotis*

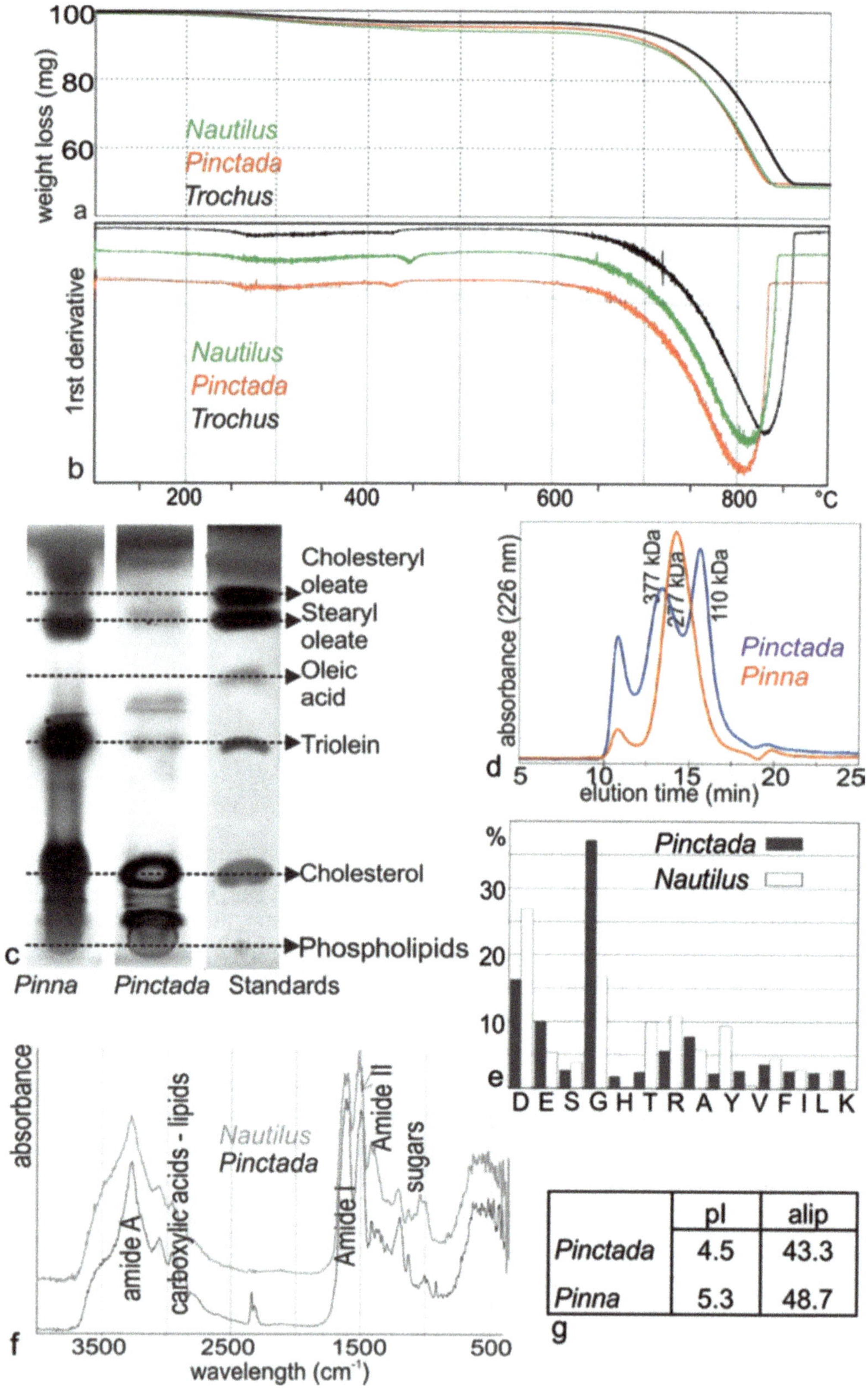

	pI	alip
Pinctada	4.5	43.3
Pinna	5.3	48.7

Fig. 36.2 (**a**, **b**) Thermogravimetric profiles showing the differences in the quantity and composition of the organic matrices in three nacreous layers. (**c**) Thin-layer chromatography showing the lipidic composition of the calcitic prisms in two bivalve shells. (**d**) Liquid chromatography of the soluble organic matrices of calcitic prisms. (**e**) Amino acid composition of the insoluble matrix of nacreous layers. (**f**) Infrared spectrometry of the insoluble organic matrix of nacreous layers. (**g**) Isoelectric point (pI) and aliphatic index (alip) of the insoluble organic matrix of calcitic prisms

suit the usual characteristics of a model. They are neither simple nor unique, so that the nacro-prismatic model concept cannot be sustained.

References

Ben Mlih A (1983) Organisation de la phase carbonatée dans les prismes de *Neotrigonia margaritacea* Lmk. C R Acad Sci Paris 296(Série III):313–318

Boggild OB (1930) The shell structure of the molluscs. D Kgl Danske Vidensk Selsk Skr, naturvidensk og mathem 9:231–326

Checa AG, Rodriguez-Navarro A (2001) Geometrical and crystallographic constraints determine the self-organization of shell microstructures in Unionidae (Bivalvia: Mollusca). Proc R Soc Lond B 268:771–778

Checa AG, Salas C, Harper EM, De Dios Bueno-Perez J (2014) Early stage biomineralization in the periostracum of the "living fossil" bivalve *Neotrigonia*. PLOS ONE 9:2. https://doi.org/10.1371/journal.pone.0090033

Cuif JP, Dauphin Y, Sorauf JE (2011) Biominerals and fossils through time. Cambridge Univ. Press, Cambridge, 490 p

Dauphin Y (2003) Soluble organic matrices of the calcitic prismatic shell layers of two pteriomorphid bivalves: *Pinna nobilis* and *Pinctada margaritifera*. J Biol Chem 278(17):15168–15177

Dauphin Y, Cuif JP, Mutvei H, Denis A (1989) Mineralogy, chemistry and ultrastructure of the external shell layer in ten species of *Haliotis* with reference to *Haliotis tuberculata* (Mollusca: Archaeogastropoda). Bull Geol Inst Univ Uppsala, NS 15:7–38

Dauphin Y, Cuif JP, Doucet J, Salomé M, Susini J, Williams CT (2003) In situ chemical speciation of sulfur in calcitic biominerals and the simple prism concept. J Struct Biol 142:272–280

Dauphin Y, Ball AD, Cotte M, Cuif JP, Meibom A, Salomé M, Susini J, Williams CT (2008) Structure and composition of the nacre – prism transition in the shell of *Pinctada margaritifera* (Mollusca, Bivalvia). Anal Bioanal Chem 390:1659–1169

Dauphin Y, Cuif JP, Salomé M (2014) Structure and composition of the aragonitic shell of a living fossil: *Neotrigonia* (Mollusca, Bivalvia). Eur J Mineral 26:485–494

Farre B, Dauphin Y (2009) Lipids from the nacreous and prismatic layers of two Pteriomorpha mollusc shells. Comp Biochem Physiol B152:103–109

Farre B, Brunelle A, Laprévote O, Cuif JP, Williams CT, Dauphin Y (2011) Shell layers of the black-lip pearl oyster *Pinctada margaritifera*: matching microstructure and composition. Comp Biochem Physiol B. https://doi.org/10.1016/j.cbpb.2011.03.001

Hovden R, Wolf SE, Holtz ME, Marin F, Muller DA, Estroff L (2015) Nanoscale assembly processes revealed in the nacroprismatic transition zone of *Pinna nobilis* mollusc shells. Nature Comm 6:10097. https://doi.org/10.1038/ncomms10097

Kocot KM, McDougall C, Degnan BM (2016) Developing perspectives on molluscan shells, part 1: introduction and molecular biology. In: Saleuddin S, Mukai S (eds) Physiology of molluscs: a collection of selected reviews. CRC Press

Mutvei H (1963) On the shells of *Nautilus* and *Spirula* with notes on the shell secretion in non-cephalopod molluscs. Arkiv Zool 16:221–227

Mutvei H (1978) Ultrastructural characteristics of the nacre of some gastropods. Zool Scr 7:287–296

Mutvei H (1979) On the internal structures of the nacreous tablets in molluscan shells. Scan Electron Microsc II:451–462

Samata T (1990) Ca-binding glycoproteins in molluscan shells with different types of ultrastructure. Veliger 33:190–201

Simkiss K (2016) Developing perspectives on molluscan shells, part 2: cellular aspects. In: Saleuddin S, Mukai S (eds) Physiology of molluscs: a collection of selected reviews. CRC Press

Suzuki M, Nagasawa H (2013) Mollusk shell structures and their formation mechanism. Can J Zool 91:349–366

Taylor JD, Kennedy WJ, Hall A (1969) The shell structure and mineralogy of the Bivalvia. I. Introduction. Nuculacae – Trigonacae. Bull Br Mus Nat Hist Zool 3:1–125

Taylor JD, Kennedy WJ, Hall A (1973) The shell structure and mineralogy of the Bivalvia. II. Lucinacea – Clavagellacea. Conclusions. Bull Br Mus nat hist Zool 22:253–294

Wise SWJ (1970) Microarchitecture and mode of formation of nacre (mother-of-pearl) in pelecypods, gastropods and cephalopods. Eclogae Geol Helv 63:775–797

Chapter 37
The Marsh's Membrane: A Key-Role for a Forgotten Structure

Jean-Pierre Cuif and Yannicke Dauphin

Abstract Recent imaging methods applied to the growing edge of the *Pinctada margaritifera* shell allow for a better appreciation of ancient structural data. Growth of the *Pinctada* shell (both lateral extension and thickness increase) is a coordinated mechanism involving a series of clearly identified steps in contrast to the prevailing concept of a direct "self-assembly" process.

Keywords Periostracal transit · Flexible shell · Layered growth mode · Marsh membrane

37.1 Introduction

In contrast to Wada (1961) or Wilbur (1964) who recognized the importance of a specific structural phase predating the prismatic layer of mollusk shells (Fig. 37.1a), most modern investigators propose microstructural schemes in which the calcite prisms and their organic envelopes are directly and simultaneously produced at the growing edges of the shells (Saleuddin and Petit 1983; Volkmer 2007; Soldati et al. 2008). These models share the surprising ability of the prisms to continue to grow after having been covered by the nacreous layer. This is also the case in the scheme initiated by Petit (1978) and repeated up to Calvo-Iglesias et al. (2016, fig. 10) who summarized the concept of a remotely controlled formation of the prismatic layer: "Molecules secreted into the extrapallial cavity would be self-assembled and they reach the shell growing area without the participation of any cell."

J.-P. Cuif (✉)
Centre de recherche sur la paléodiversité et les paléoenvironnements, CR2P – UMR 7207, Museum National d'Histoire Naturelle, Paris, France

Y. Dauphin
Institut de systématique, Evolution, Biodiversité, ISYEB – UMR 7205, Muséum national d'Histoire naturelle, Paris, France
e-mail: Yannicke.dauphin@upmc.fr

K. Endo et al. (eds.), *Biomineralization*,
https://doi.org/10.1007/978-981-13-1002-7_37

In such models, no place exists for the "innermost shell lamella" described by Marsh and Sass (1983) as "a single continuous layer which forms the inner surface of the shell … firmly attached to the mineral in the underlying calcified layer".

Here, through a microstructural approach of the growing edge of a prismatic shell layer, an attempt is made to establish a junction between the several decade-old observations clearly neglected in current literature.

37.2 Material and Methods

Adult pearl oysters (*Pinctada margaritifera*) were collected alive in Tuamotu archipelago. Young samples come from the hatchery of the Direction des Ressources Marines et Minières (DRMM, the Polynesian governmental office for pearl cultivation).

Observations were carried out with optical microscopy (natural and polarized light), scanning electron microscopy in both secondary and backscattered electron modes, and atomic force microscopy in tapping mode. X-ray diffraction measurements were performed at the ID13 beam line of the ESRF (Grenoble).

37.3 Results

37.3.1 Structure of the Flexible Shell Initiated and Developed in the Periostracal Grove

On the internal side of the periostracal film, numerous nonadjacent mineral disks are visible and regularly distributed (Fig. 37.1b, c). Every disk is growing around a non-mineralized center (Fig. 37.1d, arrows). The concentric mode of growth of the disks is visible of the outer side (Fig. 37.1e), whereas their inner side reveals a continuous granular structure (Fig. 37.1f). Using transmitted polarized light, the disks appear homogenous, each of them with a specific nuance always in the gray levels of the Newton scale (Fig. 37.1g). The single-crystal behavior of the disks is well

Fig. 37.1 (continued) disks are clearly visible (**d**: arrows); Bar 30 μm (**c**), 15 μm (**d**). (**e**) Central nodule surrounded by concentric growth layers. Bar 8 μm. (**f**) Granular appearance of the inner surface of a disk. Bar 6 μm. (**g**) Optical view of disks (transmitted polarized light). Note the homogeneity of the gray levels for every disk. Bar 15 μm. (**h–i**) Three series of nine points where X-ray diffraction was carried out on a single disk. Note the superposition of the diffraction spots (**i**). (**j–l**) Series of growing disks. Thickness does not increase during diametral growth; periostracum almost completely discarded excepted in left part of the picture. Bar 20 μm. (**m**) The flexible shell at the end of the periostracal phase, just before passage to the rigid shell status. Note the 3 μm thickness of the disks. Bar 50 μm. (**n**) Scheme of a section of the shell growing edge cut perpendicularly to shell surface. Focus is made on the transit of the disks carried on the internal side of the periostracum, from deposition of the disk organic centers (*oc*) up to the upside-down movement (*ud*, arrow) by which the disks become the initial substrates for prism growth

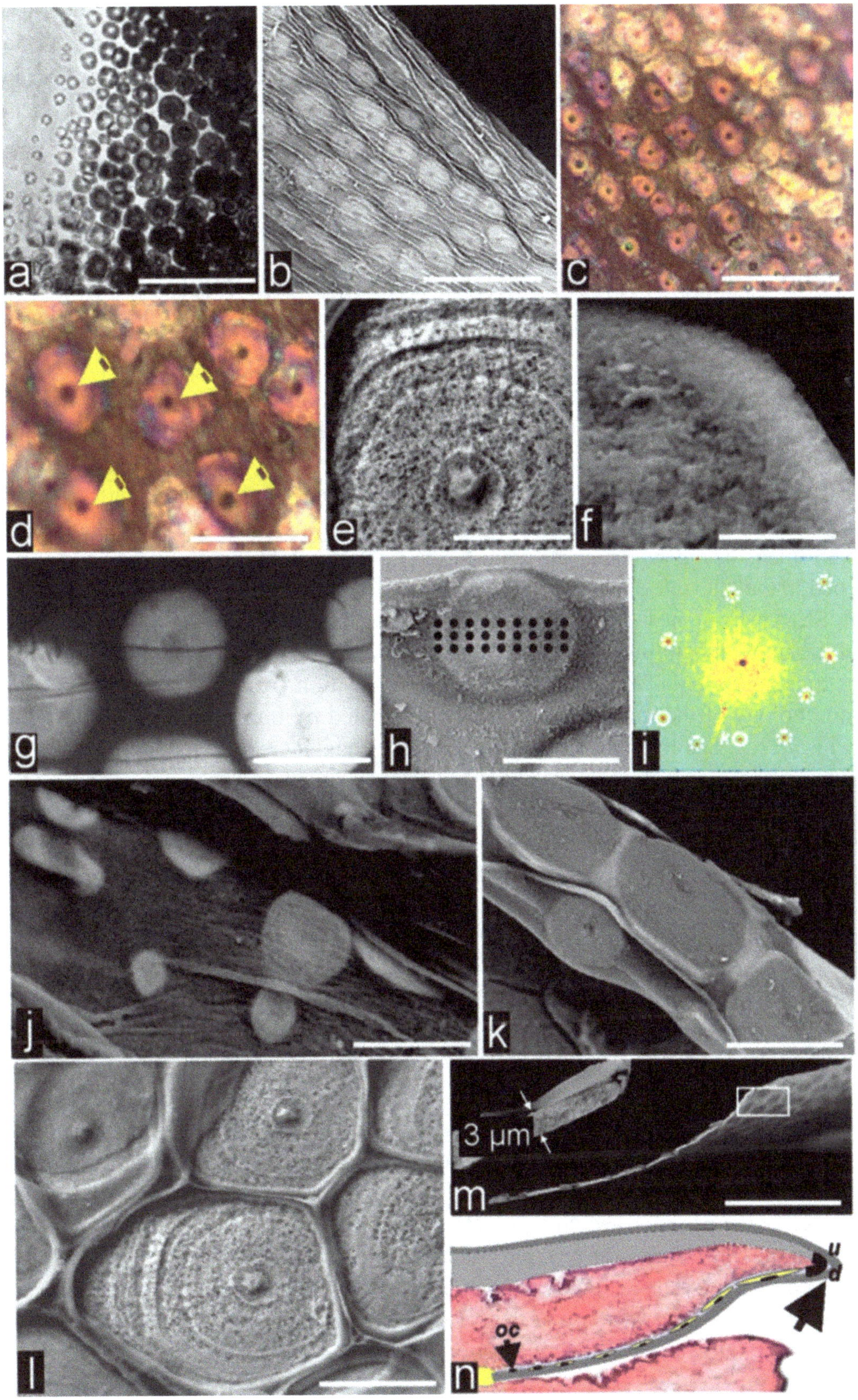

Fig. 37.1 (**a**) Wada (1961) reprinted in Wilbur (1964). Growing edge surface of a *Pinctada fucata* shell viewed in transmitted polarized light. Bar 50 µm. (**b**) SEM view of the outer surface of the periostracal membrane. Through the membrane the growing disks are visible. Note their centers. Bar 30 µm. (**c–d**) Optical view of an equivalent area (episcopic polarized light). Centers of the

established by the perfect superposition of the spots in a series of 27 X-ray diffractions in a single disk (Fig. 37.1h, i). Through their concentric growth mode during their transportation by the periostracum acting as a conveyor belt, the disks reach their maximal size, becoming in close contact at the distal end of the periostracal grove (Fig. 37.1j–m). Their thickness remains about 3–4 μm (Fig. 37.1m, n, black arrow).

37.3.2 Transition from Flexible to Rigid Shell: Occurrence of a New Growth Mode

The distal end of the periostracal transit is a turning point in shell formation. Through an upside-down movement, the disks are placed in geometrical continuity with the previously built "rigid shell." By this movement, the internal sides of the disks (with non-mineralized centers) become the outer side of the shell growing edge. The outer surface of the shell growing edge shows the roughly circular crests, the dimensions of which correspond to the final stages of the discoid units developed in the "flexible shell" stage (Fig. 37.2a).

SEM view of the internal side in the same area reveals the polygonal morphology of the mineral building units (Fig. 37.2b) whose single crystal behavior is obvious in transmitted polarized light (Fig. 37.2c). Transition from discoid to polygonal morphology of the mineral units is well illustrated by transmitted polarized light (Fig. 37.2d). The limits of the previously discoid units are still visible (Fig. 37.2d: blue arrows), while the mineral phase has been extended up to become in contact to the neighboring units (Fig. 37.2d: red arrows). This close contact between the newly formed polygonal units ensures the shell rigidity.

This developmental step shows the first occurrence of an additional component of the shell: the internal side of the crystal-like polygonal units is now covered by a continuous organic membrane (Fig. 37.2b: Mm) so that the mineral phase is sandwiched between the external periostracum and this internal organic membrane. Simultaneously, a completely different biomineralization pattern can be observed. Instead of an individual lateral extension of the disks, mineralization occurs as a synchronic process insuring a simultaneous increase of shell thickness (Fig. 37.2e). Once more, the organic film is visible at the internal side of the polygonal units (Fig. 37.2e, arrows). It is still present (Fig. 37.2f, arrows) when the repeated layered growth process leads the thickness of these calcareous units to be superior to their lateral dimensions, justifying the term "prism." Closer observations of the basal surface of the prisms leave no doubt about the presence of this well-individualized membrane (Fig. 37.2g, arrows). This membrane, permanently present at the internal surface of the prisms, exhibits a granular structure rather similar to the granular structure of the mineral phase of the prisms (Fig. 37.2h–j).

37.4 Discussion

37.4.1 Inadequacy of the "Direct Crystallization" Model to Account for Formation of the Prismatic Layer in the Pinctada *Shell*

The "molecular self-assembly process" underlying recent schemes and explicitly formulated by Calvo-Iglesias et al. (2016) cannot be applied to the outer shell layer of the *Pinctada margaritifera*. The two-phase mechanism briefly described in the present report was suggested by Wada (1961, Figure 8) and Wilbur (1964, Figure 10), who observed circular crystalline units growing "in oolitic aggregation" becoming progressively polygonal by mutual contact. The crystalline properties of the mineral units forming the "flexible shell" were established by Suzuki et al. (2013), but the presence of a non-mineralized center in each of these calcareous units basically modifies the interpretation of their formation and role.

37.4.2 Origin of the Crystallographic Individuality of the Calcite Prisms of the Pinctada *Shell*

From the deeper parts of the periostracal grove, the calcareous disks transported on the internal side of the periostracum exhibit a non-mineral center, suggesting that this organic glomerule was deposited in close vicinity to the group of cells dedicated to the formation of the periostracum itself (see histological sections in Jabbour et al. 1992). Polarization microscopy and multiple X-ray diffractions show that, in conformity to the results of Suzuki et al. (2013), the disks are crystal-like units, each of them with a specific crystalline orientation (assessed by the distinct gray levels corresponding to a 3–4 μm thickness measured by SEM; Fig. 37.1m). It can be assumed that these specific crystalline orientations take origin in the slightly diverse orientations of the organic substrates of the disks.

From this very early origin of crystallographic orientation in the transitional phase from flexible to rigid shells (Fig. 37.2d), the crystallographic orientation of the first mineral polygons forming the rigid shell relies on the crystallographic orientation of the disks after their upside-down movement. In further growth steps of the prisms, crystallographic orientation of every newly formed polygon is repeated.

Thus, conclusion arises that the long-recognized crystal-like behavior of the prisms forming the outer shell layer of the *Pinctada* is determined in the deeper part of the periostracal grove and is by no means the result of a "self-assembly process."

37.4.3 The Crystal-Like Disks as Examples of Non-Ion-by-Ion Crystallization

In the search of evidences for a biological control of crystallization, we must note that all along their growth, the freely and independently crystallizing disks exhibit a concentric layering as obvious traces of their stepping growth mode. If disk crystallization was based on an ion-by-ion mechanism, the presence of calcite faces oriented in conformity with those of crystals produced by purely chemical precipitation should appear in these distant and freely growing units. This is not the case: no exception has been observed to the circular morphology and concentric mode of growth for the crystal-like units. This provides a contrario evidence for a nonionic but biochemically controlled mode of crystallization (i.e., non-purely chemical).

37.4.4 The Marsh's Membrane as Coordinator of the Layered Growth Mode of the Prisms

Occurrence of the organic membrane covering the newly formed polygons (Fig. 37.2e) and its persistency during further development of the prisms introduce a new factor to be taken into account in the crystallization process. Its granular structure was noted from the early descriptions (Fig. 37.2k) and among the very rare mentions that have been made of this shell component. Yan et al. (2008) have well noted the time-based variability in the development of these grains, leading these authors to qualify the Marsh's membrane as a "dynamic structure." This means that the Marsh's membrane is involved in the mineralization process, a conclusion here confirmed (Fig. 37.2g–j) and by previous observations (Cuif et al. 2014).

One of the most striking features of the calcite prisms in *Pinctada margaritifera* is the microstructural change that regularly occurs after about 150 μm growth length. After an initial stage with a single crystal structure (Fig. 37.2l), the prisms become polycrystalline (Fig. 37.2m) (Cuif et al. 2011, 2014; Checa et al. 2013).

Fig. 37.2 (continued) the front raw and the changing colors revealing the increasing thickness of the polygonal units. Bar 50 μm. (**d**) Formation of the rigid shell: limits of the disks, still visible by the round-shaped trace (blue arrows), are overcome by new mineral deposits that bring the neighbor units in close contact (red arrows). Transmitted polarized light; Bar 20 μm. (**e**) The Marsh's membrane is visible at the base of the newly formed polygons (arrows). Note the decayed periostracum making visible the outer surface of the initial disks and their centers. Bar 10 μm. (**f**) The Marsh's membrane at the inner surface of young prisms. Compare to picture of the compartment lamella by Bevelander and Nakahara (1980). Bar 25 μm. (**g**) Closer view of the Marsh's membrane. Note the transversal striation and the granular structure. Bar 5 μm. (**h–j**) Aspect of the Marsh's membrane: h, SEM view, Bar, 5 μm; i, SEM view, Bar, 2 μm; j, AFM view, Bar, 150 nm. (**k**) Reprint of a Marsh figure (TEM). Note the granular pattern of the Marsh membrane, corresponding to the high-resolution SEM view here reported. Bar: 0.5 μm. (**l–m**) Thin sections (transmitted polarized light) in the upper part of prisms (up to 150 μm) and in their lower part. Note the passage from single crystal-like to polycrystalline organization. Bar: 50 μm (l) and 30 μm (m)

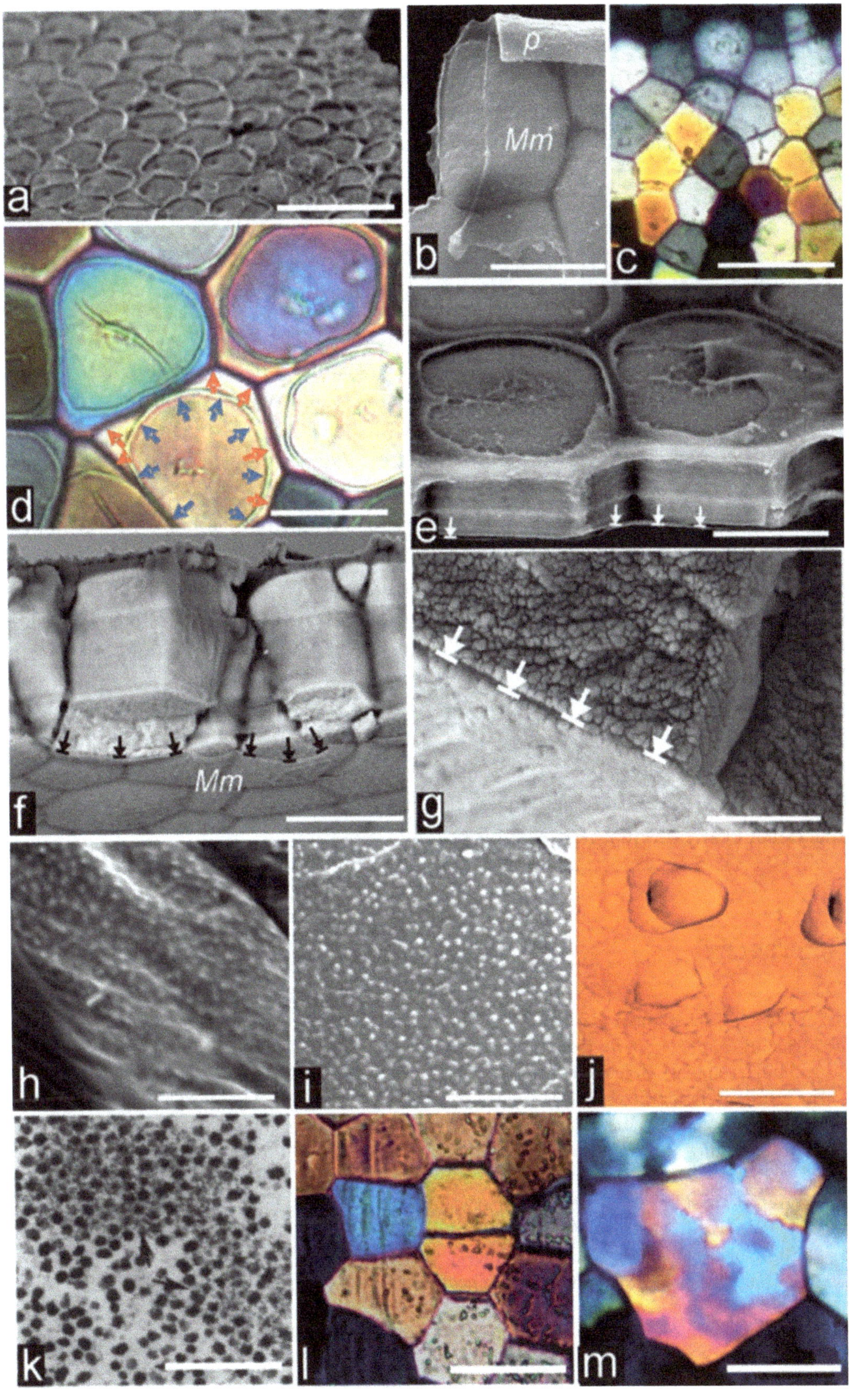

Fig. 37.2 (**a**) SEM view of the outer surface of the rigid shell at its growing edge. Bar 30 μm. (**b**) Internal side of a polygonal unit at the distal raw of the rigid shell. Mm: organic membrane. SEM view, Bar 25 μm. (**c**) Polygonal units in transmitted polarized light. Note the various gray levels in

Such a coordinated change contradicts the theory of "crystal growth competition" that postulates a selection of the best oriented crystals leading to a progressive increase of the mean diameter in a given shell.

37.4.5 *The Key Role of the Marsh's Membrane in Microstructural Evolution of the Prisms*

Pinctada calcite prisms are submitted to microstructural changes during aging (Cuif et al. 2014), and composition of both the mineral and organic phases is modified before the occurrence of nacre deposition (Cuif et al. 2011). Microstructural variations of the prisms during shell growth provide evidence for time-based genetically programmed secretion process.

What is remarkable is that the repeated back-and-forth movements of the mantle due to the rhythmic mode of life of the animal leave no trace in prism microstructure. This contrast epitomizes the key role of the Marsh's membrane in shell formation. When the animal withdraws its mantle for shell closure, the Marsh's membrane stays in place at the basis of the prismatic layer. Thus, when the mantle returns to an actively mineralizing position, growth of the microstructural units (each of them with its specific crystalline orientation) can restart without any apparent interruption.

Under many respects understanding the Marsh's membrane as an active interface between mantle secretions and shell is an important issue for both microstructural analysis and any attempt to create biomimetic materials.

References

Bevelander G, Nakahara H (1980) Compartment and envelope formation in the process of biological mineralization. In: Omori M, Watabe N (eds) The mechanisms of biomineralization in animals and plants. Tokai University Press, Kanagawa

Calvo-Iglesias J, Pérez-Estévez D, Lorenzo-Abalde S, Sánchez-Correa B, Quiroga María I, Fuentes José M, González-Fernández A (2016) Characterization of a monoclonal antibody directed against *Mytilus spp.* larvae reveals an antigen involved in shell biomineralization. PLoS One 11:1–17. https://doi.org/10.1371/journal.pone.0152210

Checa AG, Bonarski JT, Willinger MG, Faryna M, Berent K, Kania B, Gonzalez-Segura A, Pina CM, Pospiech J, Morawiec A (2013) Crystallographic orientation inhomogeneity and crystal splitting in biogenic calcite. J R Soc Interface 10:20130425

Cuif JP, Dauphin Y, Sorauf JE (2011) Biominerals and fossils through time. Cambridge University Press, Cambridge, 490 p

Cuif JP, Burghammer M, Chamard V, Dauphin Y, Godard P, Le Moullac G, Nehrke G, Perez-Huerta A (2014) Evidence of a biological control over origin, growth and end of the calcite prisms in the shells of *Pinctada margaritifera* (Pelecypod, Pterioidea). Minerals 4:815–834

Jabbour-Zahab J, Chagot D, Blanc F, Grizel H (1992) Mantle histology, histochemistry and ultrastructure of the pearl oyster *Pinctada margaritifera* (L.). Aquat Living Resour 5:287–298

Marsh ME, Sass RL (1983) Calcium-binding phosphoprotein particles in the extrapallial fluid and innermost shell lamella of clams. J Exp Zool 226:193–203

Petit H (1978) Recherches sur des séquences d'évènements périostracaux lors de l'élaboration de la coquille *d'Amblema plicata* Conrad, 1834. Thèse, Laboratoire de Zoologie, Université de Bretagne occidentale, 276 pp

Saleuddin ASM, Petit H (1983) The mode of formation and the structure of the periostracum. In: Saleuddin ASM, Wilbur KM (eds) The Mollusca. Academic, New York

Soldati AL, Jacob DE, Wehrmeister U, Hofmeister W (2008) Structural characterization and chemical composition of aragonite and vaterite in freshwater cultured pearls. Mineral Mag 72:577–590

Suzuki M, Nakayama S, Nagasawa H, Kogure T (2013) Initial formation of calcite crystals in the thin prismatic layer with the periostracum of *Pinctada fucata*. Micron 45:136–139

Volkmer D (2007) Biologically inspired crystallization of calcium carbonate beneath monolayers: a critical overview. In: Behrens P, Baeuerlein E (eds) Handbook of biomineralization: biomimetic and bioinspired chemistry. Wiley, Hoboken

Wada K (1961) Crystal growth of molluscan shells. Bull Natl Pearl Res Lab 36:703–782

Wilbur KM (1964) Shell formation and regeneration. In: Wilbur KM, Owen G (eds) Physiology of mollusca. Academic, New York

Yan Z, Ma Z, Zheng G, Feng Q, Wang H, Xie L, Zhang R (2008) The inner shell-film: an immediate structure participating in Pearl Oyster formation. Chembiochem. https://doi.org/10.1002/CBC.200700553

Chapter 38
Pearl Production by Implantation of Outer Epithelial Cells Isolated from the Mantle of *Pinctada fucata* and the Effects of Blending of Epithelial Cells with Different Genetic Backgrounds on Pearl Quality

Masahiko Awaji, Takashi Yamamoto, Yasunori Iwahashi, Kiyohito Nagai, Fumihiro Hattori, Kaoru Maeyama, Makoto Kakinuma, Shigeharu Kinoshita, and Shugo Watabe

Abstract In the current method of pearl production, the mantle fragment of a donor pearl oyster is transplanted into a host pearl oyster together with an inorganic bead (pearl nucleus). After this surgical procedure, only outer epithelial cells (OEC) in the transplanted mantle survive in a host pearl oyster and form a pearl sac to begin pearl formation. Therefore, implantation of only the OEC instead of the mantle fragment would be a possible alternative to the current procedure. To examine the potential of pearl production by implanting OEC in *Pinctada fucata*, we developed

M. Awaji (✉)
National Research Institute of Aquaculture, Japan Fisheries Research and Education Agency, Minami-Ise, Japan
e-mail: awajim@affrc.go.jp

T. Yamamoto · Y. Iwahashi · K. Nagai
Pearl Research Laboratory, K. MIKIMOTO & CO., LTD, Shima, Japan
e-mail: kenkyujo@mikimoto.com; y-iwahashi@mikimoto.com; k-nagai@mikimoto.com

F. Hattori · K. Maeyama
MIKIMOTO COSMETICS, Mie, Japan
e-mail: hattori.468@mikimoto-cosme.com; maeyama.511@mikimoto-cosme.com

M. Kakinuma
Graduate School of Bioresources, Mie University, Tsu, Mie, Japan
e-mail: kakinuma@bio.mie-u.ac.jp

S. Kinoshita
Department of Aquatic Bioscience, Graduate School of Agricultural and Life Sciences, The University of Tokyo, Tokyo, Japan
e-mail: akino@mail.ecc.u-tokyo.ac.jp

S. Watabe
School of Marine Biosciences, Kitasato University, Minami, Sagamihara, Kanagawa, Japan
e-mail: swatabe@kitasato-u.ac.jp

K. Endo et al. (eds.), *Biomineralization*,
https://doi.org/10.1007/978-981-13-1002-7_38

a cell implantation method using the pearl nucleus carrying a small pit inoculated with OEC. As a result, approximately 70% of the inserted nuclei formed the nacreous layer when the OEC were inoculated at 5×10^4 cells/nucleus. Then, OEC isolated from two genetically different types of pearl oysters that significantly differed in shell nacre color (yellowness) were mixed at four different ratios, and the prepared OEC mixtures were transplanted to investigate the effects of the blend on the yellowness of pearls to be harvested. The yellowness of harvested pearls differed significantly in accordance with the mixing ratio. Similarly, OEC isolated from two types of pearl oysters that showed a significant difference in the thickness of their shell nacre aragonite tablets were mixed at four different ratios and transplanted. Mean thickness of the aragonite tablets of the harvested pearls differed according to mixing ratio. These results suggest the method to control pearl quality by blending OEC obtained from pearl oysters genetically improved by selective breeding for traits related to pearl quality.

Keywords Pearl oyster · Outer epithelial cells · Implantation · Blending · Yellowness · Aragonite tablets

38.1 Introduction

Currently, the method of pearl production using pearl oyster *Pinctada fucata* involves transplanting a small fragment of the mantle of a donor pearl oyster into a host pearl oyster together with a small shell bead called a pearl nucleus (Masaoka et al. 2013). After transplantation, only outer epithelial cells (OEC) in the transplanted mantle fragment survive in the host pearl oyster and form a pearl sac surrounding the pearl nucleus to begin pearl formation (Awaji and Suzuki 1995). Therefore, implantation of only OEC instead of the mantle fragment would be a possible alternative to the current pearl production procedure.

Quality of a pearl is determined by various traits: size, color, luster, shape, and blemish (Jerry et al. 2012; Atsumi et al. 2014). Among these traits, color is mainly developed by the amount of yellow pigments and the interference color of pearl nacre. The amount of yellow pigment in nacre is known to be largely affected by the genetic backgrounds of a donor pearl oyster (Wada 1985). The interference color is determined by thickness of the aragonite tablets of pearl nacre, which is also affected by the genetic backgrounds of a donor pearl oyster combined with water temperature and nutritional condition of a host pearl oyster (Linard et al. 2011; Muhammad et al. 2017; Odawara et al. 2017). Therefore, if we can produce pearls by implanting OEC, it might be possible to control yellowness or the interference color of pearls by blending the OEC isolated from donor pearl oysters with different genetic backgrounds regarding these traits.

To assess the possibility of these technical improvements in pearl production, we developed a method to produce pearls by implanting OEC and examined the effects of blending of OEC isolated from donor pearl oysters with different genetic backgrounds on the yellowness and interference color of pearls.

38.2 Materials and Methods

38.2.1 Implantation of a Pearl Nucleus with Outer Epithelial Cells into a Host Pearl Oyster

OEC were separated from the mantle of a pearl oyster by the methods described in Awaji and Machii (2011). Briefly, a pallial zone of the pearl oyster mantle was excised out and washed in sterile balanced salt solution for marine mollusks (BSS, Awaji and Machii 2011) containing 1 mg/ml of kanamycin sulfate (11815-024, Thermo Fisher Scientific K.K., Yokohama, Japan) with several changes of the medium. Then the mantle strips were digested for 6 h at 25 °C with a mixture of 1.25 mg/ml of dispase (17105-041, Thermo Fisher Scientific K.K.) and 0.5 mg/ml of collagenase (034-10533, Wako Pure Chemical Industries, Ltd., Osaka, Japan) in sterile BSS buffered at pH 7.5 with 20 mM HEPES (346-01373, Wako Pure Chemical Industries, Ltd.). After the digestion, the outer epithelium on an outer side of the mantle strip was carefully peeled off using forceps under a binocular microscope. The obtained outer epithelium was washed in the buffered BSS containing 0.4 mg/ml of hyaluronidase (151272, MP Biomedicals, LLC, Santa Ana, USA) to prepare suspension of the OEC clusters (Fig. 38.1a). Cell density was determined by staining cell nuclei with 0.1% crystal violet in 0.1 M citric acid (Sanford et al. 1951). Briefly, precipitated cell clusters were incubated in 0.5 ml of the crystal violet solution for 1 h at room temperature with agitation, and the number of cell nuclei stained dark blue with the dye was counted using a hemocyte counter. For pearl production, 1 μl of OEC suspension (1–5 × 10^4 cells/μl) was inoculated into a small pit (1 mm diameter and 0.5–1.0 mm depth) of a pearl nucleus (4.5 mm diameter, Fig. 38.1b), and the pearl nucleus was inserted into a host pearl oyster, as described in Awaji et al. (2014).

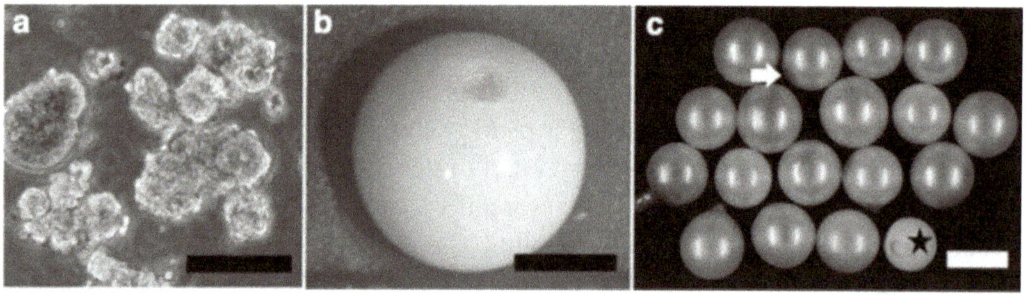

Fig. 38.1 Pearl formation by implanting outer epithelial cells isolated from a pearl oyster mantle. (**a**) Suspension of outer epithelial cell clusters prepared for implantation; (**b**) a pearl nucleus carrying a small pit; (**c**) pearls formed by the implantation of a pearl nucleus carrying a pit inoculated with outer epithelial cells. A white arrow indicates a dimple formed on the surface of a pearl at the site of a pit. A black star denotes a pearl nucleus harvested from a host oyster without pearl layers. Scale = 100 μm (**a**), 2 mm (**b**), 5 mm (**c**)

38.2.2 *Effects of the Blending of Outer Epithelial Cells on Yellowness of Pearls*

Several strains of *P. fucata* genetically different in shell nacre color have been maintained at Mikimoto Pearl Research Laboratory. Among these strains, strains Y and W are significantly different in yellowness of the shell nacre, strain Y being yellowish, while strain W being whitish. We used these two strains for the experiment. OEC isolated from these strains were blended at four different mixing ratios (Y:W = 3:0, 2:1, 1:2, 0:3) and implanted for pearl production at 6.0×10^5 cells/nucleus. The host pearl oysters were reared in Ago Bay, Mie Prefecture, for 5 months until pearl harvesting. Yellowness of the harvested pearls was measured using a fast spectrophotometric color meter (CMS-35SP, Murakami Color Research Laboratory, Tokyo, Japan) and expressed as yellowness index (YI, $YI=(1.250X-1.038Z)/Y$), where X, Y, and Z represent tristimulus values of CIE 1931 XYZ color space, as described in Awaji et al. (2014).

38.2.3 *Effects of the Blending of Outer Epithelial Cells on the Thickness of the Pearls' Aragonite Tablets*

Strains YW and BWW are genetically different in terms of thickness of shell aragonite tablets, and the interference color of shell nacre differs between these strains. OEC were isolated from these strains and blended at the same ratios as in the experiment on yellowness. The blended cells were implanted for pearl production at 5.0×10^4 cells/nucleus. The host pearl oysters were reared in Ago Bay for 5 months until pearl harvesting. Thickness of the aragonite tablets of harvested pearls was calculated from the images obtained with a color 3D laser microscope (VK-9700, Keyence Corporation, Osaka, Japan) and a scanning electron microscope (S-2380N, Hitachi High Technologies Corporation, Tokyo, Japan) using VK-H1A1 software (Keyence Corporation) and ImageJ1.50-b, respectively.

38.3 Results

38.3.1 *Pearl Production by Implantation of Outer Epithelial Cells*

Nacreous pearls could be produced by the implantation of OEC, and the inoculation of 5×10^4 cells/nucleus led to formation of aragonite layers in approximately 70% of the inserted nuclei (Awaji et al. 2014). An example of the harvested pearls is shown in Fig. 38.1c.

38.3.2 *Effects of the Blending of Outer Epithelial Cells on Yellowness of Pearls*

The harvested pearls were different in terms of yellowness (Fig. 38.2a). Blending of OEC from strains Y and W at the ratio of 2 to 1 (Y2+W1 in Fig. 38.2a, b) showed significantly higher yellowness than the 0 to 3 group (Y0+W3), and the 1 to 2 group (Y1+W2) was considered intermediate yellowness (Awaji et al. 2014). This result

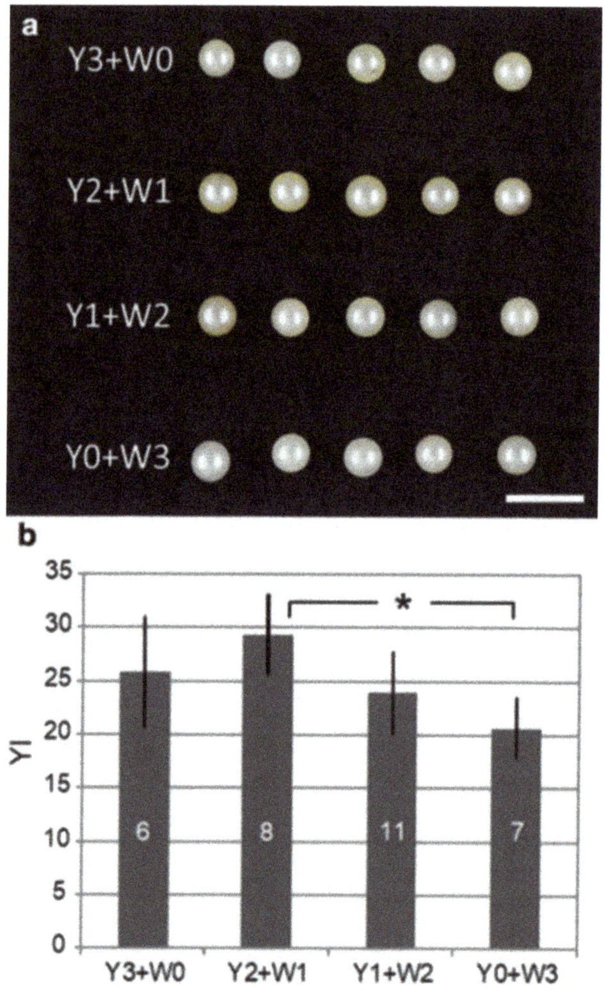

Fig. 38.2 Effects on the yellowness of harvested pearls of blending the outer epithelial cells isolated from two pearl oyster strains that significantly differed in shell nacre yellowness. The outer epithelial cells from the strains with yellow (Y) or white nacre (W) were mixed at four different ratios and transplanted into host oysters with the pearl nucleus carrying a pit. (**a**) A photograph showing difference in the yellowness of pearls harvested from four experimental groups. Scale = 10 mm; (**b**) the yellowness of the pearls expressed by the yellowness index (YI). Numbers in the columns indicate the sample size, and bars indicate 95% confidence limits of the average. An asterisk indicates a significant difference (Steel-Dwass test, $p < 0.05$). (Cited from Awaji et al. 2014)

implied that we could modify the yellowness of pearls by the blending of OEC isolated from genetically different pearl oyster strains.

38.3.3 *Effects of the Blending of Outer Epithelial Cells on the Thickness of the Pearls' Aragonite Tablets*

Blending of OEC from strains YW and BWW caused difference in the thickness of the aragonite tablets of nacre. In the observations by scanning electron microscopy, implantation of OEC from strains YW and BWW at the blending ratio of 3 to 0 (YW3+BWW0) or 0 to 3 (YW0+BWW3) resulted in significant difference in the tablet thickness, and the groups with the blending ratio of 2 to 1 (YW2+BWW1) or 1 to 2 (YW1+BWW2) showed intermediate thickness (Fig. 38.3). The surface structure of the nacreous pearls could be observed clearly with a color 3D laser microscope. On this surface, a significant difference in the thickness of the aragonite tablets was observed in accordance with the mixing ratio, with the blended groups showing intermediate thickness. These results implied that we could modify the thickness of the aragonite tablets, namely, the interference color of the pearls, by the blending of OEC.

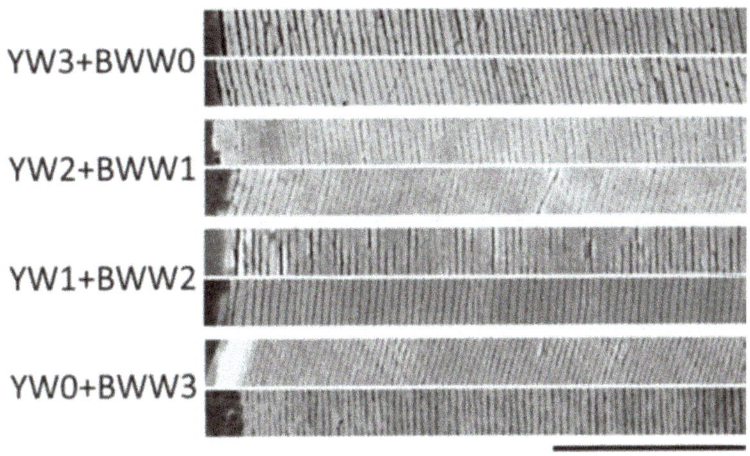

Fig. 38.3 Scanning electron microscopy images showing effects on the thickness of aragonite tablets in the pearl nacre of blending the outer epithelial cells isolated from two pearl oyster strains that significantly differed in the thickness of aragonite tablets of shell nacre. The outer epithelial cells from the strains with thick (YW) or thin (BWW) aragonite tablets were mixed at four different ratios and transplanted into host oysters with the pearl nucleus carrying a pit. Pearl surface is located to the left. Scale = 10 μm

38.4 Discussion

The obtained results indicate that we could modify the color of pearls by implanting blended OEC isolated from pearl oysters with genetically different phenotypes for pearl color traits. Intermediate phenotypes observed in the blended groups suggest that OEC isolated from two different strains can survive in a host pearl oyster to form a chimeric pearl sac after the implantation. Further studies to confirm the chimeric formation of a pearl sac by the blended OEC are needed, by using, for example, genomic DNA markers that can identify the origin of OEC (Masaoka et al. 2013). The practical use of the OEC implantation for pearl culture, however, is still challenging since a pit of a pearl nucleus remains as a dimple on the surface of a harvested pearl. OEC implantation methods without making a pit on a pearl nucleus are needed.

Pearl formation by the implantation of OEC would also serve to clarify mechanisms underlying shell and pearl formation at a molecular level in combination with gene transfection technologies. Various genes and molecules have been reported to be involved in shell formation, but details of their function have remained mostly unknown. Implantation of OEC transfected with a gene of interest for its overexpression would be a novel tool to analyze functions of the target gene. Gene transfection techniques effective for OEC are now under investigation.

For pearl oysters, breeding programs to develop superior donor and host pearl oyster strains are ongoing (Jerry et al. 2012; Wada 1985). The present studies became possible because several strains that exhibit different phenotypes for nacre color traits have been established through breeding programs. Although the use of pearl oyster strains showing different phenotypes for traits related to shell structures has been uncommon in shell formation studies, they would serve as novel tools for clarifying the mechanisms that underlie shell and pearl formation in detail.

Acknowledgment Part of this study was supported by JSPS KAKENHI Grant Numbers JP23658169, JP26292108, JP17K19282.

References

Atsumi T, Ishikawa T, Inoue N, Ishibashi R, Aoki H, Abe H, Kamiya N, Komaru A (2014) Post-operative care of implanted pearl oysters *Pinctada fucata* in low salinity seawater improves the quality of pearls. Aquaculture 422–423:232–238

Awaji M, Machii A (2011) Fundamental studies on in vivo and in vitro pearl formation – contribution of outer epithelial cells of pearl oyster mantle and pearl sacs. Aqua BioSci Monogr 4:1–39

Awaji M, Suzuki T (1995) The pattern of cell proliferation during pearl sac formation in the pearl oyster. Fish Sci 61:747–751

Awaji M, Yamamoto T, Kakinuma M, Nagai K, Watabe S (2014) Pearl formation by transplantation of outer epithelial cells isolated from the mantle of pearl oyster *Pinctada fucata*. Nippon Suisan Gakkaishi 80:578–588 (in Japanese with English abstract)

Jerry DR, Kvingedal R, Lind CE, Evans BS, Taylor JJU, Safari AE (2012) Donor-oyster derived heritability estimates and the effect of genotype environment interaction on the production of pearl quality traits in the silver-lip pearl oyster, *Pinctada maxima*. Aquaculture 338–341:66–71

Linard C, Gueguen Y, Moriceau J, Soyez C, Hui B, Raoux A, Cuif JP, Cochard J-C, Le Pennec M, Le Moullac G (2011) Calcein staining of calcified structures in pearl oyster *Pinctada margaritifera* and the effect of food resource level on shell growth. Aquaculture 313:149–155

Masaoka T, Samata T, Nogawa C, Baba H, Aoki H, Kotaki T, Nakagawa A, Sato M, Fujiwara A, Kobayashi T (2013) Shell matrix protein genes derived from donor expressed in pearl sac of Akoya pearl oysters (*Pinctada fucata*) under pearl culture. Aquaculture 384–387:56–65

Muhammad G, Atsumi T, Sunardi KA (2017) Nacre growth and thickness of Akoya pearls from Japanese and hybrid *Pinctada fucata* in response to the aquaculture temperature condition in Ago Bay, Japan. Aquaculture 477:35–42

Odawara K, Ozaki R, Takagi M (2017) Influence of the thickness of the nacreous elemental lamina of the pearl oyster *Pinctada fucata* used as donor oysters on the pearls. Nippon Suisan Gakkaishi. https://doi.org/10.2331/suisan.16-00090 (in Japanese with English abstract)

Sanford KK, Earle WR, Evans VJ (1951) The measurement of proliferation in tissue culture by enumeration of cell nuclei. J Natl Cancer Inst 11:773–795

Wada KT (1985) The pearls produced from the groups of pearl oysters selected for color of nacre in shell for two generations. Bull Natl Res Inst Aquat 7:1–7 (in Japanese with English abstract)

Chapter 39
Functional Analyses of MMP Genes in the Ligament of *Pinctada fucata*

Kazuki Kubota, Yasushi Tsuchihashi, Toshihiro Kogure, Kaoru Maeyama, Fumihiro Hattori, Shigeharu Kinoshita, Shohei Sakuda, Hiromichi Nagasawa, Etsuro Yoshimura, and Michio Suzuki

Abstract The bivalve hinge ligament is the hard tissue that functions to open and close shells. The ligament contains fibrous structures consisting of aragonite crystals surrounded by a dense organic matrix. This organic matrix may contribute to the formation of fibrous aragonite crystals, but the mechanism underlying this formation remains unclear. Recently, we showed that tissue inhibitor of metalloproteinase (TIMP) and matrix metalloproteinase (MMP) is related to the formation of the ligament in *Pinctada fucata*. BLAST search of genome database revealed that seven

K. Kubota · S. Sakuda · H. Nagasawa · M. Suzuki (✉)
Department of Applied Biological Chemistry, Graduate School of Agricultural and Life Sciences, The University of Tokyo, Bunkyo-ku, Tokyo, Japan
e-mail: asakuda@mail.ecc.u-tokyo.ac.jp; anagahi@mail.ecc.u-tokyo.ac.jp; amichiwo@mail.ecc.u-tokyo.ac.jp

Y. Tsuchihashi
Mie Prefecture Fisheries Research Institute, Mie, Japan
e-mail: tsuchy00@pref.mie.jp

T. Kogure
Department of Earth and Planetary Science, The University of Tokyo, Tokyo, Japan
e-mail: kogure@eps.s.u-tokyo.ac.jp

K. Maeyama · F. Hattori
MIKIMOTO COSMETICS, Mie, Japan
e-mail: maeyama.511@mikimoto-cosme.com; hattori.468@mikimoto-cosme.com

S. Kinoshita
Department of Aquatic Bioscience, Graduate School of Agricultural and Life Sciences, The University of Tokyo, Tokyo, Japan
e-mail: akino@mail.ecc.u-tokyo.ac.jp

E. Yoshimura
Department of Applied Biological Chemistry, Graduate School of Agricultural and Life Sciences, The University of Tokyo, Bunkyo-ku, Tokyo, Japan

Department of Liberal Arts, The Open University of Japan, Chiba, Japan
e-mail: ayoshim@mail.ecc.u-tokyo.ac.jp

K. Endo et al. (eds.), *Biomineralization*,
https://doi.org/10.1007/978-981-13-1002-7_39

MMP genes are encoded in the genome of *P. fucata*. To identify the specific MMP that may contribute to ligament formation, the expression level of each MMP was measured in the mantle isthmus, which secretes the ligament. The expression of MMP54089 increased after scratching of the ligament, while the expressions of other MMPs did not increase after doing the same operation. To identify the role of MMP54089 in forming the ligament structure, double-stranded (ds) RNA targeting MMP54089 was injected into the living *P. fucata* to suppress the function of MMP54089. Scanning electron microscopic images showed disordered growing surfaces of the ligament in individuals injected with MMP54089-specific dsRNA. These results suggest that PfTIMP and MMP54089 play important roles in the formation of the fibrous ligament structure.

Keywords Pinctada fucata · Ligament · Matrix metalloproteinase

39.1 Introduction

The components of the ligament are secreted by the mantle isthmus, which is the mantle tissue attached to the shell hinge. Bevelander and Nakahara (1969) reported that small fibrous aragonite crystals and organic frameworks are secreted from cells of the mantle isthmus and align to form long aragonite fibers. These fibers and the organic matrix are connected and transported to the shell to form the ligament microstructure. The crystals grow vertically toward the growing surface of the ligament. In a cross section of the ligament, a pseudohexagonal aragonite crystal was observed (Kahler et al. 1976; Marsh and Sass 1980), which appears to be the euhedral shape of the aragonite crystal. The diameter of the crystal is 50–100 nm, and the *c* axis is parallel to the long axis. In contrast, the *a* and *b* axes are oriented randomly. Aragonite crystals with the defect of {110} twinning were observed in the ligament (Kahler et al. 1976; Marsh and Sass 1980).

Suzuki et al. (2015) reported that the aragonite crystals in the ligament of *P. fucata* contain ligament intracrystalline peptide (LICP). LICP regulates the growth of the aragonite crystal and maintains the orientation of the *c* axis to keep the aragonite crystals small. These small aragonite crystals can be aligned in the same direction and stacked to form aragonite fibers. The mechanism by which these small crystals are gathered and arranged in the organic matrix of the ligament is still unknown. To reveal the mechanisms underlying the formation of the complicated aragonite microstructures present in the ligament, structural and functional analyses of the organic matrix between the aragonite fibers are necessary. Recently, we reported that tissue inhibitor of metalloproteinase (TIMP) was identified from the insoluble fraction of the ligament in *P. fucata* (Kubota et al. 2017). This report shows the function of matrix metalloproteinase (MMP) for the formation of the ligament.

39.2 Materials and Methods

We used the BLAST search method to identify the MMP genes. We also prepared three types of pearl oyster samples to synthesize the cDNA for the templates of RT-PCR: sample 1 received no wound as a control, sample 2 received a wound on the shell by breaking the edge of the outer side of the shell with a nipper as the non-specific injured control, and sample 3 received a wound on the ligament from the outside to the inside with a cutter. After making a wound, each oyster was cultured in about 10 L seawater for 36 h. The PCR used the following cycling conditions: 35 cycles of 30 s at 94 °C (3 min 30 s for the first cycle), 30 s at 55 °C, and 30 s at 72 °C. The expression level of each MMP was checked by agarose gel electrophoresis of the PCR products. The gel contained 0.004% ethidium bromide so that amplified DNA could be visualized. After the electrophoresis, the fluorescence of the gel was observed under the exposure of the light at the wavelength of 365 nm.

dsRNAs of MMP genes were prepared for the RNAi experiments. 30 μg of each dsRNA was dissolved with 50 μL PBS buffer and injected to adductor muscle of *Pinctada fucata*. We used four young oysters (7 cm in shell size) in this experiment, because it was necessary to observe the growth surface of the ligament. Four days after injection, the growth surface of the ligament was observed by scanning electron microscope (SEM). We observed the ligament growth edges of three individuals using SEM independently. These observations showed similar results. Table 39.1 shows the list of primers used in these experiments.

Table 39.1 Primer sequences for MMPs

21914-5	AAAGAAAACTACAGACAAAG
21914-3	GTTTTACGGCGAGGTATTAT
07860-5	AGCTACACAAAGGTATGCCT
07860-3	ATAGCATCGAATTTCATGTT
60936-5	TGGTGATGCTGACATTATGA
60936-3	TCCTCCTGGAGTTTCCAGTA
32404-5	AAGTGGTCAGATGTGACGCC
32404-3	ATCTGTCATTAAGTTTGACG
23659-5	CGTAGCGGCCCACGAGTTTG
23659-3	TTGGGGTACCCAGGTGGGGG
54089-5	AAGCTTGTCTTTCGCACCTC
54089-3	TAAAGAGTTTGTATTCCTCT
14973-5	AAAACAAGTAGAAAATGCAA
14973-5	TTAAGTAATCTCCATCGAAT
54089-5(ds)	GGGTAATACGACTCACTATAGGGAGCAGTTTAACTTAGGACCA
54089-3(ds)	GGGTAATACGACTCACTATAGGGTTAGGATCATATCCAGCGTA
14973-5(ds)	GGGTAATACGACTCACTATAGGGTCACCATTTCCAGATGTCAT
14973-3(ds)	GGGTAATACGACTCACTATAGGGTCAAAGAATATCAAAAGAGG

39.3 Results

39.3.1 MMP Genes in P. fucata

Blast search showed seven MMP genes in the *P. fucata* genomic database (Takeuchi et al. 2012): pfu_aug1.0_21.1_21914 (21914), pfu_aug1.0_1282.1_07860 (07860), pfu_aug1.0_11733.1_60936 (60936), pfu_aug1.0_14122.1_32404 (32404), pfu_aug1.0_4795.1_23659 (23659), pfu_aug1.0_14629.1_54089 (54089), and pfu_aug1.0_322.1_14973 (14973) (Fig. 39.1). Among these MMPs, some conserved domains were identified. All MMPs in the database have the MMP superfamily domain that contains the activity site of MMP. MMP21924, MMP07862, MMP32404, MMP54089, and MMP14973 have a putative peptidoglycan-binding domain. No putative peptidoglycan-binding domain is found in human MMPs. MMP21914, MMP07860, MMP23659, and MMP14973 have hemopexin-like repeat domain, which is also found in most of human MMPs. Only MMP14973 has a signal peptide in the N-terminal sequence.

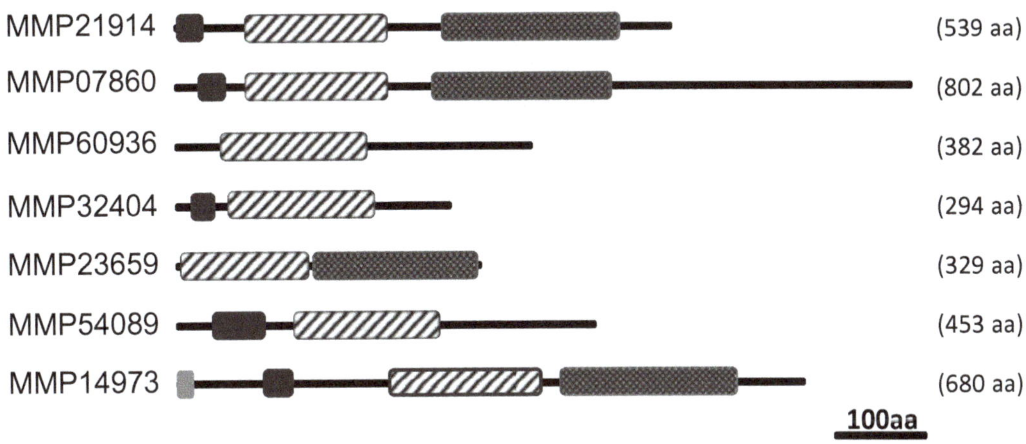

Fig. 39.1 The domain structures of MMPs from *P. fucata*. MMP21914 consists of a putative peptidoglycan-binding domain, an MMP superfamily domain, and hemopexin-like repeats. MMP07860 consists of a putative peptidoglycan-binding domain, an MMP superfamily domain, and hemopexin-like repeats. MMP60936 consists of only an MMP superfamily domain. MMP32404 contains of a putative peptidoglycan-binding domain and an MMP superfamily domain. MMP23659 consists of an MMP superfamily domain and hemopexin-like repeats. MMP54089 consists of a putative peptidoglycan-binding domain and an MMP superfamily domain. MMP14973 consists of a putative peptidoglycan-binding domain, an MMP superfamily domain, and hemopexin-like repeats. Black boxes show the putative peptidoglycan-binding domain. Dotted boxes show the hemopexin-like repeats. Slashed boxes show the MMP superfamily domain. Gray box shows the signal peptide

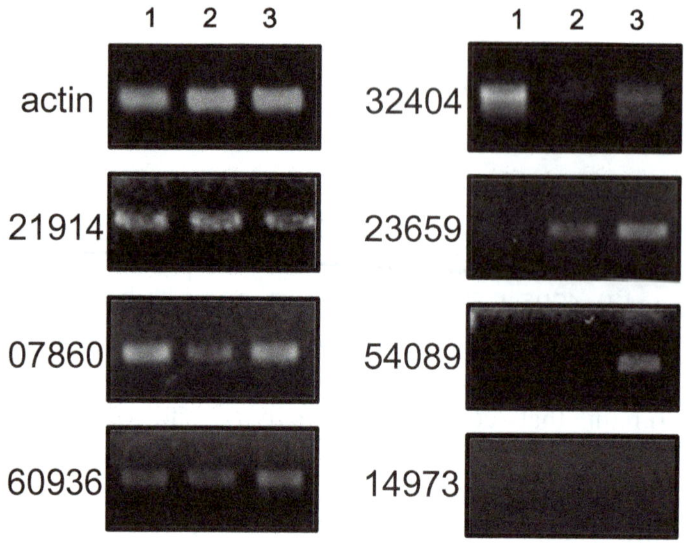

Fig. 39.2 RT-PCR analysis of MMP expression after wound treatment. (1) Unwounded control, (2) shell wounded with a nipper, (3) ligament wounded with a cutter

39.3.2 *MMP Gene Expressions in Response to Wounds*

To further investigate the expression level of each MMP in the mantle isthmus, the wound repair process was investigated, and MMP expression levels during this process were compared (Fig. 39.2). We assumed that expression of the MMP related to formation of the ligament would increase during the wound repair response of the ligament. Living pearl oysters were cultured in an aquarium for 1 week at 20 °C after the shell had been damaged by a knife. We used three treatment conditions: a control without any wounds, a wound on the shell margin, and a wound on the ligament. Significant changes in the expression levels of MMPs 32404, 23659, and 54089 were detected under these three conditions. Although the expression of MMP32404 decreased when the oyster was wounded on its shell margin, the expression levels in the control was higher than that in the ligament wound treatments, indicating that MMP32404 did not play a role in regeneration of the ligament. The expression level of MMP23659 increased after both shell margin and ligament wounds, indicating that MMP23659 has a non-specific wound-repair function in the shell. The expression level of MMP54089 increased only in the ligament wound treatment, indicating that MMP54089 plays a role specifically in regeneration of the ligament.

39.3.3 *RNAi Experiment*

To investigate the function of MMP54089 in the ligament, an RNAi experiment was performed. dsRNA targeting MMP54089 was injected into four living pearl oysters, which were then cultured in an aquarium for 4 days at 20 °C. The hinge ligament is attached to the nacreous layer of the shell (Fig. 39.3a, b). The growing edge of the ligament was observed by SEM 4 days after injection. In the control treatment of

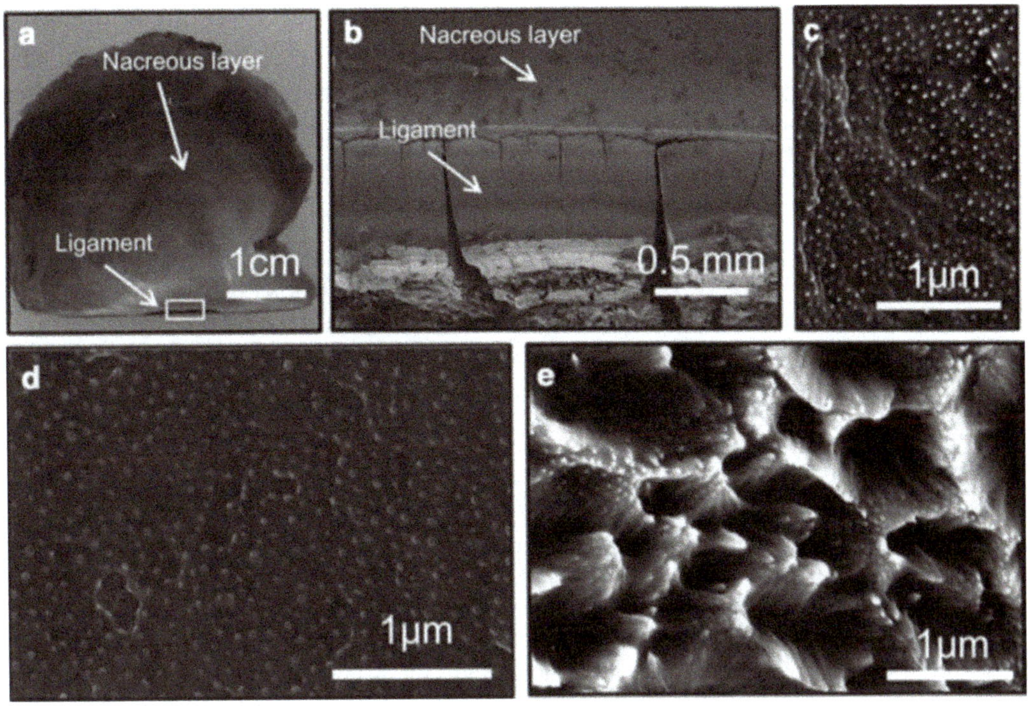

Fig. 39.3 (**a**) The shell of *P. fucata*. The white rectangle showed the region observed in (**b**). (**b**) SEM observations of the ligament and nacreous layer. (**c**) SEM observations of the surface in the ligament's growing edge in the sample of EGFP-dsRNA injection. (**d**) The surface in the ligament's growing edge in the sample of MMP14973-dsRNA injection. (**e**) The surface in the ligament's growing edge in the sample of MMP54089-dsRNA injection

(EGFP)-specific dsRNA injection, the tips of aragonite crystals were observed as white dots along the surface of the growing edge (Fig. 39.3c). Similar microstructures were observed after injections with MMP14973 dsRNA (Fig. 39.3d). In contrast, disordered microstructure was observed after MMP54089-specific dsRNA injection (Fig. 39.3e). The disordered organic matrix exhibited a wavy surface, and the aragonite crystals were not aligned, suggesting that MMP54089 plays a key role in the regulated formation of the fibrous microstructure of the ligament.

39.4 Discussion

Two hypotheses regarding the functions of PfTIMP and MMP54089 in the ligament were formulated. First, MMP54089 may degrade extracellular organic fibers to soften them and increase the space between them. The loosened extracellular organic fibers tend to adjust to the same orientation. A previous report showed that physical stress increased the activity of human MMP2 as well as its expression and also increased the toughness of a blood vessel analog in a cell-seeded collagen gel (Seliktar et al. 2003). A similar phenomenon may occur in the ligament of *P. fucata*. MMP54089 of *P. fucata* degrades extracellular organic fibers in the ligament and arranges them to regulate the direction of their growth. In the second hypothesis, MMP54089 digests proteins to prepare the peptides that contribute to calcium carbonate crystallization. A previous work suggested that amelogenin in the enamel of human teeth is digested by human MMP20, and the peptide fragments of amelogenin promote the crystallization of calcium phosphorus in the teeth (Vuk et al. 2011). MMP54089 may digest some matrix proteins such as LICP to prepare the released peptides for calcium carbonate crystallization (Suzuki et al. 2015). Further investigation is required to reveal the relationships among PfTIMP, MMP54089, extracellular organic fibers, and calcium carbonate crystallization.

References

Bevelander G, Nakahara H (1969) An electron microscope study of the formation of the ligament of *Mytilus edulis* and *Pinctada radiata Calcif.* Tiss Res 4:101–112

Kahler G, Sass R, Fisher F (1976) The fine structure and crystallography of the hinge ligament of *Spisula solidissima* (Mollusca: Bivalvia: Mactridae). J Comp Physiol 109:209–220

Kubota K, Tsuchihashi Y, Kogure T, Maeyama K, Hattori F, Kinoshit S, Sakuda S, Nagasawa H, Yoshimura E, Suzuki M (2017) Structural and functional analyses of a TIMP and MMP in the ligament of Pinctada fucata. J Struct Biol 199:216–224

Marsh M, Sass R (1980) Aragonite twinning in the molluscan bivalve hinge ligament. Science 208:1262–1263

Seliktar D, Nerem R, Galis Z (2003) Mechanical strain-stimulated remodeling of tissue-engineered blood vessel constructs. Tissue Eng 9:657–666

Suzuki M, Kogure T, Sakuda S, Nagasawa H (2015) Identification of ligament intra-crystalline peptide (LICP) from the hinge ligament of the bivalve, Pinctada Fucata. Mar Biotechnol 17:153–161

Takeuchi T, Kawashima T, Koyanagi R, Gyoja F, Tanaka M, Ikuta T, Shoguchi E, Fujiwara M, Shinzato C, Hisata K, Fujie M, Usami T, Nagai K, Maeyama K, Okamoto K, Aoki H, Ishikawa T, Masaoka T, Fujiwara A, Endo K, Endo H, Nagasawa H, Kinoshita S, Asakawa S, Watabe S, Satoh N (2012) Draft genome of the pearl oyster *Pinctada fucata*: a platform for understanding bivalve biology. DNA Res 2:117–130

Vuk U, Feroz K, Haichuan L, Halina E, Li Z, Wu L, Stefan H (2011) Hydrolysis of amelogenin by matrix metalloproteinase-20 accelerates mineralization in vitro. Arch Oral Biol 56:1548–1559

Chapter 40
Chitin Degraded by Chitinolytic Enzymes Induces Crystal Defects of Calcites

Hiroyuki Kintsu, Taiga Okumura, Lumi Negishi, Shinsuke Ifuku, Toshihiro Kogure, Shohei Sakuda, and Michio Suzuki

Abstract Mollusk shells have unique microstructures and mechanical properties such as hardness and flexibility. Calcite in the prismatic layer of *P. fucata* is extremely tough due to small crystal defects and localized organic networks inside calcites. Electron microscopic observations have suggested that such crystal defects are caused by the organic networks during calcite formation. Our previous work reported that the chitin which is the main component of organic networks and chitinolytic enzymes that bind to chitin were identified. In this article, to investigate the effects of chitin and chitinolytic enzymes on the formation of calcites, calcites were synthesized in chitin gel after treatment with chitinolytic enzymes. Chitin fibers seemed to become smooth and loosened after degradation. The crystal defects became larger as the chitin fibers became more degraded by chitinolytic enzymes in a dose-dependent manner. These results suggest that the shape of chitin fiber, which is regulated by the degradation of chitinolytic enzymes, contributes to the formation of small crystal defects.

Keywords Biomineralization · Prismatic layer · Chitinase · Chitin · *Pinctada fucata*

H. Kintsu · S. Sakuda · M. Suzuki (✉)
Department of Applied Biological Chemistry, Graduate School of Agricultural and Life Sciences, The University of Tokyo, Bunkyo-ku, Tokyo, Japan
e-mail: asakuda@mail.ecc.u-tokyo.ac.jp; amichiwo@mail.ecc.u-tokyo.ac.jp

T. Okumura · T. Kogure
Department of Earth and Planetary Science, The University of Tokyo, Tokyo, Japan
e-mail: okumura@eps.s.u-tokyo.ac.jp; kogure@eps.s.u-tokyo.ac.jp

L. Negishi
Institute of Molecular and Cellular Biosciences, The University of Tokyo, Tokyo, Japan
e-mail: lnegishi@iam.u-tokyo.ac.jp

S. Ifuku
Department of Chemistry and Biotechnology, Graduate School of Engineering, Tottori University, Tottori, Japan
e-mail: sifuku@chem.tottori-u.ac.jp

K. Endo et al. (eds.), *Biomineralization*,
https://doi.org/10.1007/978-981-13-1002-7_40

40.1 Introduction

Biominerals are biogenic mineralized tissues containing a small amount of organic matrices which regulate crystal nucleation, orientation, polymorphism, and morphology of inorganic substances (Belcher et al. 1996; Chen et al. 2008; Falni et al. 1996; Weiner and Addadi 1997). The shell of *Pinctada fucata*, Japanese pearl oyster, has two layers: prismatic and nacreous layer. The prismatic layer focused on in this study is composed of calcite prisms that are surrounded by thick polygonal organic frameworks as intercrystalline organic matrices. Each prism in the prismatic layer of *P. fucata* consists of several small calcites. Scanning electron microscope (SEM) and transmission electron microscope (TEM) analyses have revealed that each calcite contains subgrain units of several hundred nanometers divided by crystal lattice distortions known as small-angle grain boundaries (Okumura et al. 2012, 2013); however, the crystal structures of adjacent grains were continuous. Calcites that contain such crystal defects are tougher and stiffer than single calcites of another type of shell that contain no crystal defects because the defects inhibit the propagation of cracks (Olson et al. 2013). TEM observations have also revealed that organic matrices inside the small calcite of *P. fucata* prisms are localized in networks (Okumura et al. 2012). The location of the organic network correlates with the location of the crystal defects, indicating that the organic network affects the formation of the crystal defects. Our previous report clarified chitin and chitinolytic enzyme as the components of this organic network (Kintsu et al. 2017), in which we indicated that the chitin treated by chitinolytic enzymes may induce the formation of crystal defects.

In this article, we performed calcium carbonate crystallization using chitin hydrogel and chitinolytic enzymes in vitro to assess the effects of such organic matrices on lattice distortion inside the synthesized crystals.

40.2 Materials and Methods

Calcium carbonate crystallization in the chitin hydrogel. Chitin hydrogel was prepared according to the previous method (Tamura et al. 2006). The prepared chitin hydrogel was incubated with Yatalase (an enzyme complex containing chitinase and chitobiase activities from *Corynebacterium* sp. OZ-21; TaKaRa) as chitinolytic enzyme for 24 h. After incubation, chitin hydrogel was filtered and washed with 10 mM calcium chloride to remove Yatalase. The chitin hydrogel was spread on a plate and put into desiccator filled with the gas of 5 g of ammonium carbonate (Kanto Chemical) to crystallize calcium carbonate in the chitin hydrogel for 24 h. Chitin hydrogel was dissolved in 50% sodium hypochlorite to collect crystals.

Calcium carbonate crystallization using chitin nanofiber. A chitin nanofiber solution (1.1% (w/v) was prepared according to the previous report (Ifuku et al. 2010). A solution of 10 mM calcium chlorite was added to the chitin nanofiber solution, followed by calcium carbonate crystallization in the chitin nanofiber solution using the same method described above.

Fixation of chitin gel. Chitin gel was fixed by using the method of cell fixation with glutaraldehyde, osmium tetroxide, and potassium permanganate for reference with some modifications (Gunning 1965). Chitin gel was incubated sequentially in glutaraldehyde, osmium tetroxide, and potassium permanganate solution for 1 h. After fixation, the sample was dehydrated by ethanol and embedded in Spurr resin (Polysciences, Inc., USA). Sections prepared by ultramicrotome using a diamond knife.

Variance of lattice spacing determined from XRD spectra. The variance of lattice spacing in calcite crystal was estimated from peak broadening of XRD spectra using a RINT-Ultima$^+$ diffractometer (Rigaku) with graphite-monochromated Cu Kα radiation emitted at 40 kV and 20 mA according to the method reported previously (Okumura et al. 2012). The variance of lattice spacing ($\Delta d/d$) of the samples was calculated using Williamson-Hall plot (Williamson and Hall 1953) as follows:

$$\frac{\Delta(2\theta)\cos\theta}{\lambda}=\frac{(\Delta d/d)2\sin\theta}{\lambda}+\frac{0.94}{L}$$

40.3 Results and Discussion

40.3.1 Observation of Chitin Fibers by TEM

In an initial phase of prism formation, after the organic frameworks in the prismatic layer are constructed, the space surrounded by the organic framework is filled with organic gel solution composed mainly of chitin and matrix proteins; calcium carbonate is then crystallized with organic gel solution in the space. The organic gel solution such as chitin and chitinolytic enzymes we identified can develop into organic networks during calcite crystallization and affect the crystallization to form small-angle grain boundaries. Therefore, we performed an in vitro calcium carbonate crystallization experiment using chitin hydrogel and chitinolytic enzymes.

Chitin hydrogel was prepared by dissolving chitin powder in methanol saturated with calcium chloride dehydrate. To compare the differences of chitin fibers between before and after treatment with chitinolytic enzymes at concentration of 1.2 mg/mL, the chitin gels were observed by using TEM. Chitin gel was fixed according to a chemical fixation procedure for physiological tissues in order to observe in natural condition. TEM images of the chitin gels showed that a lot of chitin fibers of a few dozen of nanometer were observed in both conditions and no apparent differences of thinness and length could be seen (Fig. 40.1). However, while chitin fibers without treatment of chitinolytic enzymes became entangled with each fiber (Fig. 40.1a, b), chitin fibers with treatment of chitinolytic enzymes became smooth and loosened, not entangled (Fig. 40.1c, d), indicating that the chitinolytic enzymes may

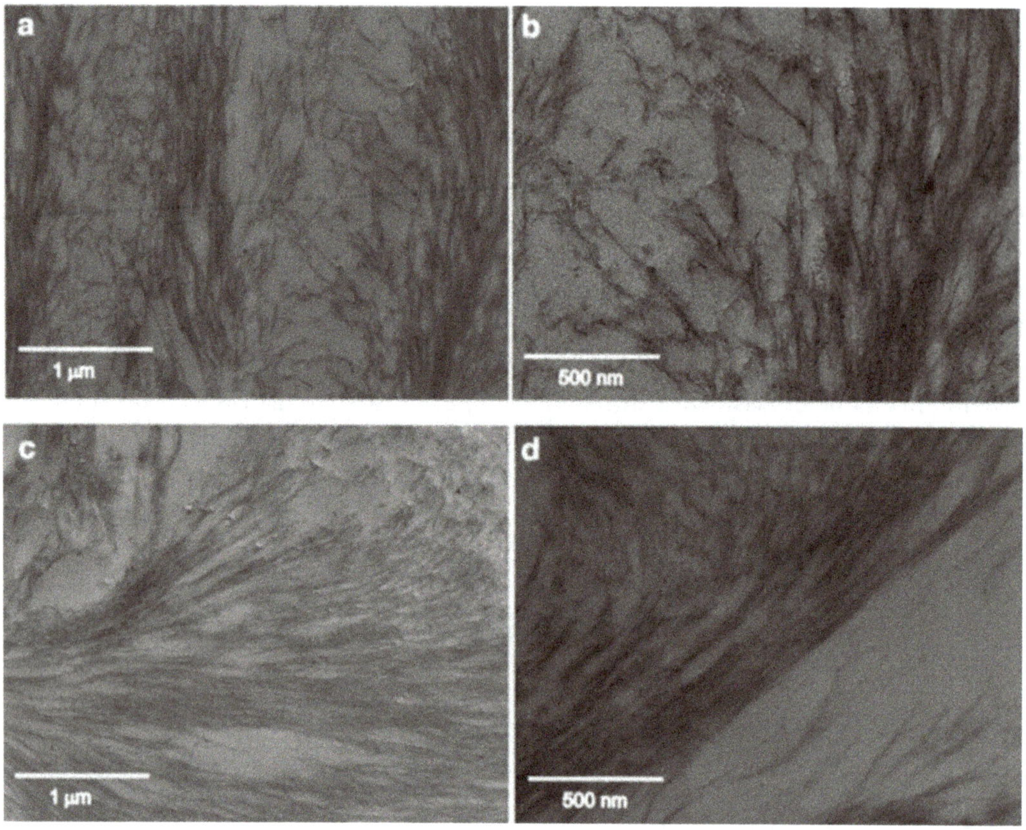

Fig. 40.1 TEM images of chitin gel. (**a**) Chitin gel before treatment with chitinolytic enzymes and (**b**) its high magnification. (**c**) Chitin gel after treatment with chitinolytic enzymes at the concentration of 1.2 mg/mL and (**d**) high magnification

degrade branched molecular chains of chitin which was getting entangled with each other. We suggest from this result that chitin fibers are loosened by chitinolytic enzymes and become such organic network as observed in the prism of *P. fucata*.

40.3.2 Synthesis of Calcium Carbonate Crystals in Chitin Hydrogel Treated with Chitinolytic Enzymes

To investigate how chitin and chitinolytic enzymes have effects on the formation of the small crystal defects in single calcites, calcium carbonate was crystallized in the chitin hydrogel with or without Yatalase which is a commercially available chitinolytic enzyme produced by a *Streptomyces* strain. After crystallization in the chitin hydrogel, calcium carbonate crystals were collected and observed by SEM. The normal shape of calcium carbonate crystals (a typical rhombohedral calcite) was formed in the chitin hydrogel without Yatalase treatment (Fig. 40.2a). In contrast, in the chitin hydrogel treated with 1.2 mg/mL chitinolytic enzyme, the shape of the crystal was completely changed and appeared to be round (Fig. 40.2b). As the concentration of chitinolytic enzymes increased, the chitin fiber became thinner, and

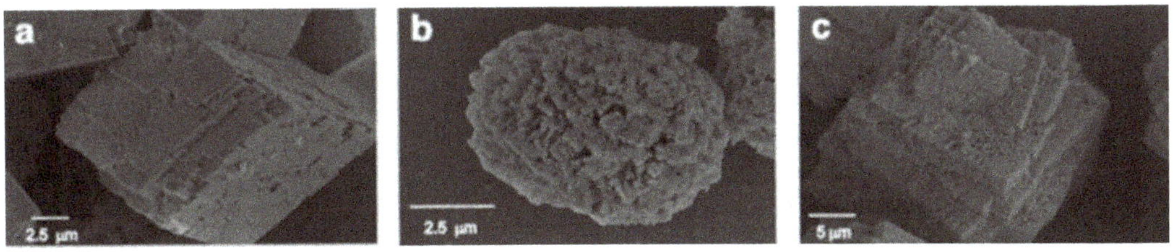

Fig. 40.2 The calcite crystals synthesized under different conditions. Calcite crystal formed in the chitin hydrogel treated with chitinolytic enzymes at concentrations of (**a**) 0 mg/mL, and (**b**) 1.2 mg/mL, and (**c**) in the chitin nanofiber solution

the surface microstructure of the calcite crystals in the chitin hydrogel changed. These results enabled us to guess that the thinness of chitin is a key factor to induce crystal defects.

Although it is indicated that thinness and length of chitin fiber are important, it is difficult to achieve a uniform thickness and length of chitin fibers using chitinolytic enzymes. Chitin nanofibers prepared by mechanical cleavage were used because the chitin nanofiber has a uniform thickness of several dozens of nanometers. Calcium carbonate was precipitated in the chitin nanofiber solution using the same method as described above without chitinolytic enzymes. SEM image of formed calcium carbonate crystals showed that chitin nanofiber can also affect crystallization and the surface microstructure became polygonal (Fig. 40.2c).

40.3.3 X-Ray Diffraction (XRD) Analyses of Calcite Crystals

To estimate the reason for the crystal defects among synthesized calcite crystals, XRD spectra of calcite samples were analyzed to calculate the variance of lattice spacing ($\Delta d/d$) as crystal defects. Figure 40.3 shows the ratio of $\Delta d/d$ gained from Williamson-Hall plots (data not shown) of each crystal synthesized in the presence of chitin pretreated with 0, 1.2 mg/mL chitinolytic enzymes, chitin nanofibers, and *P. fucata* prisms. At concentrations of 0, the $\Delta d/d$ value was very low and showed few crystal defects. In contrast, at a concentration of 1.2 mg/mL, the $\Delta d/d$ value was high, and the $\Delta d/d$ value in the chitin nanofiber was nearly equal to that observed at a concentration of 1.2 mg/mL. However, the $\Delta d/d$ value in the *P. fucata* prisms was approximately 1.7-fold higher than that observed at a concentration of 1.2 mg/mL.

These results showed that lattice distortion became larger as the chitin fiber became thinner. Although the data are not shown, TEM observation of the cross section of the calcite clarified that thinner chitin fibers were more easily embedded in calcium carbonate crystals. However, the lattice distortion ratio of synthesized calcite was still much smaller than that of prism calcite. This is perhaps because there are many acidic matrix proteins identified from the prismatic layer (Gotliv et al. 2005; Suzuki et al. 2004). Such proteins may also contribute to the increase in the lattice distortion ratio in calcite prisms.

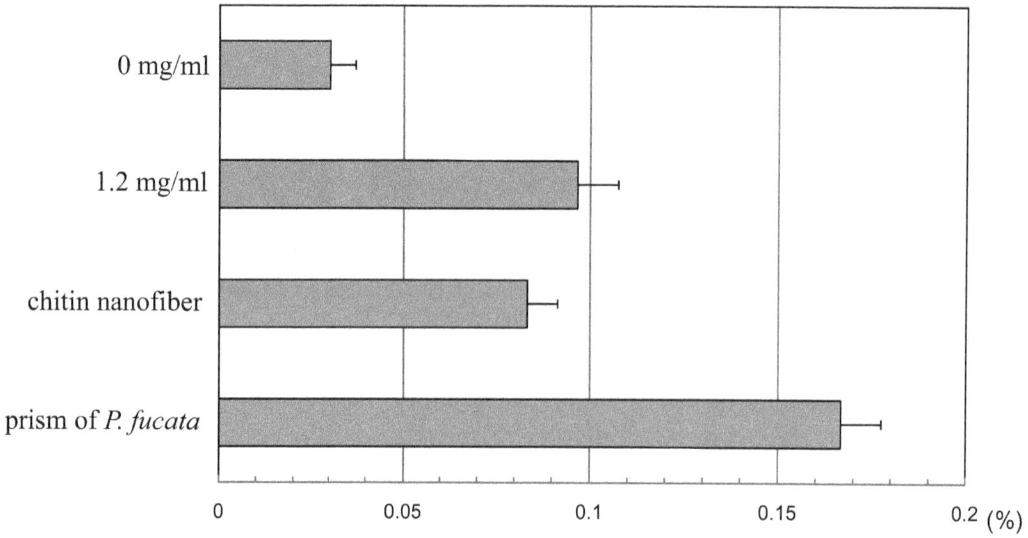

Fig. 40.3 Variance of lattice spacing calculated from Williamson-Hall plots. The synthesized calcites in the chitin hydrogel treated with chitinolytic enzymes at the concentrations of 0, 1.2 mg/mL, and in the chitin nanofiber solution, and prisms of the prismatic layer. Error bars indicate the standard deviation of the measurements ($n = 3$)

Taken together, chitin degradation plays an important role in the formation of calcite prisms in the prismatic layer. Crystal defects became larger as the chitin fibers were degraded by chitinolytic enzymes, because the increasing surface area of chitin fibers strengthens the physical and/or chemical interaction between calcium carbonate and the chitin fiber. This strong interaction may allow chitin fibers to attach to the crystal growth front in a random manner, which prevents calcium or carbonate ions from being well-oriented around crystal growth planes, leading to the crystal lattice distortion. Therefore, in the prismatic layer of *P. fucata*, the thinness of chitin fiber may be precisely regulated by chitinolytic enzyme to induce the small-angle grain boundaries. This novel mechanism may provide useful insights to the fields of biomineralization and biomimetic material engineering.

References

Belcher AM, Wu XH, Cristensen RJ, Hansma PK, Stucky GD, Morse DE (1996) Control of crystal phase switching and orientation by soluble mollusc-shell proteins. Nature 381:56–58

Chen PY, Lin AY, McKittrick J, Meyers MA (2008) Structure and mechanical properties of crab exoskeletons. Acta Biomater 4:587–596

Falini G, Albeck S, Weiner S, Addadi L (1996) Control of aragonite or calcite polymorphism by mollusk shell macromolecules. Science 271:67–69

Gotliv BA, Kessler N, Sumerel JL, Morse DE, Tuross N, Addadi L, Weiner S (2005) Asprich: a novel aspartic acid-rich protein family from the prismatic shell matrix of the bivalve *Atrina rigida*. Chem Bio Chem 6:304–314

Gunning BES (1965) The fine structure of chloroplast stroma following aldehyde osmium-tetroxide fixation. J Cell Biol 24:79

Ifuku S, Nogi M, Yoshioka Y, Morimoto M, Yano H, Saimoto H (2010) Fibrillation of dried chitin into 10–20 nm nanofibers by a simple grinding method under acidic conditions. Carbohydr Polym 81:134–139

Kintsu H, Okumura T, Negishi L, Ifuku S, Kogure T, Sakuda S, Suzuki M (2017) Crystal defects induced by chitin and chitinolytic enzymes in the prismatic layer of *Pinctada fucata*. Biochem Biophys Res Commun 489:89–95

Okumura T, Suzuki M, Nagasawa H, Kogure T (2012) Microstructural variation of biogenic calcite with intracrystalline organic macromolecules. Cryst Growth Des 12:224–230

Okumura T, Suzuki M, Nagasawa H, Kogure T (2013) Microstructural control of calcite via incorporation of intracrystalline organic molecules in shells. J Cryst Growth 381:114–120

Olson IC, Metzler RA, Tamura N, Kunz M, Killian CE, Gilbert PU (2013) Crystal lattice tilting in prismatic calcite. J Struct Biol 183:180–190

Suzuki M, Murayama E, Inoue H, Ozaki N, Tohse H, Kogure T, Nagasawa H (2004) Characterization of Prismalin-14, a novel matrix protein from the prismatic layer of the Japanese pearl oyster (*Pinctada fucata*). Biochem J 382:205–213

Tamura H, Nagahama H, Tokura S (2006) Preparation of chitin hydrogel under mild conditions. Cellulose 13:357–364

Weiner S, Addadi L (1997) Design strategies in mineralized biological materials. J Mater Chem 7:689–702

Williamson G, Hall W (1953) X-ray line broadening from filed aluminium and wolfram. Acta Metall 1:22–31

Chapter 41
Screening for Genes Participating in the Formation of Prismatic and Nacreous Layers of the Japanese Pearl Oyster *Pinctada fucata* by RNA Interference Knockdown

Daisuke Funabara, Fumito Ohmori, Shigeharu Kinoshita, Kiyohito Nagai, Kaoru Maeyama, Kikuhiko Okamoto, Satoshi Kanoh, Shuichi Asakawa, and Shugo Watabe

Abstract Many genes have been identified to participate in the shell formation so far. Nevertheless, the whole picture of the molecular mechanisms underlying the shell formation has remained unknown. In our previous study, we analyzed comprehensively genes expressed in the shell-producing tissues and identified 14 genes to be involved in the shell formation by the RNA interference (RNAi) method. In the present study, we performed further screening to find additional novel genes involved in the formation of the nacreous and prismatic layers. We here selected 80 genes from the EST data as candidates to function in the shell formation, conducted knockdown experiments by the RNAi method, and observed surface appearances on the nacreous and prismatic layers. We newly identified 64 genes that could participate in the shell formation. Taken together with our previous study, 78 genes were

---

D. Funabara (✉) · S. Kanoh
Graduate School of Bioresources, Mie University, Tsu, Mie, Japan
e-mail: funabara@bio.mie-u.ac.jp; kanoh@bio.mie-u.ac.jp

F. Ohmori · K. Maeyama · K. Okamoto
MIKIMOTO COSMETICS, Mie, Japan
e-mail: oomori.353@mikimoto-cosme.com; maeyama.511@mikimoto-cosme.com; okamoto.632@mikimoto-cosme.com

S. Kinoshita · S. Asakawa
Department of Aquatic Bioscience, Graduate School of Agricultural and Life Sciences, The University of Tokyo, Tokyo, Japan
e-mail: akino@mail.ecc.u-tokyo.ac.jp; asakawa@mail.ecc.u-tokyo.ac.jp

K. Nagai
Pearl Research Laboratory, K. MIKIMOTO & CO., LTD., Hamajima, Shima, Mie, Japan

S. Watabe
School of Marine Biosciences, Kitasato University, Minami, Sagamihara, Kanagawa, Japan
e-mail: swatabe@kitasato-u.ac.jp

K. Endo et al. (eds.), *Biomineralization*,
https://doi.org/10.1007/978-981-13-1002-7_41

supposed to function in the shell formation. These findings indicate that the combination of transcriptome and knockdown analyses is a powerful tool to screen novel genes involved in the shell formation.

Keywords EST · Knockdown · Nacreous layer · Pearl oyster · Prismatic layer · RNAi · Shell

41.1 Introduction

Many genes have been identified to participate in the shell formation so far. In classical ways, proteins were purified from shells after decalcification and their properties were analyzed. Nacrein, for instance, was purified from shells of the Japanese pearl oyster *Pinctada fucata* and characterized in detail (Miyamoto et al. 1996). Suzuki et al. (2009) employed the RNA interference (RNAi) method to elucidate possible functions of Pif discovered as an aragonite-binding protein in the shell of *P. fucata*. Knockdown of the *Pif* gene by the RNAi method induced an abnormal crystal structure of aragonite. This finding confirmed that Pif is really involved in the nacreous layer formation and proved that the RNAi method is useful to study genes involved in shell formation. We obtained the EST data of nacreous and prismatic layer-producing tissues of *P. fucata*, which contained 29,682 genes, and found novel 29,550 genes (Kinoshita et al. 2011). Genes involved in the shell formation must be contained in these genes. Thus, we compared gene expression patterns among mantle pallium, edge, and pearl sac tissues using the EST data to find genes expressed in a tissue-specific manner. We selected five genes specifically expressed in the mantle pallium, three highly expressed in the mantle pallium and pearl sac, and six specifically expressed in the mantle edge as candidates to function in shell formation. Knockdown experiments for these candidate genes induced abnormal appearances on the inner surface of the shells in the oysters (Funabara et al. 2014). These findings demonstrated that a combination of transcriptome analyses and RNAi knockdown is a powerful tool to screen genes involved in the shell formation. In the present study, we conducted further screening for genes involved in the shell formation of *P. fucata* using the above method.

41.2 Materials and Methods

We selected 195 genes having more than 200 reads from the EST data (Kinoshita et al. 2011) of the shell-forming tissues, along with 9 genes expressed similarly to those known to be involved in the shell formation from genes having less than 200 reads in the EST data. We conducted cDNA cloning of the selected genes with primers designed using the nucleotide sequences of respective genes. dsRNAs of the selected genes were synthesized using the cDNA clones as templates with a ScriptMAX™ Thermo T7 Transcription Kit (Toyobo, Osaka, Japan). About 40 μg of dsRNA/100 μl H_2O were injected into adductor muscles of 2-year-old pearl oysters ($n = 3$), followed by rearing them in artificial seawater at 23 °C for 8 days with feeding plankton once a day. The green fluorescence protein (GFP) and *Pif* genes were used as negative and positive references, respectively, to verify the RNAi experiments. Surface appearances of the prismatic and nacreous layers on the shells of the knockdown oysters were observed with a scanning electron microscope (SEM), S-4000 (Hitachi, Tokyo, Japan).

41.3 Results

41.3.1 Selection of Candidate Genes Functioning in Shell Formation

We selected candidate genes having more than 200 reads in the EST data (Kinoshita et al. 2011) to be possibly involved in the shell formation, except for 14 genes which we analyzed in our previous study (Funabara et al. 2014) (Table 41.1). cDNAs of 71 genes out of the selected 181 genes above were successfully cloned and used for synthesizing dsRNAs as templates. We selected additionally 9 genes showing expression patterns similarly to those of known shell formation-related genes such as PFMG1, KRMP1, N19, and N16 series from those having less than 200 reads (Table 41.1). cDNAs of all the nine genes were cloned and used for the synthesis of dsRNAs. A total of 80 genes were subjected to the knockdown experiments.

41.3.2 Observation of the Appearances on the Inner Surface of the Knockdown Oyster Shells

Knockdown of 64 out of 80 genes induced abnormal appearances on the inner surface of the shells (Table 41.2). Among them, 18 knockdown oysters had abnormal appearances on both the prismatic and nacreous layers, 45 only on the nacreous layers, and 1 only on the prismatic layers. The data combined with our previous study are shown in Fig. 41.1. Ninety-four genes, 80 in the present and 14 in our previous studies, contained 78 genes that are suggested to be involved in the shell formation processes. Only one gene changed the surface appearance on the prismatic layer.

41.4 Discussion

We have obtained the data of gene expression patterns and genes possibly involved in shell formation (Tables 41.1 and 41.2). It is not easy to discuss how genes play roles in shell formation based on expression patterns in the EST and knockdown data. We have only short sequences of the respective genes in the EST data. Full-length sequences or at least open reading frame (ORF) regions of the interest genes

Table 41.1 Gene expression patterns in shell- and pearl-forming tissues

Gene[a]	TPM			Total	Gene	TPM			Total	Gene	TPM			Total	Gene	TPM			Total
	ME	MP	PS	reads		ME	MP	PS	reads		ME	MP	PS	reads		ME	MP	PS	reads
1[b]	6042	6381	7207	1728	52[b]	1456	1386	93	226	104	1922	908	148	224	179	1456	1028	1129	308
2[b]	12,142	17,827	1240	24,620	53[b]	1922	1529	3099	595	105	1267	1063	805	263	187	1834	2282	0	317
3[b]	4833	4672	1351	369	54[b]	1485	1159	3238	549	106	1150	920	1933	365	188	772	1123	2396	406
4	2737	1410	5301	879	55[b]	1470	1326	2923	528	107	2329	2342	2156	589	190	903	836	805	219
5[b]	4062	4146	28	629	56[b]	1776	1529	0	250	108[b]	815	729	2535	391	191	466	430	1480	228
6[b]	3479	2449	5458	1034	57[b]	2538	2951	0	409	109	961	478	1628	282	193	1267	1195	1018	297
7[b]	3130	3644	4200	974	58[c]	2635	275	0	204	110	1616	1482	1286	374	194[c]	2751	1028	0	275
8[b]	1994	2892	185	399	59[b]	2140	2426	629	418	111[b]	1601	1864	1008	375	196	597	347	3349	432
9[b]	3261	2366	19	424	60[b]	2519	1937	1415	463	112[b]	975	1135	601	227	197	1092	1267	722	259
10[b]	2737	2892	111	442	61[b]	1529	1338	3654	612	113[c]	1019	2653	56	298	200[c]	2227	789	0	219
11[b]	3494	2844	65	485	62[b]	2373	1852	2563	595	114[b]	2504	1470	2082	520	209	189	72	1878	222
12[b]	2227	3597	315	438	63[b]	3712	2438	0	459	115[b]	1529	1302	1758	404	215	1631	1338	0	224
13[b]	3217	1972	130	400	64[b]	3217	2461	1878	630	116	2009	1517	0	265	216	932	1111	490	210
14[b]	2125	1816	3173	641	65[b]	3072	1972	0	376	118[c]	641	1924	102	216	218	670	789	860	205
15[b]	5008	3023	1739	785	66[c]	2853	48	0	200	121	830	657	1813	308	228	1325	1350	0	204
16[b]	2009	2593	5107	907	67[b]	2053	1625	3312	635	122	1077	1171	786	257	237	1194	1446	28	206
17[b]	2504	2665	4431	874	68[b]	2737	1470	2285	558	123	1077	753	1147	261	243	1529	1075	361	234
18	1732	1995	3007	611	69[b]	3523	3190	4496	995	124	728	693	1452	265	248	1441	1099	333	227
19	2533	1613	5097	860	70[b]	757	1051	833	230	125	1689	1147	2720	506	250	1296	1338	1332	345
20[b]	2038	1804	3626	683	71[b]	1878	1972	1480	454	127	1791	2246	2017	529	252	1252	1506	0	212
21	1470	1995	5190	829	72[b]	3028	143	0	220	128	1820	1852	1092	398	268	903	1016	1425	301
22[b]	2475	1697	3423	682	73	1354	2031	481	315	129	2038	1482	2044	485	272	1936	1386	37	253
23[b]	2358	2210	3830	761	74[b]	2795	2043	111	375	130	1034	1816	648	293	274	684	633	1471	259
24[b]	2198	1888	4330	777	75[b]	2562	1936	2868	648	132	1194	1565	259	241	292	903	789	1018	238
25[b]	2737	3405	0	473	76[b]	2082	1912	2646	589	133[c]	903	1804	46	218	300	611	203	1369	207
26[b]	2286	2306	4459	832	77[b]	2373	2414	65	372	134	888	930	962	243	301	1616	1290	0	219

27[c]	641	1744	3432	561	78	1441	1410	1721	403	136	1383	944	2054	396	323	1485	1147	83	207
28[b]	3669	3967	0	584	79[b]	2795	2497	2812	705	137	1237	2031	1600	428	336	1092	442	1221	244
29[b]	2417	2115	3867	761	80	2679	2139	1915	570	138	1558	1434	56	233	344	1310	1876	916	346
30[b]	2868	2270	5005	928	81[c]	364	1625	463	211	139	1893	1517	1767	448	384	859	1040	1203	276
31[c]	4586	1267	0	421	82	2053	2605	583	422	141	1252	1577	0	218	395	58	36	2618	290
32[b]	2519	3202	2877	752	83	1776	1972	851	379	143	1558	2031	65	284	399	1441	1673	333	275
33[b]	2446	1613	3719	705	84	1339	2210	453	326	145[c]	4047	167	0	292	407	1325	1517	296	250
34[b]	2067	2151	786	407	85	1689	2402	1295	457	147	1150	1398	361	235	411[c]	131	211	259	214
35[b]	4367	2784	6642	1251	86	1412	1840	546	310	148	1601	1601	0	244	3840	0	0	2812	304
36[b]	2868	2258	2655	673	87	1645	693	1878	374	150	1747	1374	2461	501	3969	0	0	1896	205
37[b]	4906	4756	0	735	88	1150	36	1147	206	152	670	442	3275	437	4121	0	0	1896	205
38[b]	1951	1685	1970	488	89	1456	2031	1610	444	154	670	609	1129	219	4600	0	0	2109	228
39[b]	2140	1995	2997	638	90	1005	621	1018	231	155	1063	741	814	223	5656	0	0	2017	218
40	3188	2485	0	427	91	1208	801	1110	270	157	1398	908	1591	344	7101	0	0	2054	222
41	3596	3465	2711	830	92[b]	1631	2342	0	308	161	1077	1804	0	225	7147	0	0	1952	211
42[b]	2795	2772	2396	683	93	2198	2449	1795	550	162	1063	645	1480	287	11,232	0	0	1961	212
43	1922	1458	3867	672	94	1514	1398	1425	375	164	1776	1792	1230	405	390[b]	1267	896	0	152
44[b]	1907	2629	194	372	95	2140	1756	2738	590	165	2024	1458	1304	402	493[b]	422	574	259	105
45[b]	1645	1649	3210	598	96[c]	437	1446	2701	443	166	2693	2019	0	354	496[b]	87	585	0	55
46[b]	2955	1900	2600	643	97	2096	1792	851	396	167	1019	1243	1489	335	1362[b]	335	36	204	48
47[b]	2636	2342	3034	705	98[c]	1194	2760	194	334	168	320	454	2785	361	3968[b]	0	550	0	4
48[b]	2198	2856	0	390	99	1893	2175	315	346	170	742	442	1175	215	4254[b]	0	0	1138	123
49	2446	2222	157	371	101	1718	2306	2211	550	171	742	382	1499	245	6605[b]	0	574	0	48
50[b]	2941	2330	3451	770	102	1310	1350	1563	372	172	495	693	1674	273	14278[b]	0	48	0	4
51[b]	2417	2103	3608	732	103	2315	2067	1832	530	176	1048	1040	749	240	16419[b]	0	0	28	55

TPM templates per million, *ME* mantle edge, *MP* mantle pallium, *PS* pearl sac

[a]Data and gene numbers from Kinoshita et al. (2011)

[b]Genes subjected to RNAi experiments in the present study

[c]Genes analyzed in our previous study Funabara et al. (2014)

Table 41.2 Appearances of the inner surface of shells injected with dsRNAs of the subject genes

Gene[a]	Prismatic	Nacreous	Gene	Prismatic	Nacreous	Gene	Prismatic	Nacreous
1	n	a	39	a	a	79	a	a
2	a	a	42	n	a	92	a	a
3	a	a	44	n	a	108	n	a
5	n	a	45	n	a	111	n	a
6	a	a	46	a	a	112	n	a
7	a	a	47	n	a	114	a	n
8	a	a	48	n	a	115	n	n
9	n	a	50	n	a	390	n	n
10	a	a	51	n	a	493	n	n
11	a	a	52	n	a	496	n	n
12	n	a	53	n	a	1362	n	n
13	a	a	54	n	n	3968	n	n
14	a	a	55	n	a	4254	n	n
15	a	a	56	n	a	6605	n	a
16	n	a	57	n	a	14,278	n	n
17	n	a	59	a	a	16,419	n	n
20	n	a	60	n	a	27[b]	a	a
22	n	a	61	n	n	31[b]	a	a
23	a	a	62	n	a	58[b]	n	a
24	n	a	63	n	a	66[b]	n	a
25	n	a	64	n	n	81[b]	a	a
26	n	a	65	n	a	96[b]	a	a
28	n	a	67	n	n	98[b]	a	a
29	a	a	68	n	a	113[b]	n	a
30	n	a	69	n	a	118[b]	n	a
32	n	a	70	n	a	133[b]	n	a
33	n	a	71	n	n	145[b]	n	a
34	n	a	72	n	n	194[b]	a	a
35	n	a	74	n	a	200[b]	n	a
36	a	a	75	n	a	411[b]	n	a
37	n	a	76	n	n			
38	n	a	77	n	a			

n normal appearance, *a* abnormal appearance
[a]Gene numbers from Kinoshita et al. (2011)
[b]Data from Funabara et al. (2014)

are required to discuss their function. To determine the full-length sequences, it is reasonable that we choose genes in descending order of the numbers of their reads in the EST data. We can also search the genome database for their gene models by BLAST searching using the EST sequence data (Takeuchi et al. 2012).

Many studies on shell formation-related proteins have focused on those secreted from mantle tissues into shells. This way is incapable of analyzing regulatory

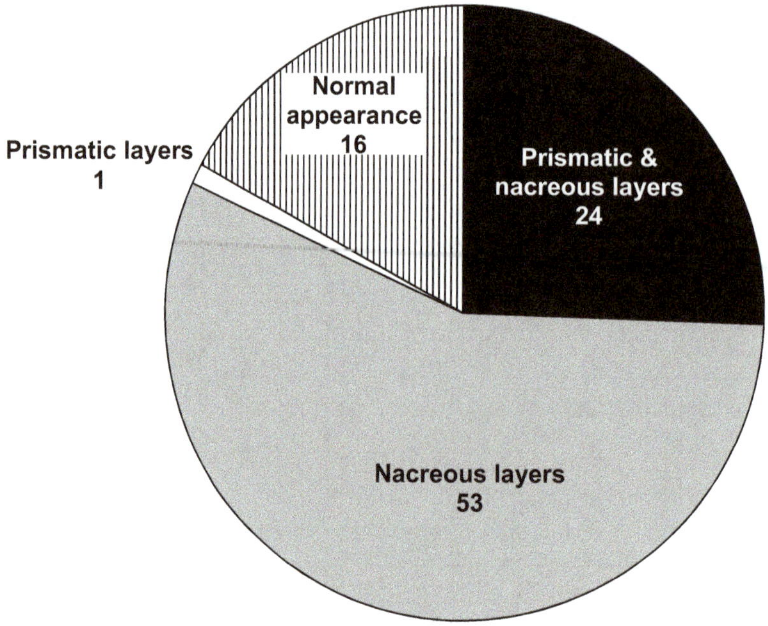

Fig. 41.1 The numbers of individuals having normal and abnormal appearances on the inner surface of the shells of the Japanese pearl oysters *Pinctada fucata* subjected to the RNAi experiments as observed by SEM. "Prismatic and nacreous layers," "nacreous layers," "prismatic layers," and "normal appearances" indicate individuals having abnormal appearances on "both the prismatic and nacreous layers," "only on the nacreous layers," "only on the prismatic layers," and "normal appearances" on the shell inner surface, respectively. Numerals indicate the numbers of the genes

pathways to form shells. We found in our previous study that some shell formation-related genes encoded proteins lacking a signal peptide, suggesting that such cytoplasmic proteins function in shell formation together with secretory ones (Funabara et al. 2014). We have not determined the full-length sequences for the newly identified 64 genes to be involved in shell formation yet. They may contain cytoplasmic proteins which function in shell formation. The combination of transcriptome and knockdown analyses would give us some useful information on the shell formation processes from genes to shells.

References

Funabara D, Ohmori F, Kinoshita S, Koyama H, Mizutani S, Ota A, Osakabe Y, Nagai K, Maeyama K, Okamoto K, Kanoh S, Asakawa S, Watabe S (2014) Novel genes participating in the formation of prismatic and nacreous layers in the pearl oyster as revealed by their tissue distribution and RNA interference knockdown. PLoS One 9:e84706

Kinoshita S, Wang N, Inoue H, Maeyama K, Okamoto K, Nagai K, Kondo H, Hirono I, Asakawa S, Watabe S (2011) Deep sequencing of ESTs from nacreous and prismatic layer producing tissues and a screen for novel shell formation-related genes in the pearl oyster. PLoS One 6:e21238

Miyamoto H, Miyashita T, Okushima M, Nakano S, Morita T, Matsushiro A (1996) A carbonic anhydrase from the nacreous layer in oyster pearls. Proc Natl Acad Sci U S A 93:9657–9660

Suzuki M, Saruwatari K, Kogure T, Yamamoto Y, Nishimura T, Kato T, Nagasawa H (2009) An acidic matrix protein, Pif, is a key macromolecule for nacre formation. Science 325:1388–1390

Takeuchi T, Kawashima T, Koyanagi R, Gyoja F, Tanaka M, Ikuta T, Shoguchi E, Fujiwara M, Shinzato C, Hisata K, Fujie M, Usami T, Nagai K, Maeyama K, Okamoto K, Aoki H, Ishikawa T, Masaoka T, Fujiwara A, Endo K, Endo H, Nagasawa H, Kinoshita S, Asakawa S, Watabe S, Satoh N (2012) Draft genome of the pearl oyster *Pinctada fucata*: a platform for understanding bivalve biology. DNA Res 19:117–130

Chapter 42
Gene Expression Patterns in the Mantle and Pearl Sac Tissues of the Pearl Oyster *Pinctada fucata*

Shigeharu Kinoshita, Kaoru Maeyama, Kiyohito Nagai, Shuichi Asakawa, and Shugo Watabe

Abstract The shell of pearl oysters consists of two distinct layers, nacre and prismatic. Mantle is the tissue involved in the shell formation, and its ventral part (mantle edge) forms the prismatic layers, whereas the dorsal part (pallium) forms the nacre. In pearl culture, mantle grafts from the pallium of donor are transplanted into the recipient. Then pearl sac is formed by proliferation of epithelial cells from the grafted mantle to form pearls. It has been reported that gene expression patterns are different between mantle edge and pallium in accordance with their distinct functions in the shell formation. However, it is not well addressed whether gene expression is identical or not between two nacre-forming tissues, pallium and pearl sac. Here, we examined expression patterns of known genes related to nacre and prismatic layer formation in mantle edge, pallium, and pearl sac of *Pinctada fucata*. Although the pallium and pearl sac have the same function in terms of nacre formation, various genes were not expressed identically to the respective tissues, suggesting that shell matrix proteins differently function in the formation of shell nacre and pearls.

Keywords *Pinctada fucata* · Pearl · Shell nacre · Prismatic layer · Gene expression · RNA-seq

---

S. Kinoshita (✉) · S. Asakawa
Department of Aquatic Bioscience, Graduate School of Agricultural and Life Sciences, The University of Tokyo, Tokyo, Japan
e-mail: akino@mail.ecc.u-tokyo.ac.jp; asakawa@mail.ecc.u-tokyo.ac.jp

K. Maeyama
Mikimoto Pharmaceutical CO., LTD, Ise, Mie, Japan
e-mail: maeyama.511@mikimoto-cosme.com2

K. Nagai
Pearl Research Laboratory, K. MIKIMOTO & CO., LTD., Hamajima, Shima, Mie, Japan
e-mail: k-nagai@mikimoto.com

S. Watabe
School of Marine Biosciences, Kitasato University, Minami, Sagamihara, Kanagawa, Japan
e-mail: swatabe@kitasato-u.ac.jp

K. Endo et al. (eds.), *Biomineralization*,
https://doi.org/10.1007/978-981-13-1002-7_42

42.1 Introduction

The shell of pearl oysters consists of two distinct layers: inner nacre and outer prismatic layers composed of aragonite and calcite crystals, respectively. The forming processes of these different shell layers are thought to be regulated by proteins secreted from epithelial cells in mantle tissues. The ventral part of the mantle (mantle edge) forms the prismatic layers, whereas the dorsal part (pallium) forms the nacreous layers. These two regions secrete different repertoire of shell matrix proteins. In pearl culture, mantle grafts from the pallium region of donor oyster are transplanted with spherical nuclei into the recipient oysters. Pearl sac is formed by proliferation of mantle epithelial cells originating from the mantle graft from which various proteins are secreted to form the nacre surrounding nuclei.

Pearl consists of nacre or "mother of pearl" and is formed inside the body of pearl oysters; thus the nature of shell nacre and pearls is considered to be identical. On the other hand, our previous study clearly showed differences in the expression levels of several shell matrix protein genes between pallium and pearl sac (Wang et al. 2009). Inoue et al. (2010) investigated the expression of six shell matrix protein genes and showed that some of them were not expressed identically in pearl sac and mantle center (nacre-forming region), although a significant correlation was observed in their expression patterns between the two tissues. To analyze molecular mechanisms underlying the shell and pearl formation, it is important to examine whether gene expression patterns are different or not between pearl sac and mantle. Here, we compared expression pattern of known genes related to nacre (nacreous genes) and prismatic layer formation (prismatic genes) in mantle edge, pallium, and pearl sac of pearl oyster *Pinctada fucata* by using our previous RNA-seq data (Kinoshita et al. 2011).

42.2 Materials and Methods

42.2.1 *Sample Preparation*

Mantle and pearl sac tissues were collected from four individuals of *P. fucata* maintained at the Mikimoto Pearl Research Laboratory, Mie, Japan. Mantle pieces were grafted to all individuals for pearling 5 months before sampling. The mantle edge and pallium regions were separated from the mantle. Pearl sacs were collected from gonad of pearl oysters, and contaminated recipient tissues were carefully trimmed. All tissues, pallium, mantle edge, and pearl sacs used in this study were collected at the same time.

42.2.2 RNA-Seq Analysis

mRNAs were purified from tissues. 3′-fragment sequencing was performed using the GS FLX 454 system (Kinoshita et al. 2011). After quality trimming of raw reads, a de novo assembly using MIRA assembler ver. 2.9.45x1 and the BLAST Clust program from NCBI was used to assemble the reads. Known nacreous and prismatic gene sequences were searched from assembled contig data set using the local blastn and tblastn algorithms. Expression levels of gene sequences were expressed by transcripts per million (TPM). Hierarchical cluster analysis was performed by CLUSTER3.0 using Euclidean distance.

42.3 Results and Discussion

42.3.1 Clustering of Expression Patterns in Three Shell-Formation Tissues for the Known Nacreous and Prismatic Genes

Although many studies have identified genes and proteins that are related to nacre and prismatic layer formation, the information on their functions has been limited. Among the genes previously reported, we selected 10 nacreous and 14 prismatic genes (Table 42.1). Based on the expression patterns of these nacreous and prismatic genes, hierarchical clustering analysis among three tissues, mantle edge, pallium, and pearl sac, was performed. As shown in Fig. 42.1, pallium and pearl sac were clustered in the same node and separated from the mantle edge, well in accordance with their functions in the nacre formation or prismatic layer formation.

42.3.2 Expression of Known Nacreous and Prismatic Genes

Most nacreous genes examined in this study were expressed predominantly in the pallium (Table 42.1). Among them, MSI60, MSI25, and Pif177 showed the highest expression in the pallium, suggesting their importance in the nacre formation. In contrast, two nacreous genes, *ACCBP* and *CaLP*, were expressed in the mantle edge more than in the pallium, suggesting their additional roles in the prismatic layer formation. On the other hand, N66, PFMG1, and N19 family members were detected only in pallium or pearl sac.

Table 42.1 The expression levels of known nacreous and prismatic genes

	TPM		
	ME	P	PS
Nacreous genes			
MSI60	131	2115	259
MSI25	29	406	120
Pif177	44	872	37
Nacrein	1019	2623	56
N66	0	36	0
PFMG1	0	36	0
ACCBP	146	96	0
CalP	553	466	56
N19-1	0	48	0
N19-2	0	0	28
Prismatic genes			
Aspein	4062	4146	28
Prismalin-14	1252	1577	0
KRMP1	3217	1972	13
KRMP3	3494	2844	65
KRMP4	1907	2629	194
Prismin	3669	3967	0
Prisilkin-39	641	442	0
Shematrin1	1456	1386	93
Shematrin2	4833	4672	1351
Shematrin3	379	36	0
Shematrin4	29	0	0
Shematrin5	408	1517	0
Shematrin6	4906	4756	0
Shematrin7	903	370	0

TPM transcripts per million, *ME* mantle edge, *P* pallium, *PS* pearl sac

Meanwhile, the expression levels of most known prismatic genes did not differ between the pallium and mantle edge (Table 42.1). Shematrin5 was expressed in the pallium much greater than in the mantle edge. These prismatic genes may also play roles in the nacreous layer formation. This is consistent with our previous report that knockdown of prismatic genes affects the shell nacre formation in *P. fucata* (Funabara et al. 2014). Jackson et al. (2010) also showed that prismatic genes such as shematrins and KRMPs are important in the formation of the shell nacre in *P. maxima*. These prismatic genes except for shematrin2 were marginally detected in pearl sacs (Table 42.1).

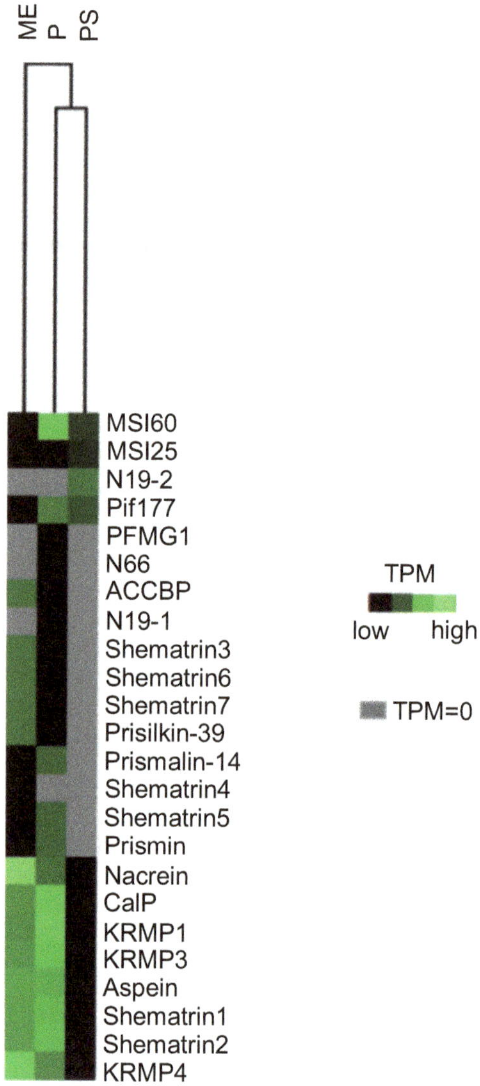

Fig. 42.1 Hierarchical clustering of expression patterns in three shell-formation tissues for known nacreous and prismatic genes. *ME* mantle edge, *P* pallium, *PS* pearl sac. Explanation about color is needed

Although the pallium and pearl sac have the same function in terms of nacre formation, our data indicate that the expression patterns of various nacreous genes are not identical, though similar to each other, between the two tissues. In addition, most prismatic genes analyzed in this study showed high expression levels in both mantle edge and pallium but only marginally in pearl sac. One possibility is that contaminating tissues surrounding the pearl sac decreased the expression of shell formation-related genes in our pearl sac preparation. Nevertheless our data suggest different composition of shell matrix proteins between the shell nacre and pearls, and the importance of the gene expression analysis in the pearl sac to address molecular mechanisms underlying the pearl formation.

References

Funabara D, Ohmori F, Kinoshita S, Koyama H, Mizutani S, Ota A, Osakabe Y, Nagai K, Maeyama K, Okamoto K, Kanoh S, Asakawa S, Watabe S (2014) Novel genes participating in the formation of prismatic and nacreous layers in the pearl oyster as revealed by their tissue distribution and RNA interference knockdown. PLoS One 9:e84706

Inoue N, Ishibashi R, Ishikawa T, Atsumi T, Akoki H, Komaru A (2010) Gene expression patterns and pearl formation in the Japanese pearl oyster (*Pinctada fucata*): a comparison of gene expression patterns between the pearl sac and mantle tissue. Aquaculture 308:68–74

Jackson DJ, McDougall C, Woodcroft B, Moase P, Rose RA, Kube M, Reinhardt R, Rokhsar DS, Montagnani C, Joubert C, Piquemal D, Degnan BM (2010) Parallel evolution of nacre building gene sites in molluscs. Mol Biol Evol 27:591–608

Kinoshita S, Wang N, Inoue H, Maeyama K, Okamoto K, Nagai K, Kondo H, Hirono I, Asakawa S, Watabe S (2011) Deep sequencing of ESTs from nacreous and prismatic layer producing tissues and a screen for novel shell formation-related genes in the pearl oyster. PLoS One 6:e21238

Wang N, Kinoshita S, Riho C, Maeyama K, Nagai K, Watabe S (2009) Quantitative expression analysis of nacreous shell matrix protein genes in the process of pearl biogenesis. Comp Biochem Physiol B Biochem Mol Biol 154:346–350

Part IX
Appendix

Chapter 43
Selected SEM and TEM Images by Late Dr. Hiroshi Nakahara

Mitsuo Kakei

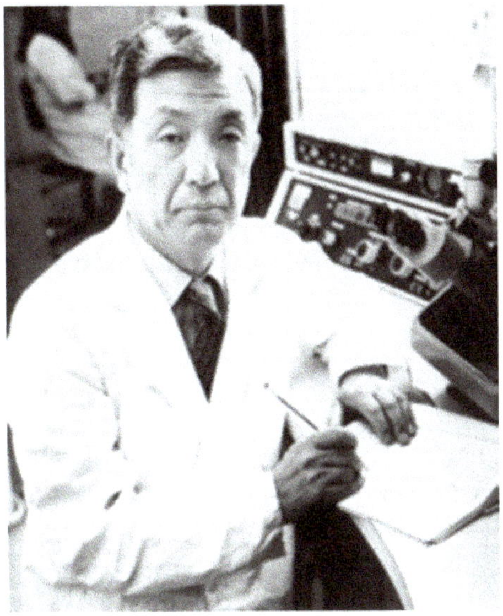

Dr. Hiroshi Nakahara (1928–2001)

Abstract The following SEM and TEM images were taken by late Dr. Hiroshi Nakahara many years ago, left unpublished, and shown on the screen during lunch-times in the symposium. He graduated from the course of zoology of the Faculty of Sciences, University of Hokkaido, and studied abroad in the University of New York and School of Dentistry, University of Texas. After returning home, he taught oral anatomy at Meikai University, School of Dentistry (former Josai Dental University). Using electron microscopes both SEM and TEM, he studied the mineralization processes of a variety of shellfish as well as vertebral hard tissues such as tooth enamel, dentin, and bone.

Keywords Bone · Ligament · *Monodonta confusa* · Nacreous layer · Otolith · Pearl · *Pinctada fucata* · Prismatic layer · Tooth enamel

M. Kakei (✉)
Tokyo Nishinomori Dental Hygienist College, Tokyo, Japan
e-mail: mkakei@jcom.home.ne.jp

K. Endo et al. (eds.), *Biomineralization*,
https://doi.org/10.1007/978-981-13-1002-7_43

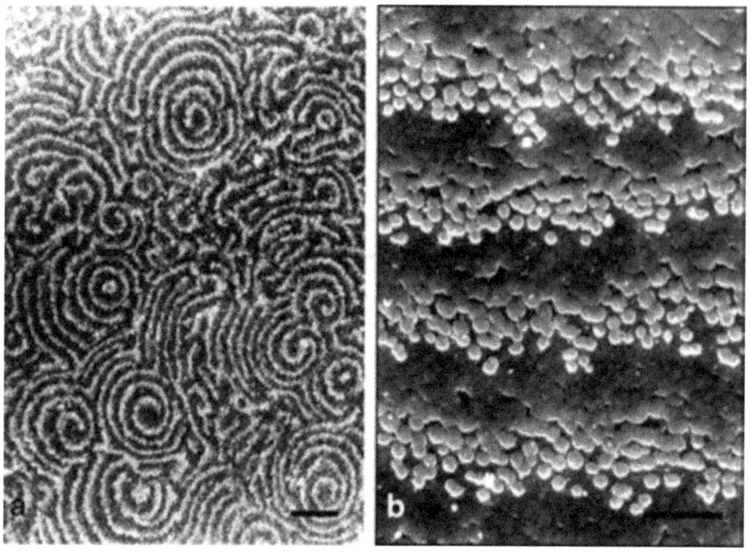

Fig. 43.1 SEM of growing surface of cultured pearl in *Pinctada fucata*. Spiral patterns are distributed across the surface (**a**). Aragonite tablets are arranged (**b**) (bars: **a** = 20 μm, **b** = 10 μm)

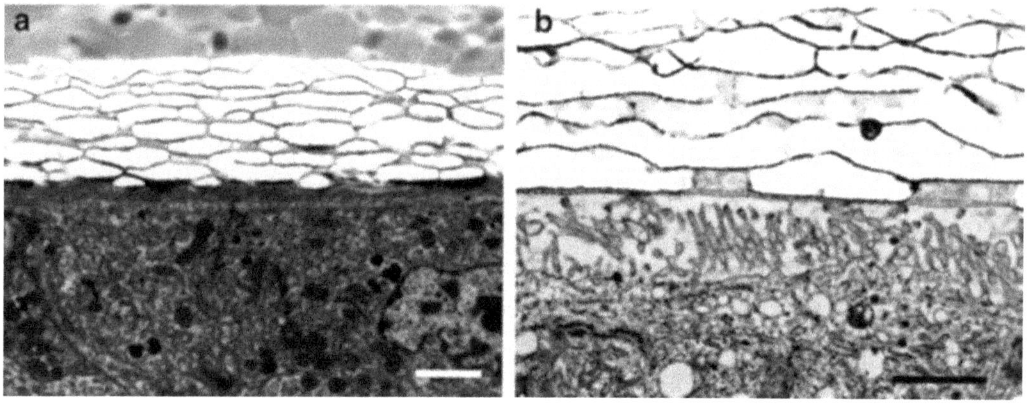

Fig. 43.2 TEM of nacre formation of *Pinctada fucata*. Growing surface of bivalve nacre is protected from being exposed to seawater by periostracum (bars: **a**, **b** = 2 μm, double staining)

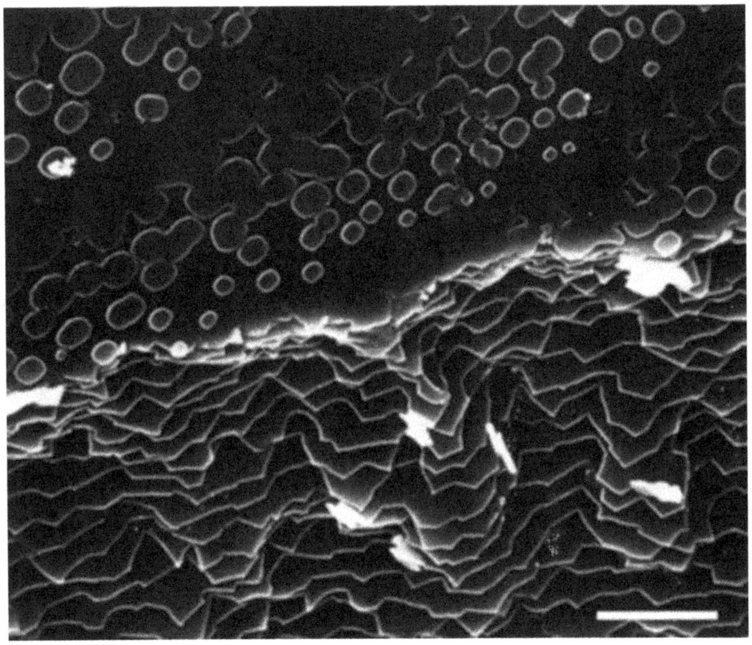

Fig. 43.3 SEM of the growing surface of nacreous layer of *Pinctada fucata*. The growing surface shows stepwise structure (bar: 5 μm)

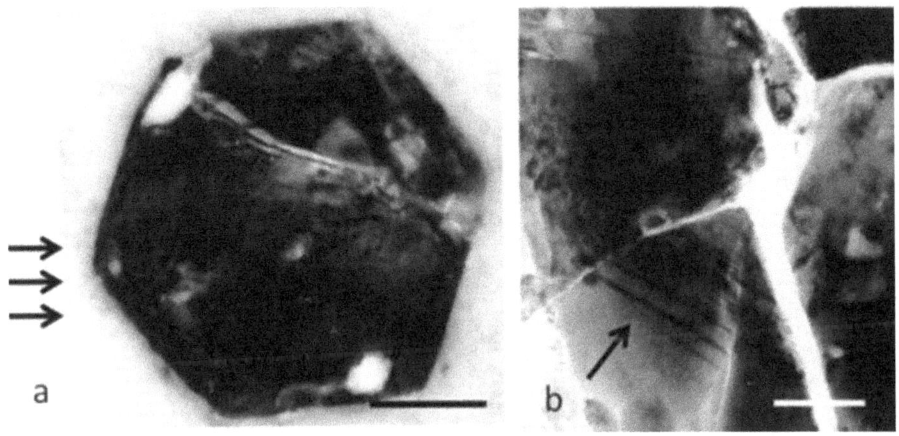

Fig. 43.4 TEM of a crystal in the nacreous layer of *Pinctada fucata*. Flat cut sections show polysynthetic twin (arrows) (bars: **a**, **b** = 500 nm)

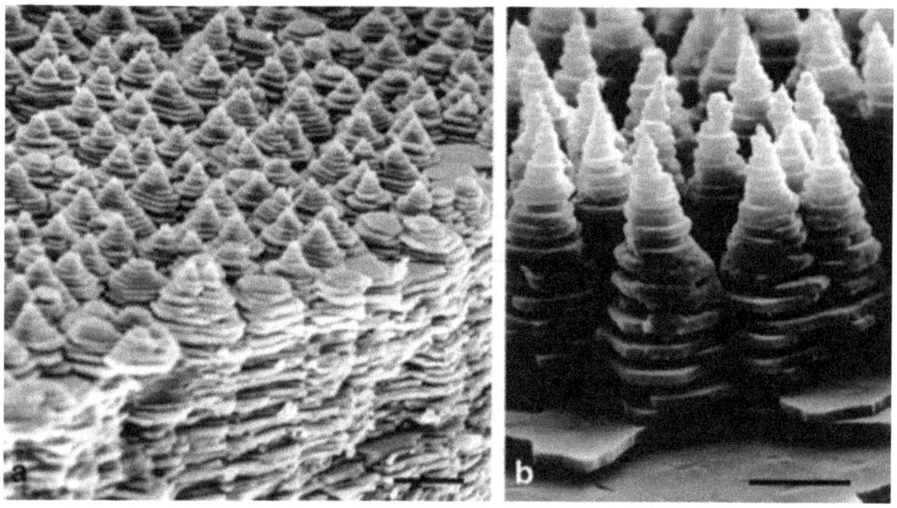

Fig. 43.5 SEM of growing surface of nacreous layer of *Monodonta confusa*. After treatment with sodium hypochlorite solution, columnar arrangement of tablets shows pyramid-shaped stacks (bars: **a** = 10 μm, **b** = 5 μm)

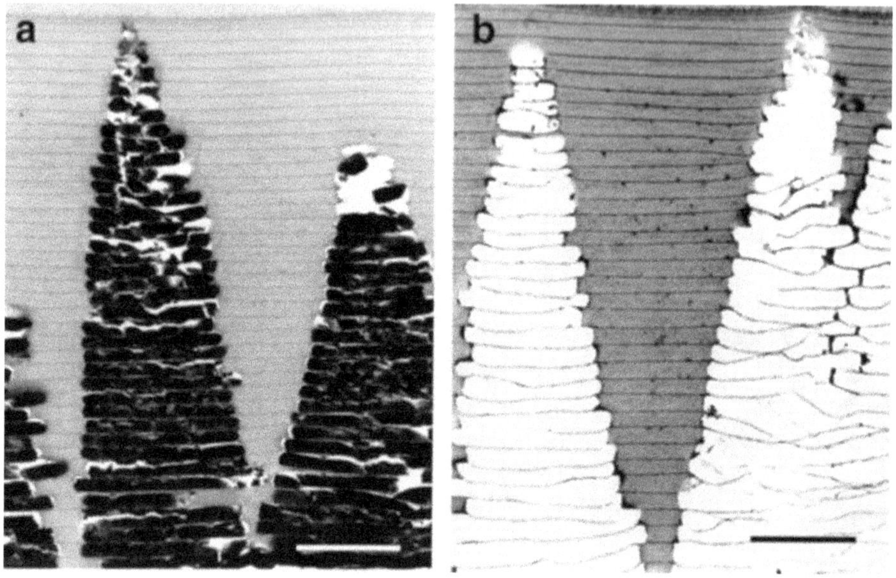

Fig. 43.6 TEM of growing surface of nacreous layer of *Monodonta confusa*. Tablets of crystals are created between the interlamellar matrix of sheets. (**a**) No staining, (**b**) double staining (bars: a, b = 5 μm)

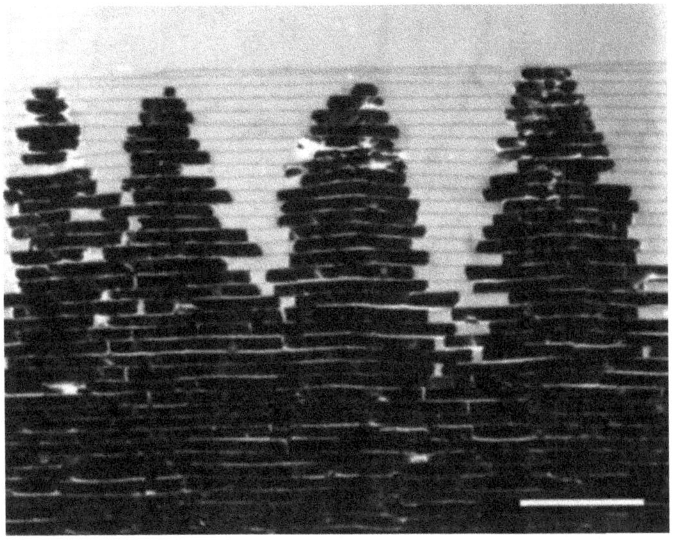

Fig. 43.7 TEM of growing surface of nacreous of *Sulculus diversicolor supertexta*. Crystals of snail nacre are arranged in the brick wall type, reinforcing the structural strength (bar = 5 μm)

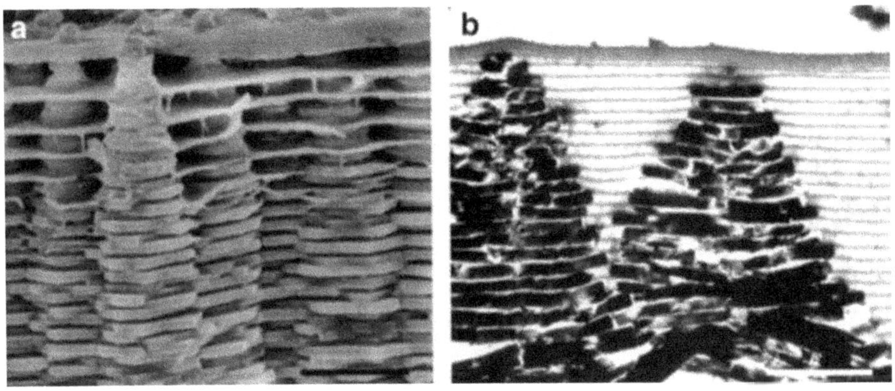

Fig. 43.8 SEM (**a**) and TEM (**b**) of the interlamellar matrix sheets of nacre of *Batillus cornutus*. Surface sheets cover the top of aragonite stacks (bars: **a** = 5 μm, **b** = 4 μm)

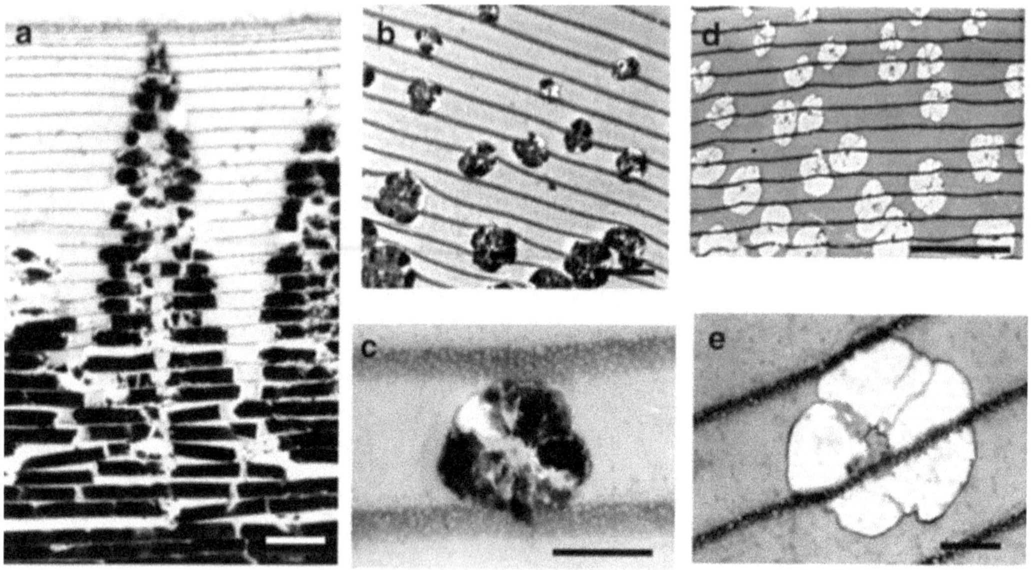

Fig. 43.9 TEM of nacre formation of *Calliostoma unicum*. (**a**) Central portion of the pyramid-shaped stacks shows empty space. (**b–e**) Sections were nearly parallel to the surface. Each tablet is divided into sectors (**b** and **c**). Organic cores remained at the center of stacks in the stained sections (**d** and **e**) (bars: **a** = 2.2 μm, **b** = 5 μm, **c** = 10 μm, **d** = 10 μm, **e** = 1 μm)

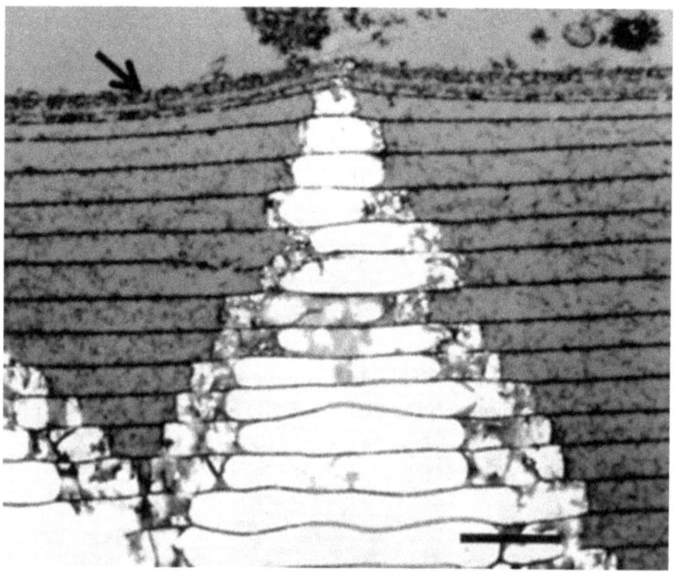

Fig. 43.10 TEM of nacre formation of *Batillus cornutus*. Thick surface sheet (arrow) is only formed in the gastropods and protects the developing nacre surface from seawater (double staining, bar = 10 μm)

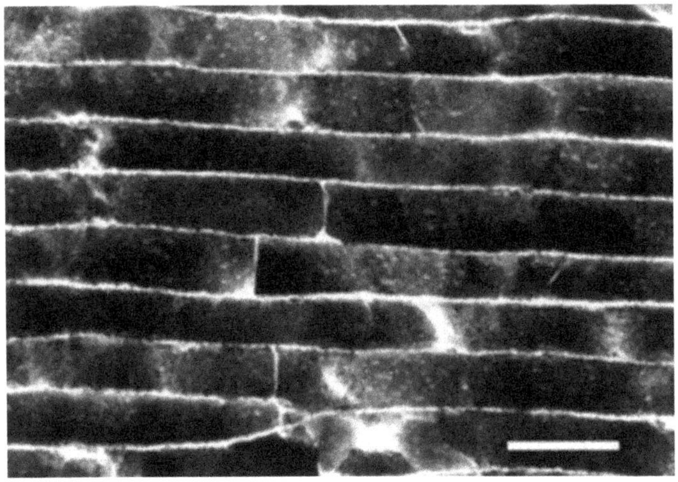

Fig. 43.11 TEM of transverse plane of nacreous layer of *Haliotis*. Brick wall-type structure enhances the structural strength (bar = 1 μm)

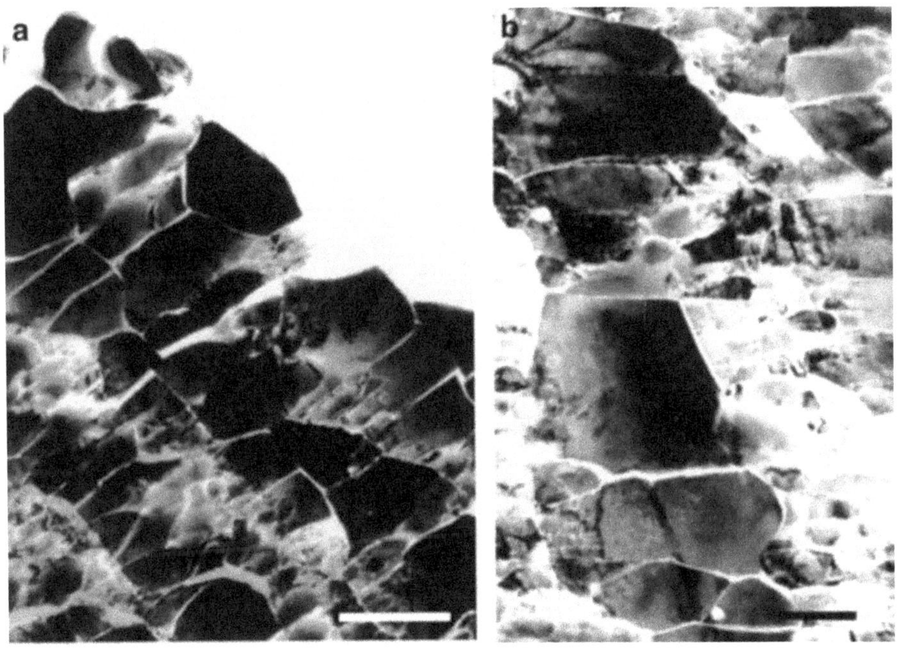

Fig. 43.12 TEM of nacre of *Lithophaga*. Flat-cut crystals are observed without staining (bars: **a** = 2 μm, **b** = 1 μm)

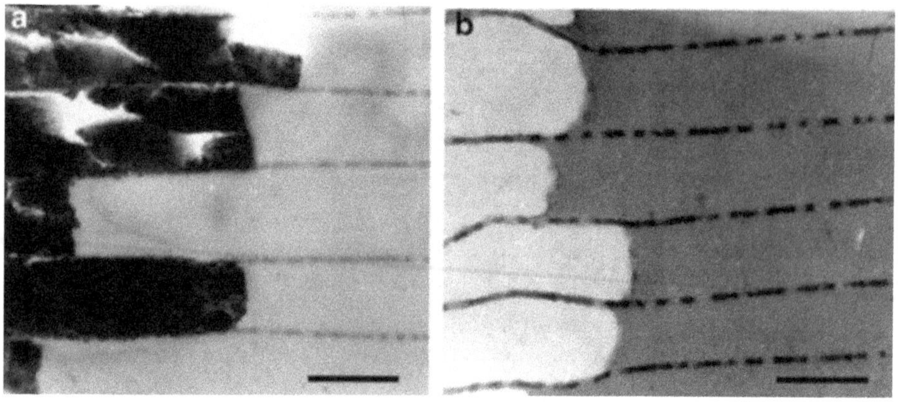

Fig. 43.13 TEM of nacre of *Sulculus diversicolor supertexta*. Thin sections show holes in the interlamellar matrix of organic sheets. (**a**) No staining, (**b**) double staining (bars: **a**, **b** = 1.0 μm)

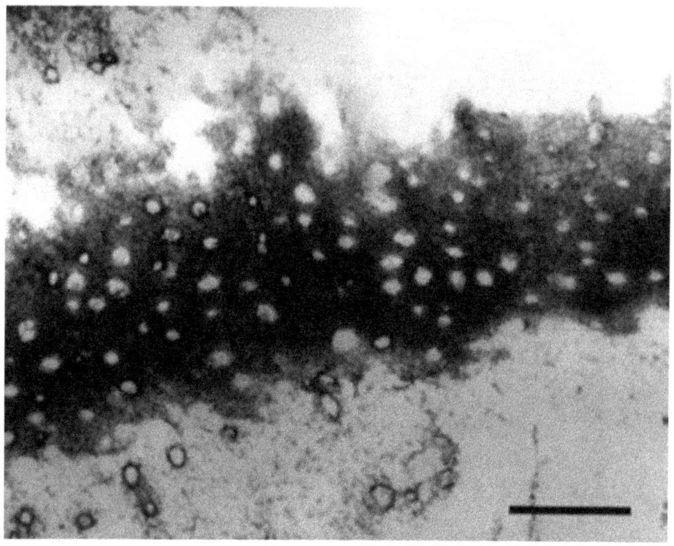

Fig. 43.14 TEM of the organic sheet of nacre of *Batillus cornutus*. Holes in the sheets are clearly observed in section cut to nearly parallel to the interlamellar matrix of sheets (bar = 250 nm)

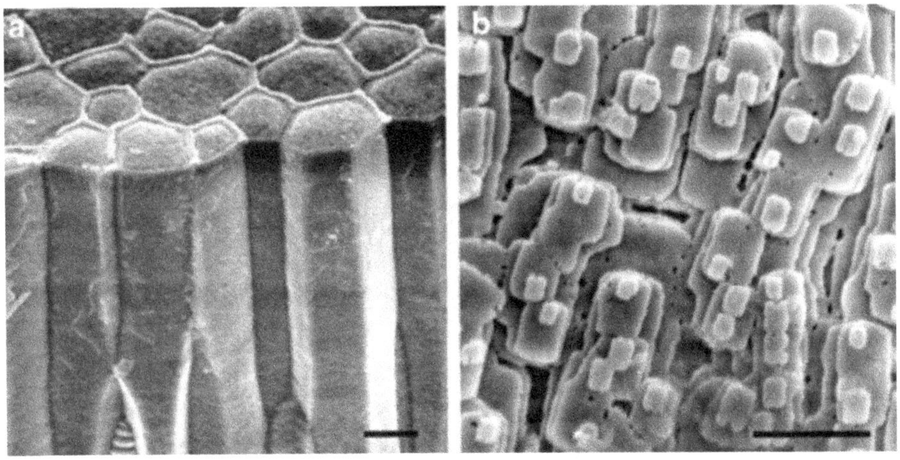

Fig. 43.15 SEM of the prismatic and nacreous layers of *Atrina pectinata*. Crystals of bivalve prismatic layer are arranged in a columnar fashion. (**a**) Crystals of the prismatic layer show rectangular shape. (**b**) Crystals of the nacreous layer (bars: **a** = 10 μm, **b** = 5 μm)

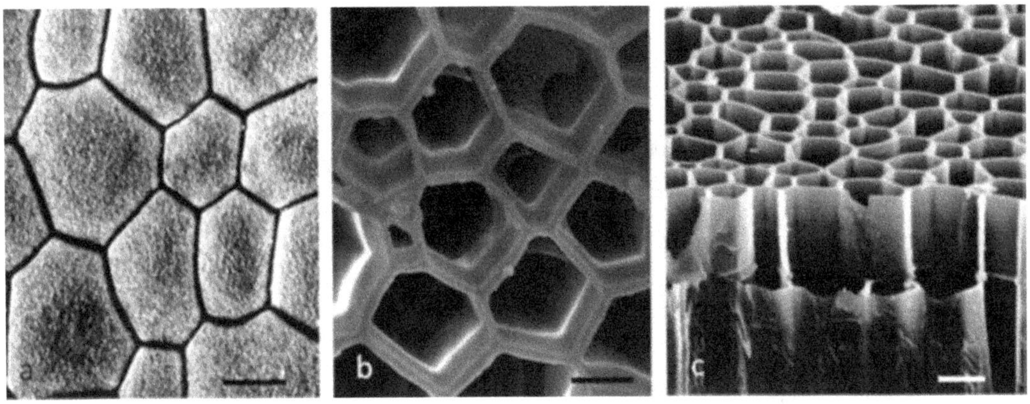

Fig. 43.16 SEM of the prismatic layer of *Pinctada fucata*. After acid treatment of (**a**), interprismatic layers remain as shown in Figs. (**b**, **c**). (**a**) Before decalcification, (**b, c**) after decalcification (bars: **a**, **b**, **c** = 10 μm)

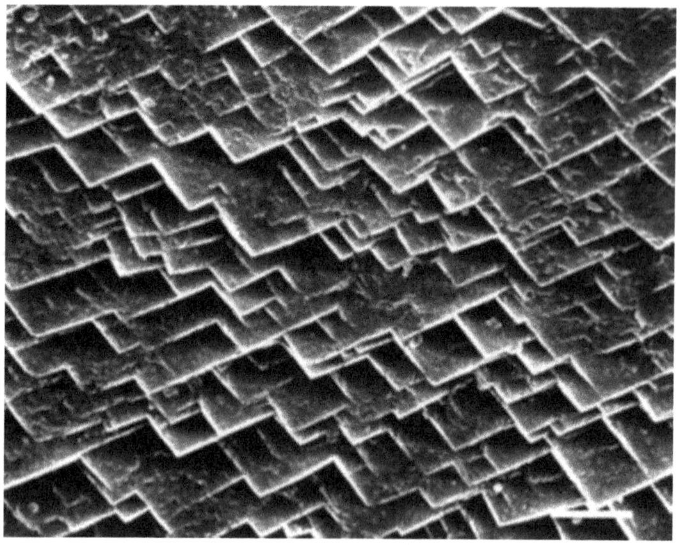

Fig. 43.17 SEM of the prismatic layer of *Cellana toreuma*. Imbricated pattern of mineral plates is observed (bar: 2 μm)

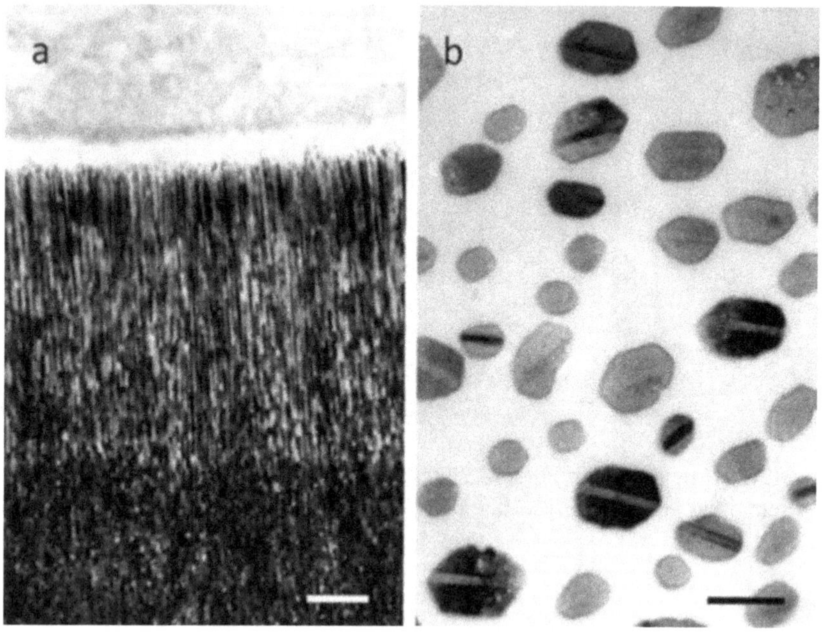

Fig. 43.18 TEM of aragonite crystals in the ligament of *Meretrix lusoria*. (**a**) Longitudinal section of crystals runs parallel with each other. (**b**) Cross section of the crystals shows hexagonal structure (bars: **a** = 2 μm, **b** = 1 μm)

Fig. 43.19 Cross section of aragonite crystals in the ligament of *Neotrigonia* sp. Arrows indicate the polysynthetic twin structure (bar: 200 nm)

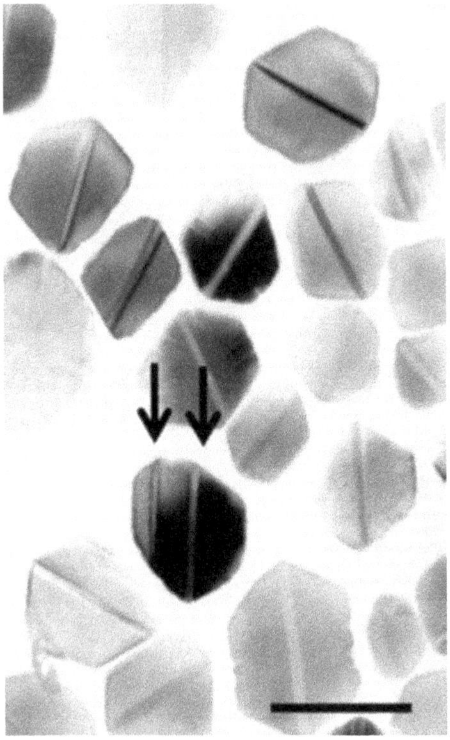

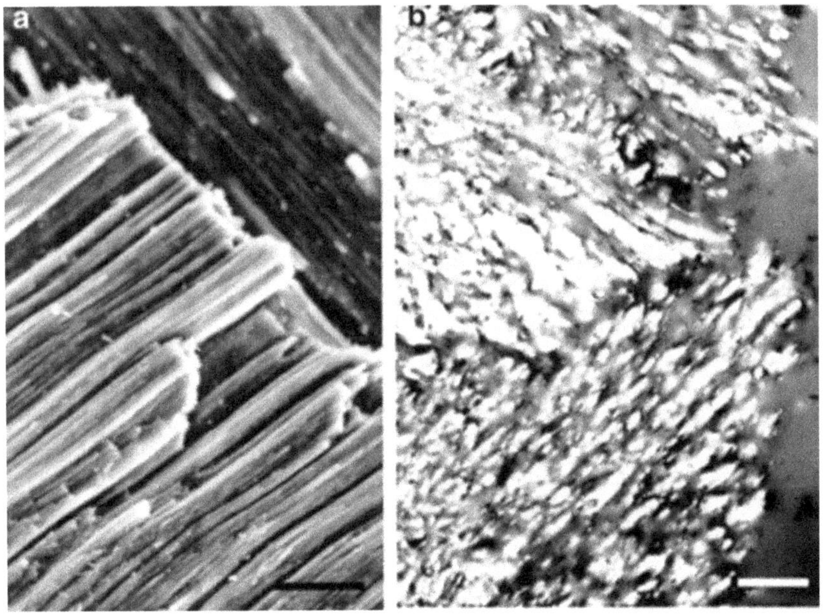

Fig. 43.20 SEM (**a**) and TEM (**b**) show the crossed lamellar structure of *Strombus gigas* (**b** double staining) (bars: **a** = 10 μm, **b** = 1 μm)

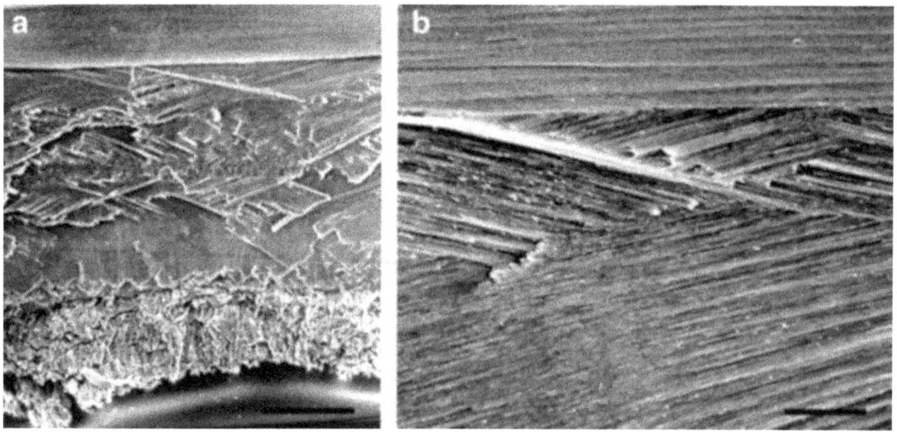

Fig. 43.21 SEM of the fracture surface of *Patelloida saccharina*. Long and thin aragonite crystals form a cross-lamellar structure (bars: **a** = 100 μm, **b** = 10 μm)

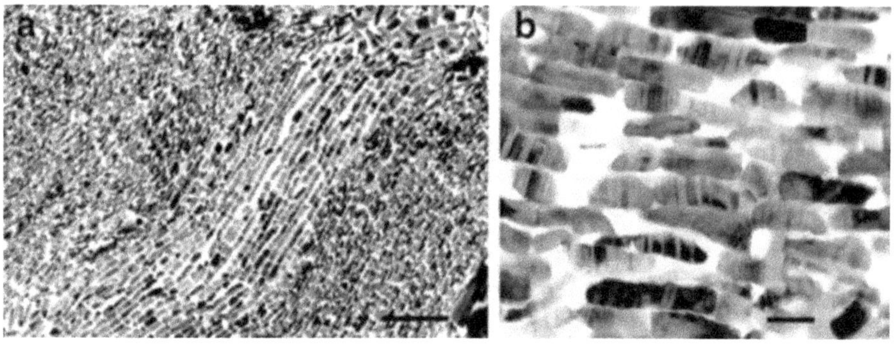

Fig. 43.22 TEM of aragonite crystals of *Patelloida saccharina*. (**a**) The cross section shows rectangular shape. (**b**) Crystals show twin pattern (bars: **a** = 1 μm, **b** = 110 nm)

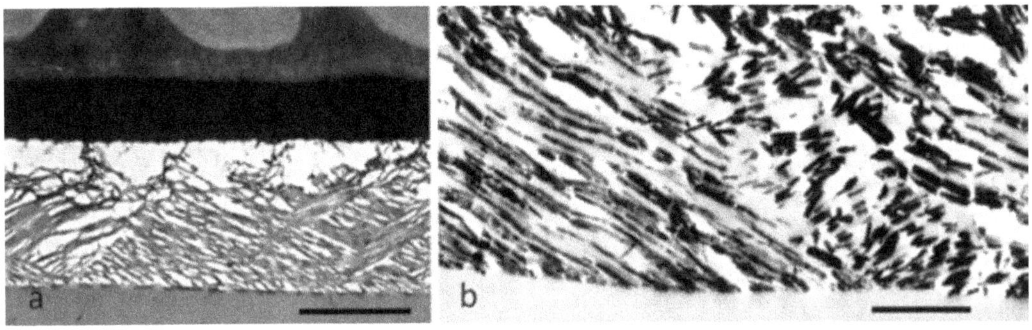

Fig. 43.23 TEM of shell of *Euhadra peliomphala*. The shell shows crossed-lamellar structure (**a** double staining, **b** no staining, bars: **a** = 5 μm, **b** = 2 μm)

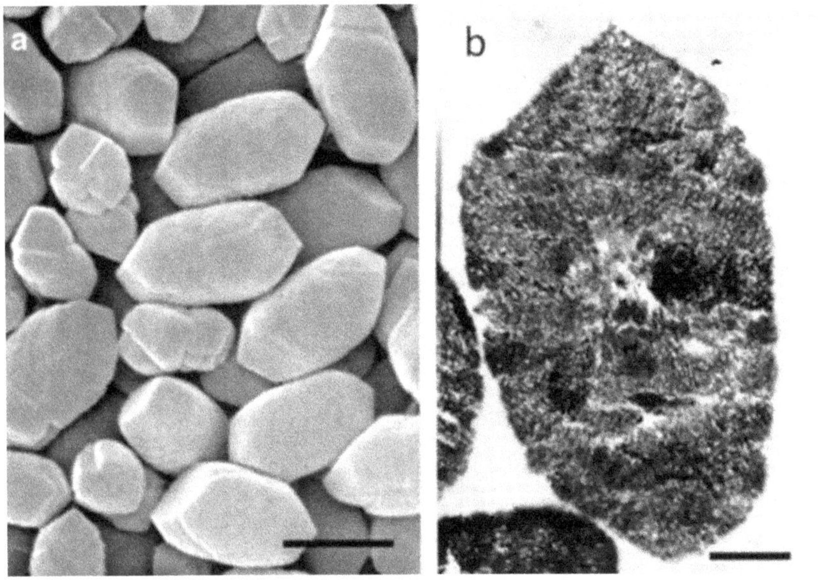

Fig. 43.24 SEM and TEM of otoliths of mouse. (**a**) SEM of both ends shows triangular in shape, and side view looks like cylindrical shape. (**b**) TEM of thin section without staining demonstrates that fine road-like crystals are arranged in a radial pattern (bars: **a** = 1 μm, **b** = 540 nm)

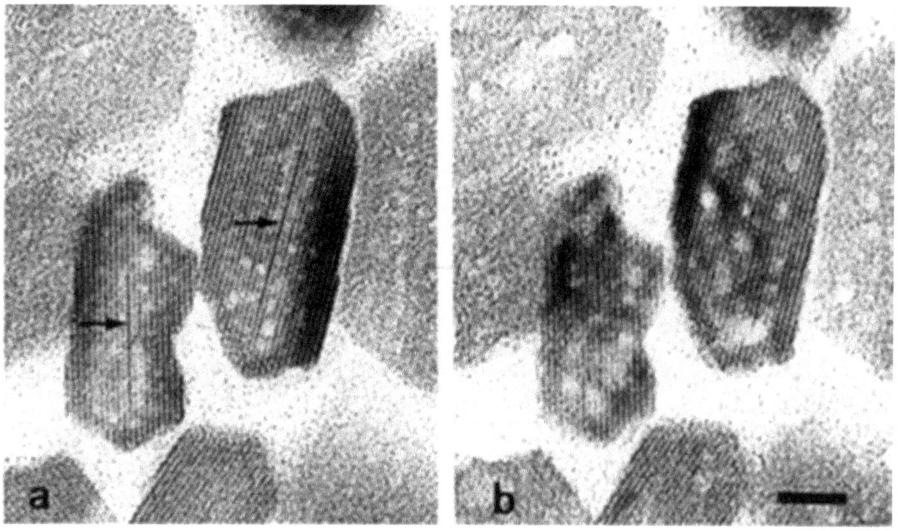

Fig. 43.25 TEM of apatite crystals of the rat tooth enamel. Central dark lines (arrows) do not create two lattice lines after electron beam exposure, showing a different physical property of octacalcium phosphate (**a** before beam damage, **b** after beam damage, bar = 10 nm)

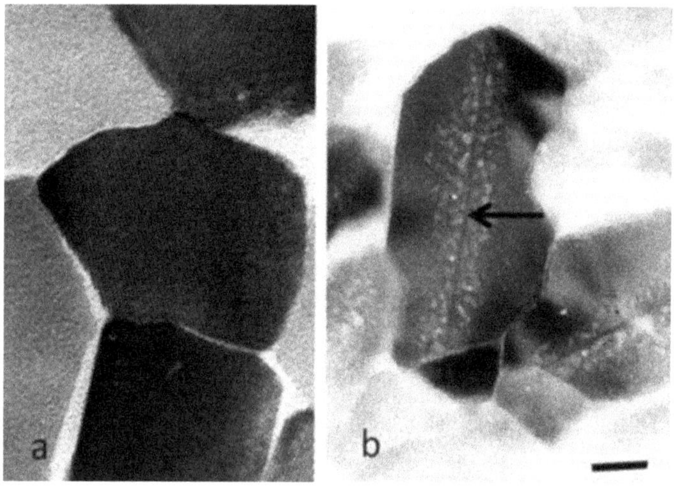

Fig. 43.26 TEM observations of shark enameloid (**a**) and rat tooth enamel (**b**) crystals. Cross sections show two different crystal characters, indicating two different mechanisms of crystal formation. Arrow: central dark line (CDL) (bar = 10 nm)

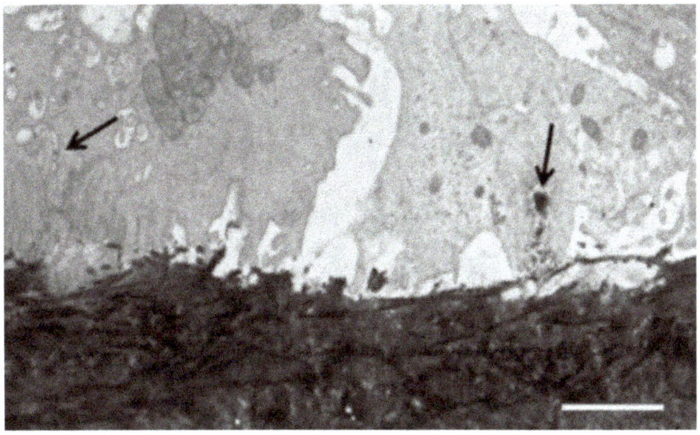

Fig. 43.27 TEM of bone resorption by osteoclast in rat. Arrows show that bone crystals were resorbed by endocytosis (bar = 2 μm)

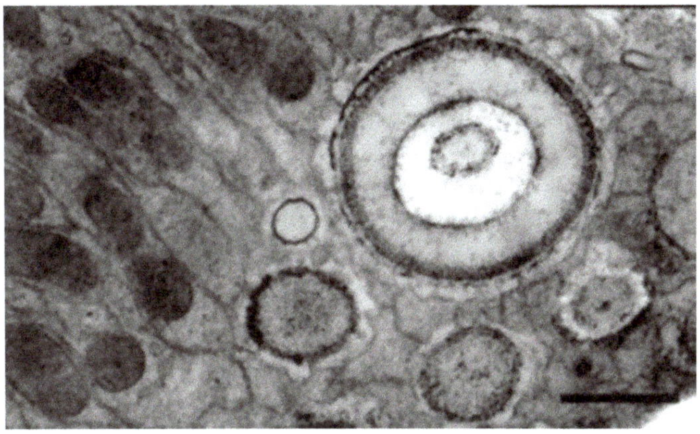

Fig. 43.28 TEM of Malpighian tubule of *Drosophila melanogaster*. Minerals of calcospherite are formed (bar = 1 μm)

Correction to: TEM Study of the Radular Teeth of the Chiton *Acanthopleura japonica*

Mitsuo Kakei, Masayoshi Yoshikawa, and Hiroyuki Mishima

Correction to:
Chapter 2 in: K. Endo et al. (eds.), *Biomineralization*, https://doi.org/10.1007/978-981-13-1002-7_2

In the original version of chapter 2, references 5 and 12 were incorrect. In this version, references 5 and 12 are corrected. The corrected references have now been added in the Chapter which reads as follows:

Reference 5

Weaver JC, Wang Q, Miserez A, Tantuccio A, Stromberg R, Bozhilov KN, Maxwell P, Nay R, Heier ST, DiMasi E, Kisailus D (2010) Analysis of an ultra hard magnetic biomineral in chiton radular teeth. Materialstoday 13 (1–2):42–52

Reference 12

Nemoto M, Wang Q, Li D, Pan S, Matsunaga T, Kisailus D (2012) Proteomic analysis from the mineralized radular teeth of the giant Pacific chiton, *Cryptochiton stelleri* (Mollusca). Proteomics 12:2890–2894

The updated online version of this chapter can be found at
https://doi.org/10.1007/978-981-13-1002-7_2

K. Endo et al. (eds.), *Biomineralization*,
https://doi.org/10.1007/978-981-13-1002-7_44

www.ingramcontent.com/pod-product-compliance
Lightning Source LLC
LaVergne TN
LVHW082112200926
848484LV00008B/1942